excellent - scallops - 309

excellent - chicken enchelada - 334

343

try - pizza rice casserole - —

(left over rice)

chicken brased in wine - — — 327

D0572509

F

THE *New* AMERICAN DIET

by

Sonja L. Connor, M.S., R.D.
and
William E. Connor, M.D.

A Fireside Book
Published by Simon & Schuster Inc.
New York London Toronto Sydney Tokyo

Fireside
Simon & Schuster Building
Rockefeller Center
1230 Avenue of the Americas
New York, New York 10020

Library of Congress Cataloging in Publication Data
Connor, Sonja L.
    The new American diet.
    Includes index.
    1. Low-fat diet.   2. Low-fat diet—Recipes.
3. High-carbohydrate diet.   4. High-carbohydrate
diet—Recipes.   I. Connor, William E., 1921–
II. Title.
RM237.7.C64   1986   613.2′6   86-3737
ISBN 0-671-54324-5
ISBN 0-671-66375-5 Pbk.

The authors are grateful for permission to reprint the following figures
and tables.

Figures 3 and 4, p. 23: Reprinted from Connor, W. E. "The
Relationship of Hyperlipoproteinemia to Atherosclerosis: The Decisive
Role of Dietary Cholesterol and Fat," in Scanu, A. M. (ed.), *The
Biochemistry of Atherosclerosis* (N.Y.: Marcel Dekker, Inc., 1979),
pp.379–80, by courtesy of Marcel Dekker, Inc.
    Table 1, p. 38: Reprinted from Connor, W. E. and Connor, S. L.
"The Dietary Treatment of Hyperlipidemia: Rationale, Technique and
Efficacy," in Havel, R. J. (ed.), *Lipid Disorders*, Med. Clin. North.
Am. 66:485 (Philadelphia: W. B. Saunders Company, 1982), by
courtesy of W. B. Saunders Company.
    Table 3, pp. 74–75: Reprinted from Connor, W. E. and Connor, S.
L. "The Dietary Prevention and Treatment of Coronary Heart
Disease," in Connor, W. E. and Bristow, J. D. (eds.), *Coronary Heart
Disease: Prevention, Complications, and Treatment* (Philadelphia:
Lippincott Co., 1985), p. 52, by courtesy of J. B. Lippincott
Company.
    Figures 20 and 24, p. 96, p. 108: Reprinted from Connor, W. E.
and Connor, S. L. "The Dietary Prevention and Treatment of
Coronary Heart Disease," in Connor, W. E. and Bristow, J. D. (eds.),
Coronary Heart Disease: Prevention, Complications and Treatment
(Philadelphia: Lippincott Co., 1985), p. 53, by courtesy of J. B.
Lippincott Company.
    Figure 21, pp. 98–99: Connor, S. L., Gustafson, J. M. and
Vaughan, S. R. "Promoting dietary change: Demonstrating
Reduction of Dietary Fat." Copyright The American Dietetic
Association. Reprinted by permission from *Journal of the American
Dietetic Association*, Vol. 85:345, 1985.

Tables 3, 4, 5, 7, pp. 74, 75, 76, 77, 116 and Figure 25, p. 113.
Reprinted from Connor, S. L., Gustafson, J. G., Artaud-Wild, S. M.,
Flavell, D. P., Classic-Kohn, C. J., Hatcher, L. F., and Connor, W. E.,
"The Cholesterol/Saturated-fat Index: An Indication of the
Hypercholesterolaemic and Atherogenic Potential of Food. The
Lancet 1: 1229–1232, 1986.
    Figure 22, pp. 102–3: Vaughan, S. R., Connor, S. L. and
Gustafson, J. G. A Calendar of Dietary Changes. Copyright *Journal of
Nutrition Education*, Vol. 15:58, 1983.
    Table 6, p. 104: Reprinted from Connor, W. E. and Connor, S. L.
"The Dietary Prevention and Treatment of Coronary Heart Disease,"
in Connor, W. E. and Bristow, J. D. (eds.), *Coronary Heart Disease:
Prevention, Complications, and Treatment* (Philadelphia: Lippincott Co.,
1985), p. 54, by courtesy of J. B. Lippincott Co., Philadelphia.
    Table 18, p. 168: Reprinted from Statistical Bulletin January–June
1983. Copyright 1983 Metropolitan Life Insurance Company. By
courtesy of Metropolitan Life Insurance Company, New York.
    Table 19, p. 170: Reprinted from Burton, B. T., Foster, W. R.,
Hirsch, J. and Van Itallie, T. B. "Health Implications of Obesity: An
NIH Consensus Development Conference." *International Journal of
Obesity*, Vol. 9:155, 1985. By courtesy of John Libbey & Company
Limited, London, England.
    Figures 33 and 34, p. 196: Reprinted from Connor, S. L., Connor,
W. E., Sexton, G., Calvin, L., and Bacon S. "The effects of age,
body weight and family relationships on plasma lipoproteins and lipids
in men, women and children of randomly selected families."
Circulation, Vol. 66:1294, 1982. By permission of the American Heart
Association, Inc., Dallas.
    Figure 35, p. 197: Reprinted from Connor, S. L., Connor, W. E.,
Henry, H., Sexton, G. and Keenan, E. J. "The effects of familial
relationships, age, body weight, and diet on blood pressure and the 24
hour urinary excretion of sodium, potassium, and creatinine in men,
women, and children of randomly selected families." *Circulation*, Vol.
70:81, 1984. By permission of the American Heart Association, Inc.,
Dallas.

ACKNOWLEDGMENTS

Some of the concepts for this book originated years ago in the dreams of a group of young research scientists at the University of Iowa, Drs. Daniel B. Stone, Mark L. Armstrong and William E. Connor. They had been inspired by their friends and senior mentors, Dr. William B. Bean, Dr. Walter Kirkendall, Dr. Emory Warner and Dr. Jeremiah Stamler. The first translation of their ideas and scientific research into a practical dietary approach to disease prevention occurred in 1966 with the publication of *A Low Cholesterol Diet Manual* by Jacqueline Allen Lichty, Joan Hady Bickel, Daniel B. Stone and William E. Connor. This book was the forerunner to *The Alternative Diet Book* (1976). Martha M. Fry and Susan L. Warner collaborated with us in the writing and recipes were contributed by Joan Bickel, Merlynn Bennion, Patricia Greiner, Mary Ann Reiter, Linda Snetselar, Karen A. Smith, Linda S. Solen, Maria C. Urban, Laura Vailas, Jamie S. Wene and the University of Iowa Dietetic Interns. A cookbook, *Best From The Family Heart Kitchens* was produced under our direction by the nutrition staff of the Family Heart Study and published in 1981. Editors were Nancy Becker and Joyce R. Gustafson. Contributors included Susan Algert, Sabine M. Artaud-Wild, Sandra R. Bacon, Carolyn Classick, Donna P. Flavell, Lauren F. Hatcher, Holly J. Henry, Martha P. McMurry, Chere B. Pereira and Susan R. Vaughan.

The *New American Diet* represents the culmination of over twenty-five years of research. We are particularly grateful to members of the Family Heart Study nutrition staff, named at the beginning of Part Three of this book, for developing recipes that appeal to a broad spectrum of tastes and for their skills in translating our dietary concepts into creative practical suggestions. Special appreciation goes to David Rorvik, Joyce Gustafson, Sabine Artaud-Wild and Carolyn Classick-Kohn, who contributed greatly to the preparation of this book. Appreciation is also accorded to other members of the Family Heart Study staff for their contributions (Drs. Joseph Matarazzo, Timothy Carmody, Cheryl Brischetto, Jack Hollis, Steven Fey, Diane Pierce, Robert McLellarn, Gerdi Weidner, Lyle Calvin, Gary Sexton, Roger Illingworth and William Morton and Barbara Healy), to the 233 families who helped in the refinement of the dietary concepts and recipes, and to Marcia Hindman and Patricia Schade for their skills in the precise preparation of this manuscript.

Finally, these concepts would never have come to fruition without the several decades of past research support, now gratefully acknowledged, from the National Heart, Lung and Blood Institute and the Clinical Research Centers of the Division of Research Resources of the National Institutes of Health, and the American Heart Association, including the Iowa and Oregon Affiliates, and financial support of these institutions by U.S. taxpayers.

To our colleagues, the children and adults of the Family Heart Study, and our patients— their inspiration and contributions have made this book possible.

CONTENTS

PART THREE: THE COOKBOOK

INTRODUCTION

The New American Diet Is for Everybody

It is usually the "simplest" ideas that are considered the most revolutionary. Only a few years ago the idea that *one* diet could prevent, to a significant degree, *all* of the major diseases of both over- and under consumption was considered utopian by many and absurd by some. But, in fact, the New American Diet detailed in this book does exactly that. It is, as this book documents, the most effective type of diet that can be devised, based upon present scientific and medical knowledge, for the prevention of atherosclerosis and coronary heart disease, stroke, hypertension (high blood pressure), diabetes mellitus, several forms of cancer and a number of other disorders. It is, in addition, ideally suited for gradual weight loss and is, we are convinced, the most promising diet available for long-term weight maintenance once target weight is achieved.

The New American Diet involves gradual alteration of the current American diet through careful, programmed changes in the high-fat, high-cholesterol, low-complex carbohydrate, high-salt diet that is presently eaten in the United States and in Western Europe. It is this typical Western-world diet which, as we will demonstrate, has become a major contributor to premature death and disease.

The New American Diet Is Market-Tested and People-Friendly

What sets the New American Diet apart from others, in addition to its unified approach to preventing disease, is its genesis in controlled experimental and clinical scientific research. It is a way of eating which we have determined, through scientific study, may not only help you live longer (because it can help prevent many life-threatening diseases) but is also a diet that *you can live happily with.*

We concluded long ago that no matter how good a diet is on paper it is worthless if people won't use it. Hence, we have devoted many years determining to what extent people can and will change to new ways of eating. Many are now recommending the kind of low-fat, high-complex carbohydrate diet that we helped pioneer, develop and refine over nearly thirty years. But it is one thing to advise people what to eat in a general way, quite another for them actually to do it—and *like* it. In our program, we have put it all together, to provide not only the what and the why but also the *how*—and to do so in ways that people can understand and utilize not just for weeks or months but for years and lifetimes.

Perhaps the most important of the studies that have permitted us to formulate a genuinely people-friendly dietary program was our recently concluded Family Heart Study. We studied the ability of randomly selected families—of *typical* Americans—to change their eating habits along lines scientifically demonstrated to help produce disease-preventive results. In short, this five-year study, involving researchers from the disciplines of medicine, nutrition, psychology, statistics and nursing, sought to find out just how many and what kind of desirable dietary changes typical Americans could comfortably make.

Never before has a dietary program been people-tested in quite this fashion. This unique study has allowed us to further fine-tune our program in ways that make it "friendlier" than ever. We are all beneficiaries of the experiences of the 233 families that participated in our study. Those experiences, which are still being minutely analyzed, have contributed a great deal to our current program and will no doubt contribute to its further refinement in years to come.

When we launched the Family Heart Study the question uppermost in our minds was: No matter how slowly they might progress, will people stick with this program? Will they keep on trying? Any progress, after all, is better than none. We knew that the drop-out rate in many scientific studies using random samples is very high. At the end of five years, the drop-out rate in our study totaled only 10 percent of the families and only 20 percent of the individuals—all of which we consider remarkable. The families progressed at different rates, of course, but almost all made progress. Many made notable progress. The group as a whole completed what we call Phase One of the program; some arrived at or near the end-point of goals of Phase Two, and others went all the way to the end of Phase Three, which confers maximum benefits.

The benefits from achieving even the Phase One goals you'll be learning about shortly can be substantial. Projections from national data indicate that adherence to Phase One goals of our program could save approximately 250,000 lives in the United States alone over an eight-year period. And those projections are based only on the data related to heart disease. Adherence to Phase Two goals could be expected to save approximately 500,000 lives, while adherence to Phase Three goals could save approximately 1 million lives in eight years. And, again, those figures are only for cardiovascular disease. In reality we believe the program can save far more lives because of its additional protective effects against cancer, hypertension, diabetes, and so on.

How We Got There

This diet program is *not* one of those overnight sensations. We have been a long time arriving at where we are today. It all began more than twenty-five years ago when one of us (William Connor) was caring for a man with incapacitating heart disease. Dr. Connor, then taking specialty training in internal medicine at the University Hospitals in Iowa City, was appalled when his patient, only thirty-nine years old, abruptly and without warning had a fatal heart attack. A picture of one of this man's obstructed coronary arteries is shown in figure 1 on page 20.

It was just at that time that the connection between dietary cholesterol and fat and coronary heart disease was being established, though not widely accepted, in medical circles. In the course of his investigations, Dr. Connor had observed the very high levels of fat in the blood of his patient. He also knew that this patient ate a diet high in fat, as did so many Americans. It seemed a reasonable postulation to him that if people would simply eat less fat their blood levels of fat might diminish, too, and heart disease might thus be reduced.

This was unconventional thinking for the time. But it was just such thinking that eventually caused Dr. Connor to reorient his career goals. After graduating from the University of Iowa he became a practitioner of medicine where he was increasingly distressed by the premature deaths of so many from coronary heart disease. And he couldn't dismiss the notion that diet was having a lot to do with these deaths.

He decided not to continue with private practice but instead to enter the budding field of coronary heart disease research and prevention. He set as his goal the design of a diet that would lower blood fat concentrations in experimental animals and then in humans. He hoped that this would help prevent the buildup of fat and cholesterol in the walls of arteries and that this in turn would prevent coronary heart disease.

This early work was pursued with the help of a research fellowship from the American Heart Association. Dr. Connor and his many associates began to isolate the different factors in the diet that he thought might be implicated in heart disease, especially cholesterol which some other researchers had completely discounted as being of any importance, focusing on saturated fats instead.

By the early 1960s, Dr. Connor and his colleagues had formulated the chemical composition for a New American Diet that they believed, on the basis of their experiments and those of many other scientists, would help prevent many of the hundreds of thousands of deaths that occur in the United States each year as a result of coronary heart disease. But the "diet" was just that—a list of chemicals okay for animals but not practical for humans.

Needed at that point were dietitians to help translate that list into foods people would actually want to eat. A number of dietitians participated in this pioneering research effort, among them a feisty young woman named Sonja (later to become Mrs. Connor) who, when she learned the details of the project, was offended by the very idea that the "good foods" of life—eggs, butter, dairy products and meat—were to be limited in the emerging New American Diet. It took her a year—while she worked in another laboratory —before she decided Dr. Connor was really on the leading edge of nutritional research, after all, and that she wanted to be part of the action.

She and the other dietitians weren't about to settle, however, for skinned broiled chicken breast and dry baked potatoes as representing a low-fat diet. One could do a whole lot better than that, they figured, and still conform to the disease-prevention requirements of the New American Diet. They set about to devise exciting and appetizing recipes, launching a tradition that continues to the present day. It was Sonja Connor who developed the concept of phased change, central to the sophisticated behavior modification technique we were to explore years later. It was her idea, and that of another dietitian, Martha McMurry, that diet should be treated not as some temporary disturbance in life but instead as a change in life-style, something you gradually and *permanently* adapt to.

Meanwhile, an impressive array of scientists had gathered at the University of Iowa to establish, under a multimillion-dollar grant from the National Heart, Lung, and Blood Institute, a major center for the study of atherosclerosis, the process by which the arteries become clogged and narrowed, leading to heart attacks and strokes. Dr. Connor was named director of this new center. He and his colleagues, including Sonja Connor, published numerous papers on their findings, many of which further documented the link between diet and disease. Dr. Connor and several dietitians traveled to other parts of the world to investigate, firsthand, the dietary habits of different cultures, including the Tarahumara Indians of Mexico and others who have a very low incidence of heart disease (and who also eat foods very low in fat and cholesterol).

In 1975, the Connors left Iowa to establish a similar program at the medical school of the Oregon Health Sciences University. There they, along with Dr. Joseph Matarazzo, chairman of the Department of Medical Psychology, Oregon Health Sciences University, Dr. Lyle Calvin, statistician and dean of the Graduate School, Oregon State University, and a cadre of staff members, launched the Family Heart Study. Dr. Connor and his associates also initiated research into the effects certain fish oils can have on cholesterol and other blood lipid concentrations. Discoveries related to fish oils, discussed in more detail later in this book, have been the subject of many scientific papers, as well as news accounts in *The New York Times, Time* magazine, etc.

Where We—and *You*— Are Going

In part 1 of this book we will document the need for a New American Diet. More than 1 million people are dying every year from heart disease and strokes in the United States alone. And that does not include the other diseases of over- and underconsumption which our dietary program will also help to prevent as well.

In part 2 we tell you in greater detail just what the New American Diet is and what it can do. If you follow our program through to its conclusion you will have a good chance of reducing your blood cholesterol levels by as much as 20 percent or more. The impact of this can be enormous. Dr. Daniel Steinberg, chairman of an advisory panel of the National Institutes of Health, recently concluded that if Americans as a whole could be persuaded to change their diets so that they have just 10 percent less cholesterol in their blood, then ultimately 100,000 fewer of them would die each year. For every 1 percent reduction in blood cholesterol, you reduce your coronary heart disease risk by 2 percent. The disease-prevention properties of our diet cannot yet be so clearly quantified with respect to some of the other diseases and disorders, such as various cancers, but there is good evidence that this diet program could have significant, positive impact there, as well.

The last chapter of part 1 is a quiz which will help you determine how well you measure up to the New American Diet goals. By taking this quiz at the beginning you will be able to find out where you need to go and, by taking the quiz at certain intervals again later on, you'll be able to determine how far you have come and get ideas about making further changes.

Part 2 provides you with all of the details you will need to make the New American Diet a *permanent* part of your life. You'll meet a number of families who have made use of the diet. We hope their stories will inspire you and help suggest ways you, too, can make the diet work within your own household.

Then it's into the program itself, which proceeds in a gradual, three-step progression. To help make the transition to a lower-fat, lower-cholesterol, lower-salt, higher-complex carbohydrate way of eating easier and tastier, we provide a number of new concepts and aids. Phase One of the program focuses on substitutions, a process through which you are able to keep old favorite recipes but modify them in ways that most family members will readily accept. Phase Two takes you a step further, introducing a number of new recipes, particularly delicious ethnic recipes (Oriental, Mexican, Mediterranean, etc.) that are easily adapted to New American Diet goals. In Phase Three you advance to what we call "a new way of eating."

Throughout our program, however, you will continue to use many of the foods you are familiar with, and even though the New American Diet deemphasizes meat it is by no means a vegetarian diet. At the end of our program you will derive only about 20 percent of your total calories from fat, instead of the present 40 percent. Fiber and complex carbohydrate intakes, on the other hand, will increase considerably. Total protein intake remains stable. Your salt intake will also be dramatically reduced and your potassium intake increased.

You'll find sample one-week meal plans for each of the three phases of the diet program as you go along. You'll also find numerous other meal and recipe suggestions, including many quickies for, among others, those who presently excuse their high-fat eating on grounds they haven't time to fix anything complicated. The New American Diet cookbook section includes some of the easiest/fastest-to-prepare meals around, as well as a lot of more exotic, gourmet fare.

Part 2 includes a detailed chapter on weight loss and weight maintenance. We pro-vide you with what we believe is the most sensible available weight-loss approach. More important, however, is the fact that the New American Diet provides you with your best chance of keeping your weight where you want it once you've shed the excess pounds. You'll learn why this diet concept fights the yo-yo effect so many dieters experience (constantly losing and regaining weight and often regaining more than they lost!). Obesity is one of the serious diseases of overconsumption, and the New American Diet is designed to combat it. This chapter provides weight-loss/maintenance regimens for both men and women, as well as advice on exercise which can be of considerble additional aid to weight control.

Another chapter in part 2 covers all those special situations that can make any dietary change difficult. These include eating out, entertaining, holidays, camping trips, pregnancy and breast feeding, feeding of infants and vegetarianism. The New American Diet is easily adaptable to all of these situations.

The final chapter in part 2 provides advice on medical tests that you might, optionally, want to have at some point to monitor your progress. These include tests for cholesterol and other blood fats, as well as for blood pressure. You'll find that our definitions of what is "normal" and what is "healthy," in terms of the results of these tests, is sometimes at variance with what some others still consider acceptable. Many individuals, for example, are still told that certain blood cholesterol levels, which we are confident pose real risks, are within "the normal range."

Part 3 is the cookbook, a collection of more than three hundred extensively tested and carefully analyzed recipes that conform to New American Diet goals. These are the product of many years of evaluation and refinement. Every recipe in this book has been used many, many times by our extensive dedicated staff and by our patients and study families. No recipe gets included in our program unless it meets the standards of the diet. One major criterion, apart from all of the nutritional considerations, is that *a lot of people have to like it!*

We believe that the New American Diet is the best dietary choice you can make. It provides fare that is not only healthy but is also highly varied and exciting as well. Moreover, it is a way of eating that can be enjoyed by and be of benefit to *the entire family.* It does not demand radical change but instead encourages gradual change—the kind of change that, once made, can last for a lifetime. The potential health benefits of our diet can be enormous, particularly if started relatively early in life, but even if begun well into middle age or later the benefits can still be very substantial.

Whether you are young or old, male or female, in good health or in poor health, trim or overweight, the New American Diet is a diet for you to consider.

PART

1

Why A "New" Diet?

1

Why Should We Change Our Present Diet?

Too Much of a Good Thing

The current American diet is the envy of much of the world. Most Americans have plenty to eat all year round. Even those of more limited economic means usually eat more than enough to prevent the sort of nutritional deficiencies that still afflict large segments of the world. Not only do we have a lot to eat, but we also have an abundance of the sort of food people covet most: meats, eggs, dairy products, sweets, ice cream, pastries and fried foods—most laced with lots of salt.

For decades, the American diet has been regarded as the kind of diet on which our children can grow big and strong. The present American diet—with a heavy emphasis on

the benefits of animal protein—seemed ideal. This thinking was cemented with the discovery of the vitamins and the vital roles they play in human health. In reality, however, the sort of diet that has evolved in this country is at considerable variance with human dietary tradition. The Chinese and Japanese built their cultures on diets of rice; the Babylonians and the Egyptians, the Romans and the Greeks built theirs on diets of wheat. The staple foods of the Mayas, Incas and Aztecs of the Americas were corn and beans. We have made a special study of the Tarahumara Indians of Mexico who eat a similar diet. It is worth noting that these great civilizations developed with the people consuming largely cereals, fruits and vegetables.

Meat, which has become our everyday fare, was reserved for the feast in many other cultures or simply was used in very small quantities as a condiment. So were sugar, fat and salt which historically have been scarce. Even in Western societies until recently only the rich had the means to consume much meat. Bread and potatoes were the basic foods most people used.

It is in the nature of humans to feast whenever possible. The problem—at least in this country—is that our affluence and our technology have now made it possible for almost all of us to feast *every day.* And that is exactly what most of us do, consuming amounts of meat, fat, sugar and salt which by historic standards are enormous.

When infectious diseases killed a great many of us at relatively early ages, we didn't have to worry about the long-range effects of our diet. It was enough that this was a diet that prevented the sort of frank nutritional deficiencies that caused stunted growth, deformities and death, especially in the very young, throughout so much of the world. But with infectious diseases now substantially controlled, we are living longer and are finding that the feast that worked so well for us in the past is now disabling and killing us in astonishing numbers in our forties, fifties, and sixties, the decades which should be our most productive.

More and more of us, faced with the grim but instructive realities of the medical statistics related below, have come to realize that we have overindulged in a good thing. The diseases that plague us today are not for the most part those of dietary deficiencies but rather of dietary *excesses.*

The key to establishing a New American Diet—a new standard—is, first, to show what is wrong with the old standard diet and, second, to propose an alternative that *modifies* rather than banishes what has worked in the past. Our present diet is not intrinsically bad. It is only in its excesses that it creates so much serious havoc. It's got out of kilter and needs tuning, and, in some instances, the sort of *fine tuning* that only recent medical discoveries make possible. And, fortunately, as we will see, technology can work *for* us as well as against us. Modern food technologies are providing greater choices and availability of all types of foods than ever before. The challenge, which this book aims to help you meet, is to choose wisely and well.

But, before we proceed to a scientifically sound New American Diet we are convinced Americans *can* gradually adopt and live with, let us look to see just where and to what extent the present diet has brought us to grief. Perhaps then we'll all understand the need for intelligent change.

The Diseases of Over- (and Under-) Consumption

Unlike most of the rest of the world, most Americans—those of us in the United States, at least—as well as most Europeans are now living without food shortages. We have moved from a deficiency of food to an excess of foods of all kinds. The quest for material abundance, though a desirable goal that has alleviated much human misery, has resulted in a dramatic departure from the traditional patterns of food consumption people had adapted to over a period of thousands of years. Some foods, previously scarce, are now overconsumed, such as meat, dairy products and fats. Other foods, high in bulk and low in caloric density, are now underconsumed by the traditional standard (e.g., beans, potatoes, whole grains). Still other foods are now highly refined and processed, producing foods of high caloric density and characterized frequently by the addition of salt, sugar and/or fat. Most of the doughnuts, pastries, crackers, pretzels, cookies, cakes and chips and some of the packaged cereals we consume in such large quantities are among the many foods that fall into this last category.

As a result of this highly significant shift in our pattern of food consumption, there has arisen a new spectrum of diseases in which nutritional factors are either the prime causes or else are major contributors. The diseases of *overconsumption* which we now associate with the current American diet are:

Atherosclerosis, coronary heart disease
  and stroke
Hypertension
Obesity
Diabetes mellitus (adult onset)
Gallstones
Cancers of the colon, breast, uterus,
  prostate, ovary and pancreas
Venous thrombosis (blood clots)
Dental caries (cavities)
Cirrhosis of the liver

The diseases of *underconsumption* of certain nutrients include:

Constipation
Diverticular disease
Appendicitis
Hemorrhoids
Hiatus hernia
Varicose veins of the legs
Cancer of the colon (associated with
  overconsumption, as well)
Venous thrombosis (blood clots,
  associated with overconsumption, as
  well)

After reviewing this daunting list of maladies associated with diet, many people would initially react with despair. They assume that many *different* diets might have to be devised in order to deal with each of these diseases individually. In fact, however, the nutritional factors that contribute to these diverse diseases are remarkably similar. Thus, *one* diet —which this books details—can be remarkably effective in helping to prevent *all* of these diseases. The factors in the current American diet which are associated with diseases of *overconsumption* are *excessive intakes* of cholesterol, saturated fats, total fat, calories, sugar, salt and alcohol. The factors which are associated with the diseases of *underconsumption* are *insufficient intakes* of complex carbohydrates, fiber, potassium and other substances contained in fruits, vegetables and cereals (grains).

Let's look more closely at the diseases listed above and examine the evidence linking our current diet to these disorders.

ATHEROSCLEROSIS, CORONARY HEART DISEASE AND STROKE

Despite the fact that the death rate from coronary heart disease has been declining for the past decade, heart attacks still kill more than half a million people in the United States *each year.* Coronary heart disease remains the number one single cause of death. Some *1.5 million* people in this country are expected to have heart attacks in the next twelve months. More than a third of those will prove fatal. Between *five and six million* people in the United States have been diagnosed as having coronary artery disease, and at least 27 million people are thought to have high blood cholesterol levels. The cost of all this disease is staggering, not only in terms of human tragedy, but also in terms of medical bills, lost productivity and wages. The National Heart, Lung, and Blood Institute puts the current tab at $60 *billion per year.*

The fact that so much of this disease can be prevented gives rise to both despair and hope—despair because, despite growing publicity, too few people still understand what can be done to stop or slow this scourge; hope because so much *can* now be done—if only word can be spread far enough, fast enough and clearly enough.

Coronary heart disease is characterized by fatty deposits which build up in and obstruct the coronary arteries. It is through these vital arteries that flow the blood-borne oxygen and energy which the heart muscle requires to serve as an adequate pump. The disorder that underlies and precedes strokes and heart attacks is called *atherosclerosis,* derived from the Greek words *athera* and *sklerosis,* meaning gruel and hardening. Like a thick gruel, fatty deposits, composed in large part of cholesterol, build up inside artery walls, narrowing and hardening them as scar tissue and calcium are also deposited. (Figure 1 shows a coronary artery that is atherosclerotic. Figure 2 shows another coronary artery that is healthy.) A disorder, experienced as pain in the chest, called angina pectoris may be the first signal that the coronary arteries are narrowing. For others, however, the first manifestation of coronary heart disease may also be the last— a sudden and fatal heart attack, caused by a blood clot—a coronary thrombosis—that completely obstructs an already narrowed vessel and leads to a stoppage of the heartbeat. *Stroke* refers to the same process, except that here it is the brain, rather than the heart, that is starved of blood and oxygen because of the atherosclerotic narrowing of the arteries in the head and neck. Some strokes are

caused by brain hemorrhage from hypertension. Some 170,000 Americans die of stroke each year. Other Americans have atherosclerosis of the arteries which supply the legs and feet with blood.

Because of all the media attention that has focused on heart-transplant operations and bypass surgery, many lay people and even some doctors have concluded that such procedures provide an answer to heart disease. This is unfortunate, for apart from the limited availability, enormous cost and uncertain outcome of these operations, surgery does not address the root causes of heart disease. At-

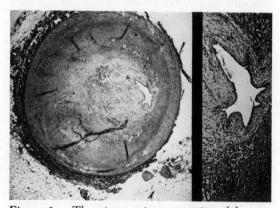

Figure 1. *The microscopic cross section of the almost completely obstructed coronary artery of a thirty-nine-year-old man who died suddenly from coronary heart disease. The enlargement on the right shows the tiny opening that remained in this artery.*

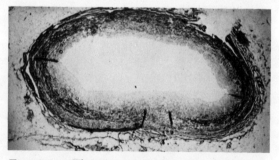

Figure 2. *The microscopic cross section of a normal, healthy human coronary artery.*

tention must be refocused on measures that can *prevent* heart disease. Diet is among the most important of these.

While many now agree that cholesterol and certain fats—notably the "saturated" fats—are implicated in these diseases, there has been some resistance, which is now weakening, however, to the idea that the fats and cholesterol we consume in our *diets* are largely responsible for coronary heart disease and other atherosclerotic disorders. Skeptics have suggested that genetic defects affecting the ways in which the body processes these substances must be at fault. It is now recognized that these genetic defects are responsible for only a *small* minority of people who ultimately develop coronary heart disease. Many have been loath even to consider that several of the foods we currently most cherish—and consume in great quantities—such as eggs, meat, butter and cheese, might be among the principal culprits. After all, these are the very foods we have come in recent decades to regard as the most "nutritious" and certainly the most desirable. Even today there persists the feeling that a diet with only small or moderate amounts of these foods is a diet that exposes us to protein, vitamin and mineral deficiencies.

The truth is, however, that there is no *dietary* requirement for cholesterol and saturated fat. The body *does* need a certain amount of these substances but it synthesizes what it needs from other sources. (Cholesterol helps provide a fatty insulation for nerves, is a necessary component of all cell membranes and is a vital part of bile, a substance that helps digest fats, and of the sex hormones.) Similarly, there is no foundation in fact for the idea that foods rich in cholesterol and saturated fats cannot be replaced in the diet by equally good foods containing

small or even nonexistent quantities of fat and cholesterol. We'll show how this can be done in a very palatable way later on in this book.

Now, however, let's look briefly at the four main lines of evidence, dating from 1908 to the present, that demonstrate an association between dietary cholesterol and saturated fats and the atherosclerosis that is killing us in such appalling numbers: (1) the worldwide epidemiological data which involve studies of large populations of people in different countries; (2) animal experiments; (3) studies in humans; and (4) pathologic/autopsy studies.

The Epidemiological Evidence. The findings here are clear-cut. Those populations which consume lots of fat and cholesterol have a significantly higher incidence of atherosclerosis than those populations that consume diets relatively low in saturated fats and cholesterol. The Finns, for example, were found in one early study of several nations to have the fattiest diet of all. They also had the highest concentrations of cholesterol in their blood and the highest incidence of heart disease. The United States came in second in terms of fat and cholesterol in the diet and in the rate of heart disease. Coronary heart disease has been rare, however, in Japan where the diet typically has been low in fat and cholesterol. But when Japanese migrate to the United States and adopt *our* diet, their incidence of atherosclerosis and heart disease escalates dramatically—to *ten times* what it had been in their own country. The concentration of cholesterol that can be found in their blood—after relocating here—can also be shown to rise consistently in direct relationship to increased fat/cholesterol intake.

An equally instructive example exists in the Tarahumara Indians who live in the

Sierra Madre Occidental Mountains of Mexico. These hardy people, whom we have personally studied in depth in their own habitat, are renowned for their remarkable abilities as long-distance runners. Many of them run races of two hundred miles. They eat a diet that would horrify most American athletes. In contrast to those of us in this country who derive 40 percent of our total calories from fat, the Tarahumaras get only 12 percent of their total calories from fat. (Most of their calories come from complex carbohydrates in the form of beans and corn.) Their daily cholesterol intake is less than 100 milligrams per day—which again is in sharp contrast to our own typical intake of 400 to 500 or more milligrams daily.

The large difference in dietary intakes of fat and cholesterol between our culture and that of the Tarahumara is reflected in similarly marked differences in blood concentrations of cholesterol. The typical Tarahumara adult has about 125 milligrams of cholesterol in each 100 milliliters of blood, whereas the typical U.S. adult has over 200 milligrams of cholesterol per 100 milliliters of blood. This striking difference is evident even among children. Tarahumara youngsters have cholesterol readings of about 116 milligrams per 100 milliliters versus 182 milligrams per 100 milliliters among U.S. children. And while heart disease is rampant in this country, it is almost unheard of among the Tarahumaras.

The data related to diet and death rates from coronary heart disease have now been analyzed for forty different countries, revealing strong positive relationships between the consumption of certain nutrients, heart disease and death. The dietary factors that correlate most strongly are dietary cholesterol, animal protein, animal fat, total fat, saturated fat, dairy products and total calories. On the other hand, such factors as complex carbohydrates (starches and fiber) and vegetable protein correlate negatively with coronary heart disease.

Efforts have repeatedly been made to refute the data linking dietary cholesterol with the elevated blood concentrations of cholesterol that attend coronary heart disease. These efforts, however, have been seriously flawed. One flaw is that they have concentrated on trying to find links—or the lack of them—among populations within a country where food consumption patterns are quite uniform overall—as, for example, they are in the United States. In such circumstances as prevail in the United States, the typical dietary intake of cholesterol is already *at or above* the disease ceiling for coronary heart disease. Thus, comparing these intakes with the intakes of those who consume even greater quantities of cholesterol is not going to yield any important distinction, either in terms of blood levels of cholesterol or incidence of heart disease. If one finds any notable, individual differences here they are due to individual metabolic and genetic factors and not to dietary cholesterol per se.

The famous Framingham (Massachusetts) diet/heart study is sometimes cited as evidence that diet is not a cause of coronary heart disease. But, in fact, the Framingham study showed only that there was no correlation between dietary intake of cholesterol and heart disease *among those Americans whose intakes of fat and cholesterol were already very high to begin with* and thus were above the ceiling at which useful distinctions could be made.

But compare the U.S. epidemiological data with that of countries where daily dietary intake is five, six, seven times *lower* than it is here and you will observe, as we have already seen, *remarkable* differences in the incidence of atherosclerosis, stroke and coronary heart disease. The worldwide epidemiological data strongly suggest that high-cholesterol, high-fat diets are not only causes but are *major* causes of these diseases. Still, epidemiological data are only *suggestive*. They must be confirmed by direct studies in animals and in people.

There is one epidemiological exception which must be mentioned because it carries an important lesson. The Greenland Eskimos eat a high-fat, high-cholesterol diet of seal and fish—almost completely animal food. Do they have coronary disease as expected? No, they do not. The reason is that seal and fish contain large quantities of a remarkable group of fatty acids called omega-3 fatty acids. These protect against coronary disease. We will have more to say about them later. This exception stresses that the kind of fat eaten is most important.

The Animal Experiments. Some very instructive and exciting results have been obtained during the last eight decades of animal experimentation related to the study of atherosclerosis. Nearly every aspect of human atherosclerotic disease has now been reproduced in various animals through the feeding of diets high in cholesterol and fats. These human diseases have now been reproduced in this fashion in monkeys and other subhuman primates, in rabbits, chickens, guinea pigs, prairie dogs and mice.

We can all derive considerable hope from several of these animal experiments in which it has been shown that some of the damage that diets high in cholesterol and fat can do can be *undone* by reverting to a low-cholesterol/low-fat diet and sticking to it. In rhesus monkeys, for example, severe atherosclerosis has been induced through high-fat, high-cho-

lesterol feeding, so severe, in fact, that the coronary arteries were 60 percent or more blocked. These monkeys had very high blood cholesterol levels, up to 700 (fig. 3). After thirty-six months of treatment with a cholesterol-free diet, however, and a lowering of the blood cholesterol level to 140, these same animals underwent tremendous improvement. Their coronary arteries had only about 20 percent blockage (fig. 4). Not *all* damage can be undone, however, so primary prevention through the sort of gradual dietary modification we propose in this book remains our first concern.

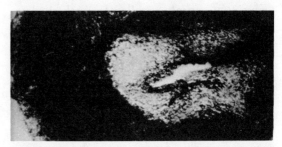

Figure 3. *The nearly completely blocked coronary artery of a rhesus monkey fed a high-cholesterol (egg yolk) diet for seventeen months. Blood flow is restricted to the small opening in the center.*

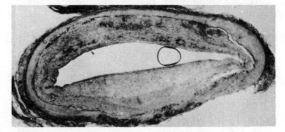

Figure 4. *The coronary artery of a monkey fed a low-fat, low-cholesterol diet for thirty-six months. This artery was previously largely obstructed, as in figure 3. Now the obstruction is much reduced, showing that dietary intervention can reverse the atherosclerotic process to some extent even after it is well-established. The circular structure in the opening of the artery is a bubble and is of no significance.*

Studies in Humans. Many of the animal dietary experiments related above have now been, in part, replicated in humans. Over the past twenty years more than two dozen separate human experiments have demonstrated that the amounts of cholesterol and saturated fat which we eat have decisive effects on blood concentrations of cholesterol and upon a fat-protein particle called LDL (low-density lipoprotein). High-fat, high-cholesterol diets not only produce more cholesterol in the blood but also increase the LDL, which is the "bad guy" with regard to the development of atherosclerosis. It is this cholesterol-carrying particle that the artery wall picks up. Another fat-protein particle is called HDL (high-density lipoprotein). This is known as the "good guy" because one of its functions is to help carry cholesterol from the tissues out of the body.

There are other factors that affect HDL and LDL. Gender is one of them. Men typically have less of the protective HDL and more of the potentially dangerous LDL than do women, a fact that undoubtedly helps explain why there are 60 percent fewer heart attacks among women than men in the United States, particularly before the menopause. Exercise may also influence the HDL to LDL ratio, but diet remains the primary variable over which we have any control.

A particularly ambitious long-term study involving 3806 men was recently concluded under sponsorship of the National Heart, Lung, and Blood Institute. This ten-year study—The Lipid Research Clinics Primary Prevention Trial—was designed to see what effects reduced levels of cholesterol in the blood would have upon the risk of developing coronary heart disease. The assumption, based on all the other evidence, was that this reduction would confer considerable protec-

tion, but since the issue remained controversial the Institute wanted to try to settle it. A definitive study using diet alone would have required an extremely large number of participants because it is difficult to get a sufficient number of people to change to, and comply with, a strict dietary regimen over a long period of time. The cost of such a study had been estimated as high as one billion dollars. Thus the Institute opted to use a nonabsorbable cholesterol-lowering drug along with a diet moderately restricted in cholesterol and fat.

The results were clear-cut. The men who received the drug-and-diet regimen had much lower blood cholesterol and LDL levels and had an incidence of heart attacks 19 percent lower than expected. The rate of *fatal* heart attacks was 24 percent lower than expected. (The control subjects, men who received placebos but some dietary modification, meanwhile, had much less LDL lowering and many more fatal and nonfatal heart attacks.) The study provides convincing, additional evidence that reduced blood cholesterol and LDL levels decrease the risk of developing coronary heart disease. For every 1 percent reduction in blood cholesterol there was, this study concluded, a 2 percent reduction in coronary heart disease risk. Changes at any point in life were thought to be beneficial, but the earlier the changes were made, the better.

The Institute, extrapolating from the results of this and other studies of the sort we've been discussing, concluded that *diet alone* can be of considerable value in reducing heart disease risks—especially among the 35 million to 49 million men and women in this country who presently have "moderately" elevated cholesterol levels. (We'll have more to say later about what blood cholesterol levels are desirable for men and women in different age groups based on our own research as well as that of others.)

There are human studies that claim to refute the idea that dietary cholesterol has any real effect on blood concentrations and disease incidence. These studies, which cause great confusion not only among lay people but also among many doctors, uniformly fail to recognize the significance of what we call *threshold* and *ceiling* amounts of dietary cholesterol. Starting with a baseline diet that is *cholesterol-free,* the amount of dietary cholesterol necessary to show a measurable increase in the amount of cholesterol in the blood is called the threshold amount. Above that threshold, increases in the blood will continue to be noted in direct relationship to increases in dietary intake of cholesterol *up to* a point we call the ceiling amount. If you add more cholesterol to the diet above the ceiling amount, you will *not* observe a further increase in blood concentrations even if the dietary increases are enormous.

Each species almost certainly has its own threshold and ceiling levels. Our own work and the experimental literature suggest that, in humans, the threshold is about 100 milligrams of cholesterol per day. The ceiling, for many of us, appears to be about 300 to 400 milligrams per day. Thus, since most of us in the United States are consuming 400 *or more* milligrams of cholesterol daily, *no* experimental effect will show up in blood studies unless care is taken to first establish a base-line diet that mandates an intake of 100 milligrams or less of cholesterol per day. When this is done, the correlations we are talking about become dramatically evident, showing that diet can have profound effects on the amount of cholesterol in our blood.

Just because the blood cholesterol level does not rise beyond the ceiling as you continue to eat more dietary cholesterol, does not mean that you can eat all the eggs or other cholesterol-rich foods that you like without any harmful effects. On the contrary. Studies have shown that much of this additional cholesterol is still absorbed into the body and must be processed. Any cholesterol that comes into the body can add to the storage of cholesterol in the body, particularly in the arteries. Even though the blood cholesterol might not rise further, the additional cholesterol from food will contribute to the accumulation of more cholesterol in the body and should therefore be avoided.

It isn't just the cholesterol, however, that does all the damage. It's also the amount and type of fat. (Cholesterol itself is a fatty-like substance found only in foods of animal origin.) Numerous studies have confirmed that diets high in the sort of saturated or hard fats that are found in most meats, high-fat dairy products and in three vegetable fats (coconut oil, palm oil and chocolate) increase the risk factors for atherosclerosis. Other studies have shown that polyunsaturated fats (such as those found in most vegetable oils) can actually lower cholesterol concentrations in many people. Fish oils with their content of polyunsaturated omega-3 fatty acids also have a lowering action upon the blood fats.

Insufficient intake of fiber and complex carbohydrates, indirectly, and excessive intake of calories and salt, more directly, may also play roles in the development of coronary heart disease and stroke. We'll have more to say about each of these factors, including cholesterol and all of the various types of fat, in subsequent chapters.

Protein is of lesser importance in a direct sense. Animal protein, for example, is usually associated with both cholesterol and saturated fat. Vegetable protein, on the other hand, is present in foods like cereals and breads which are low in fat content, high in fiber and complex carbohydrates like starch. Some studies even show that vegetable protein may actually have a blood-cholesterol-lowering effect compared to animal protein.

Pathologic/Autopsy Studies. When the coronary arteries of people who have died of coronary heart disease are examined at autopsy, atherosclerosis is confirmed in nearly every case. And the atherosclerotic plaques invariably consist primarily of cholesterol and associated scar tissue. The origin of this cholesterol in the atherosclerotic plaque is from the blood. This has been well documented both in humans and in animal studies. The artery wall does not manufacture that much cholesterol itself. Instead, the cholesterol infiltrates into the artery in the form of lipoprotein particles, particularly LDL, from the blood. Furthermore, cholesterol from the diet has been tagged and been found itself to enter the arterial wall.

In all instances, the infiltration of cholesterol from the blood into the artery wall to form the atherosclerotic plaque occurs *only* when the cholesterol level is considerably elevated over what human beings normally have when *not* consuming the American diet, that is, cholesterol levels of 140 to 160 milligrams per 100 milliliters. Cholesterol which comes into the artery wall may also *leave* the artery wall when the plasma cholesterol is lowered. In this instance, there is an outward flux. We should always consider that the atherosclerotic plaques in the arterial wall are mobile and constantly are interchanging molecules of cholesterol with the blood. This biochemical information gives us hope that *changing* the amount of cholesterol in the blood in the *downward* direction may also

lower the amount of cholesterol in the arterial wall and thus offer a treatment possibility for people with atherosclerotic plaques.

Conclusion. All of the lines of evidence that we have been discussing highlight the decisive role of cholesterol and fat, much of it derived from our present diet, in the development of atherosclerosis, stroke and coronary heart disease. Our conclusion, based upon the best evidence available at this time, is that significant atherosclerosis and the diseases that follow from it will *not* occur if the blood levels of cholesterol can be maintained at *between 160 and 180 milligrams per 100 milliliters or lower over much of the lifetime of the individual.* Even in the event, however, that moderate to advanced atherosclerosis has already set in, a diet and/or other intervention that similarly helps significantly lower blood concentrations of cholesterol will help prevent further damage and can even be expected to reverse *some* of the existing damage over a period of time.

On the basis of the atherosclerosis findings alone, it can be stated that a modification of the standard American diet is urgently needed. Autopsies on American servicemen killed in Korea and Vietnam revealed significant atherosclerosis even in those in their early twenties.

The average blood level of cholesterol that is still considered "normal" in this country is much too high. Just because more than half of the U.S. population has blood cholesterol concentrations of 200 milligrams or higher doesn't make this "normal" or "healthy." We have only to look at this country's disability and death rates from coronary heart disease to know that something is *very abnormal.* The data cited above indicate that a primary source of trouble is our diet.

An advisory panel of the National Institutes of Health (NIH) has now concluded that the best available scientific evidence proves "beyond a reasonable doubt" that the reduction of the blood cholesterol can significantly lower the risk of heart attack. If Americans as a group can be persuaded to change their diets so that they have just 10 percent less cholesterol in their blood, then ultimately 100,000 fewer of us will die each year from heart disease. (The New American Diet detailed in this book can reduce blood levels of cholesterol *considerably more* than 10 percent.)

"We think all Americans are at unnecessarily high risk of heart disease largely because of the kind of diet we eat," concluded Dr. Daniel Steinberg of the University of California, San Diego, chairman of the NIH advisory panel that examined all the relevant evidence. *All Americans.* That's quite a sweeping statement, yet it's one we agree with wholeheartedly and it's something we've been saying for years. The panel endorsed across-the-board dietary changes, something we have long advocated. The changes we propose are detailed in this book.

HYPERTENSION

The current, standard American diet frequently contributes to high blood pressure, or hypertension as it is medically known. As in the case of coronary heart disease, the dietary influences are many. The most important of these are excessive sodium, too much alcohol and excessive calories and insufficient potassium.

We know that hypertension, which currently afflicts 37 million people in the United States and is associated with an increased risk of heart disease and fatal heart attacks as well as strokes, is very rare in children but may be found in more than 20 percent of the adult population over the age of forty. That blood pressure rises continuously with age suggests that environmental factors, such as diet, may contribute significantly to the incidence of this disorder. The epidemiological evidence is especially strong that adding salt to foods as well as eating foods already high in salt are the factors most likely to contribute to the age-related tendency to develop hypertension.

Sodium is the substance in salt responsible for this influence. One can readily produce high blood pressure in laboratory animals, such as the rat, by feeding them salt or sodium. (Some strains of rats are more susceptible than others, indicating that there are genetic factors in hypertension, as well.)

Another dietary mineral—potassium—may help *protect* against hypertension. Recent studies suggest that calcium and other minerals may also have some protective influence, but more research will have to be done before this is fully demonstrated.

Excessive consumption of calories and alcohol have both been related to the development of high blood pressure. The alcohol relationship is particularly interesting since many people try to justify their intake on grounds that alcohol "relaxes" them. The best evidence suggests that alcohol elevates blood pressure. Obesity, resulting from more calories consumed than burned, is also definitely linked to hypertension.

The most important element in the dietary prevention and treatment of hypertension, however, is the decrease of sodium and an increase in potassium intake. Our program promotes a gradual reduction of the amount of salt that is added to foods at the table and in cooking, as well as in the intake of foods that come from the store with salt already added. You will find details in subsequent chapters. Our program also promotes an increase in the intake of dietary potassium through the increased eating of foods of more natural and unprocessed origin. (Processed foods usually have added salt, and much of the potassium naturally present in the food has been removed in the processing.) Our program helps to prevent the development of obesity and can be used in a gradual weight loss program, as detailed later in this book. Weight loss alone lowers blood pressure in many cases. The reasons for this have not been well documented but is in part related to reduced sodium intake. As for alcohol, those with hypertension or a tendency for it, are advised to restrict consumption to no more than one drink two or three times a week.

OBESITY

Continual excessive caloric intake characterizes the American diet. This caloric excess is particularly in the form of fat and other "calorically dense" items such as sugar and alcohol. Just as important are the reduced levels of physical activity in our daily lives. Obesity is associated with an increased risk of certain types of cancer, hypertension and cardiovascular disease. There is also a relationship to the type of diabetes which develops in adults.

DIABETES MELLITUS

The type of diabetes that typically afflicts adults is related to both sugar and fat metabolism. Overweight is also a contributing factor. The correction of obesity, in some instances, is all that is required to completely control maturity-onset diabetes. In general, the same sort of diet that will help protect against atherosclerosis will similarly help protect against diabetes. The diabetic condition also predisposes to coronary heart disease and to stroke.

GALLSTONES

The commonest form of gallstones is composed primarily of cholesterol, which is a normal constituent of the bile that the gallbladder produces. Obesity and high-cholesterol, high-fat diets are strongly associated with the formation of these gallstones in the gallbladder because cholesterol is too high in amount in the bile to remain in solution. It then precipitates out to begin a stone.

CANCERS

Less is known about dietary influences in cancer than in many of the other diseases discussed above, but because cancer afflicts so many people and with such serious consequences a great deal of research is now being devoted to probable and possible associations between diet and cancer. The evidence linking diet and some cancers is compelling enough that the National Academy of Sciences published a book compiling the relevant data (*Diet, Nutrition and Cancer*, National Research Council, National Academy Press, Washington, D.C., 1982) and is continuing to study the link.

It is estimated that 40 percent of all cancers in men and 60 percent of all cancers in women may be attributable to dietary factors. The various forms of cancer account for about 20 percent of all the deaths in the United States. And since cures have proved elusive, emphasis in recent years has shifted toward prevention. Apart from getting people to stop smoking (the cause of 25 percent of all cancer deaths in the United States), the next most important thing we can do in the preventive effort is to encourage modification of diet. Fortunately, the same New American Diet that we propose to fight heart disease and obesity can be expected to help prevent many cancers as well.

A number of intestinal cancers are, not surprisingly, related to the food we eat. These cancers include malignancies of the stomach, pancreas, colon and rectum. Cancer of the colon is the second most common cancer in both men and women. It has been linked to excessive fat and cholesterol intake and to insufficient fiber in overly refined diets. It is not surprising either, then, that those populations that have a high incidence of coronary heart disease also have a high incidence of colon cancer. The role of fiber in helping to protect against some cancers is discussed later. Cancers of the pancreas and rectum are also related to fat consumption.

Unlike cancers of the pancreas, colon and rectum, stomach cancer has markedly *decreased* in incidence over the past several decades, and, once more, we can find a dietary reason for this. Stomach cancer has been linked to the salting and pickling of foods, once common in food preservation. When refrigeration was not available, salting and pickling were the only ways of preserving many foods for any length of time. Now, of course, that has changed, and the incidence of stomach cancer has plummeted. Salt's role in cancer has to do with the changes it induces in the internal environment of the stomach and in the formation of cancer-causing chemicals called nitrosamines.

Cancer of the breast is the commonest malignancy in women, and it has been associated with the amount of fat in diet. Here, too, is a cancer that correlates very strongly with the occurrence of coronary heart disease in various countries. In Japan, for example, both cancer of the breast and coronary heart disease are much less common than in the United States. How fat promotes breast cancer remains to be elucidated, but in experimental animals fed a high-fat diet more cancer of the breast developed than would otherwise have been expected.

Study of the migration of populations also shows the apparent effect of diet on breast cancer. Japanese women living in Japan have a low incidence of this disease, but those Japanese women who have migrated to the United States have the same incidence of breast cancer as do American women in general. The primary change in life-style is the adoption of a high-fat diet. The National Cancer Institute and others are investigating the preventive potential of a low-fat diet with respect to this cancer.

Cancer of the ovary has been related to the amount of fat in the diet, as well, whereas cancer of the body of the uterus is linked to obesity. Fat cells in obese individuals have the capacity of converting an adrenal hormone into another sex hormone that apparently promotes this uterine cancer. Cancer of the prostate, so common in men, is like cancer of the breast in that it occurs most frequently in those countries consuming a high-fat diet and having a high incidence of coronary heart disease.

All of these cancers related to the American diet we think of as potentially preventable. What a marvelous thing this would be. Just as cancer of the stomach is now decreasing, so *can* cancer of the breast, prostate, ovary, pancreas, and colon also decrease. We look for this to happen in the future if Americans change their dietary habits as we know many will once they understand the possible benefits for making such changes.

Once more it can be seen that the current American diet exposes us to increased risks of getting one form or another of a major family of diseases—the cancers. It does this through *overreliance* on fatty foods, cholesterol and calories derived from overrefined, overprocessed foods. It also does this through *underreliance* on foods that provide fiber, vegetables and fruit. The same dietary factors that predispose us to cancer also predispose us, as demonstrated earlier, to atherosclerosis, stroke and coronary heart disease.

VENOUS THROMBOSIS

These blood-clotting disorders are linked with diets high in fat and with obesity. Blood clot formation is more likely to occur from saturated fat in the diet and to be inhibited by polyunsaturated fat, especially the omega-3 fatty acids from fish.

DENTAL CARIES

Tooth decay is clearly associated with the high sugar content in the standard diet.

CIRRHOSIS OF THE LIVER

Cirrhosis of the liver is linked to excessive alcohol consumption in animals and humans. Alcohol is toxic to the liver cells.

Diseases of Underconsumption

The American/Western European diet is low in fiber (indigestible carbohydrate of plant origin which reaches the colon relatively intact). Traditionally, fiber *has* been a major component of the human diet—up until recently when refined and processed foods with a low fiber content began to predominate. Those who get a lot of fiber in their diets have softer stools that are larger in volume and which pass through the system more rapidly. Fiber prevents constipation and may prevent other medical problems such as hemorrhoids, appendicitis, and diverticulosis. Furthermore, when feces transit through the bowel more rapidly there is less time and opportunity for potential cancer-causing substances to be in contact with the inner lining of the large bowel and initiate cancer.

Summary

Overall, the trouble with the current American diet can be summed up as follows: "too much," on the one hand, and "too little" on the other. Too much fat, especially of the saturated variety, too much protein from animal sources, too much carbohydrate from overprocessed sources, including too much sugar, too much salt, too much alcohol, too much food with too little fiber and too little room left over for fresh fruits and vegetables, whole grains and beans.

The result of all this is *too much disease* in the form of heart attacks, strokes, elevated blood pressure, cancer, diabetes, gallstones, liver disorders and so on. And *too few healthy people*, particularly after the age of forty-five.

A change is clearly needed—one that we can *live* with both in the sense of healthier, longer lives and in terms of a diet that we can *enjoy*. In the following chapter, we'll tell you about the diet we believe achieves these goals.

2

THE NEW AMERICAN DIET

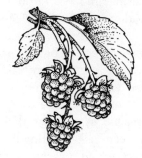

What It Is/What It Can Do

The New American Diet is a low-fat, low-cholesterol and high-carbohydrate diet. That in itself may not seem like news. Our own research—spanning three decades—has helped contribute to the vast amount of research indicating that such a diet could have very significant health benefits. The diet we propose here is the result of those thirty years of experience. Our program differs in that we have been personally involved in the basic research related to diet, atherosclerosis and coronary heart disease and have intensively studied the other diseases of over- and under-consumption and have formulated a *unified* dietary approach to best combat *all* of them.

Heretofore there has been a plethora of specialized diets that put all their eggs in one basket. Thus there are "high-fiber" diets, "low-fat" diets, "high-carbohydrate" diets, fruit diets, vegetarian diets, etc. There are also diets that are aimed exclusively at individual diseases. Unfortunately, these diets, while emphasizing some valid findings, often miss or ignore other findings that really should be taken into account if a lifelong diet program is to be offered. An example here would be a diet devised to combat breast cancer that stresses overall reduction of fat without offering ways to make sure that cholesterol and salt are also adequately reduced or fiber adequately increased.

Our experience has allowed us to create a diet program that takes all diseases into consideration, and does not focus on one disease or on one food element such as "fat-free" or "salt-free" or "sugar-free." Instead, we have been able to devise a diet that has the best possible combination of all foods and nutrients, given our current state of knowledge. Out of all of this, as indicated above, we have discovered that *one* diet or eating style offers the best hope we have of preventing and treating the diseases and disorders discussed in the preceding chapter.

When it comes to diseases, we have *all* become so fragmented or specialized in our thinking that at first blush it seems remarkable that a single diet could protect against many of the major diseases that plague us. But, with a little reflection, it will seem astonishing if it were otherwise. Nature would have to be capricious indeed to require a multiplicity of different diets in order for us to survive the many different challenges that have confronted us in the course of our evolution. Or, looked at from a somewhat different perspective, we can see that people would almost have had to find the one optimal or near-optimal diet in order to survive as they have done.

We pretty well know now what that near-optimal diet is—or, rather, *was.* That goes in the past tense because most of us in the Western world have drifted away from that diet in modern times. That drift has cost us dearly, as documented in the preceding chapter. It is only in recent times that entire cultures have attained sufficient affluence to derive so much of their food intake from animal sources.

The goal of the New American Diet is to restore many of the basic components of the diet that sustained our ancestors while at the same time utilizing modern technology to ensure that we retain the variety and convenience in foods that we have become accustomed to in the present era. Armed with

both the knowledge and the technology that we now have, it is actually possible for us to eat a diet that is just as healthy as that of our forebears but one that is far less monotonous and is actually more varied, tasty and interesting.

And here, finally, is what sets the New American Diet apart: It was designed to be acceptable to people of *all* kinds, for their entire *lifetimes,* and not just for a few weeks or months. Ours is not a crash diet or a fad diet —those are all, without exception, failures in the long run—but instead is a gradual program that amounts to a permanent change in eating life-style. Though benefits can begin to accrue from the diet almost immediately, it is a diet that individuals and especially whole families (wherein the basic eating habits are acquired) learn to eat over a period of weeks, months and years. Ultimately, *you* determine the pace at which you progress, though we will provide you with goals and objectives that will let you know what you are achieving at each phase of the diet.

Many diet programs are dictatorial. They tell you what you *must* do and when you *must* do it. The trouble with this approach is that it retains its power only very briefly. Forced to switch abruptly to tastes and textures that are unfamiliar, doled out in caloric-restricted quantities, the typical dieter finds the going gets tough very quickly and soon throws in the towel, disgusted with what has become unpalatable and monotonous fare. That's why, as scientific studies prove, the recidivism (backsliding) rate for these diets is in many instances *100 percent.* That's also why people who want to lose weight so often drift from one diet program to another, continually losing and gaining weight in what has been called "the rhythm method of girth control." That label may be a joke, but the effect of that kind of eating is anything but funny. It may actually be far less dangerous to retain some excess weight than it is to lose it continually and then regain it.

The New American Diet is not just guesswork or the product of some small, unscientific trial. Our diet has its foundations in the worldwide population studies, in experimental and clinical data summarized in the preceding chapter and in studies we and others have conducted, most notably the Family Heart Study (see Introduction and subsequent chapters for more details).

As noted in the Introduction, the Family Heart Study was the first (and to date the only) study designed to determine whether the eating patterns of *randomly selected* families could be altered in ways that would demonstrably reduce their risks of developing coronary heart disease (and other diseases of over- and underconsumption) over a long period of time. If the goal is to determine scientifically what the *general* population and, specifically, *typical* families *are* and *are not* willing to do in terms of modifying their diets, then random selection of families is of vital significance. Had we accepted volunteers we would have biased our study at the outset, for volunteers would clearly be more highly motivated than nonvolunteers to make the desired changes.

By using families we selected at random we created a unique living laboratory in which we were able to further fine-tune our diet by paying close attention to the individual tastes of typical families. No matter how "healthy" a diet may be, it will do no good whatever if people can't find foods to eat that they like. Our objective, then, really was to see to what extent typical, generally healthy people were

willing to change their dietary habits *now* in order to avoid health problems *in the future*.

The program of lifelong dietary modification which is at the heart of the New American Diet is the product of what we have learned in studies like this one. Our diet, we believe, is scientifically sound and is one that Americans and others in the Western world can successfully adapt to and maintain for long periods of time—we believe for life.

Goals of the New American Diet

The New American Diet provides delicious and even gourmet foods, all laboratory and field tested, which are low in cholesterol, fat and especially saturated fat, reduced in salt and sugar and plentiful in bulk or fiber. The diet is designed to be tasty and full of variety without sacrificing our ultimate goal: good health throughout life.

Among the goals that will help us prevent the diseases of overconsumption are:

1. To decrease the cholesterol content of food.
2. To reduce intake of saturated fats.
3. To reduce the total amount of fat intake.
4. To increase intake of complex carbohydrates and fiber, such as whole grains, breads, potatoes, beans, pastas, cereals, rice, fruits and vegetables.
5. To reduce salt intake.
6. To reduce intake of added sugars.
7. To keep alcohol consumption low.
8. If overweight, to reduce total food intake, especially consumption of foods high in fat and sugar and low in bulk.

Those are the *general* goals of the diet. But, more specifically, the objectives are these:

— To reduce the average U.S. cholesterol consumption from 400 to 500 milligrams per day to less than 100 milligrams per day.
— To reduce fat intake by about one-half, so that only 20 percent, rather than the current average of 40 percent, of all calories are derived from fat, three-fourths of which are "invisible" in the current American diet.
— To decrease *saturated* fat intake by two-thirds so that instead of getting 14 percent of our calories from this type of fat we will only get 5 or 6 percent from this source.

THE NEW AMERICAN DIET GOALS

EAT TWICE AS MUCH COMPLEX CARBOHYDRATE

Eat 2 to 5 servings at each meal (bread, cereal, pasta, potatoes, etc.)
Eat 3 to 5 cups legumes each week
Eat 2 to 4 cups vegetables each day

REDUCE TOTAL FAT INTAKE BY ONE-HALF

Avoid fried foods
Reduce fat in baked goods by one-third
Limit added fat to 2-4 teaspoons/day (margarine, mayonnaise, salad dressing)
Use peanut butter as a meal item, not snack
Use nuts sparingly, as a condiment

REDUCE SATURATED FAT INTAKE BY TWO-THIRDS

Limit red meat or cheese to twice a week
Use only low-fat milk, yogurt and cheeses
Limit ice cream and chocolate to once a month
Avoid coconut, palm and hydrogenated oils
Replace butter, lard, and drippings with oil or tub margarine

REDUCE CHOLESTEROL CONSUMPTION BY ONE-HALF TO THREE-FOURTHS

Eliminate egg yolks
Avoid organ meats
Limit daily "meat" consumption to 6 ounces fish, clams, oysters or scallops or 3 ounces red meat, poultry, crab, shrimp or lobster

EAT HALF AS MUCH REFINED SUGAR

Reduce sweetener used in baked goods by one-third
Limit sweets to one serving per day (pop or sweetened drinks or candy or dessert)
Drink water to satisfy thirst

REDUCE SALT CONSUMPTION BY ONE-HALF

Add no salt at the table
Cook with Lite Salt or reduced sodium soy sauce
Use no salt added canned products or choose fresh or frozen
Limit regular canned soup, vegetables or entrées to once a month

MAINTAIN IDEAL BODY WEIGHT

For most Americans this means a life-style adjustment of 200 Calories per day

Choose low-fat, high-fiber foods
Aerobic activity (30 minutes, 5 days a week)

Figure 5. *The New American Diet goals depicted in terms of food intake.*

— To increase carbohydrate intake from the present 45 percent of total calories to 65 percent with emphasis on increased intake of complex carbohydrates and fiber.
— To decrease the intake of refined sugar, from 20 percent of calories to 10 percent.
— To cut salt intake substantially—by half or more.

What these objectives mean in terms of food is illustrated in figure 5.

Step by Step: The Three Phases of the Diet

The goals and objectives outlined above are to be achieved gradually. The New American Diet proceeds through three major phases (fig. 6), each of which will be explored in far greater detail in part 2 of this book:

PHASE ONE

Here, instead of being introduced abruptly to entirely new recipes, the individual is instructed in improving old favorites and in modifying, in general, the meals he, she or the family currently enjoys. Some of these modifications and substitutions are very simple. People discover, for example, that many familiar recipes calling for egg yolks can be made to work—and remain tasty—through a reduction or even complete elimination of egg yolks, while increasing the use of egg whites. A Cholesterol-Saturated Fat Index

(CSI), which we have developed in our laboratories, is utilized in this phase, providing a whole new, very useful way of comparing foods, making it much easier for a person to select lower-fat cheese, frozen desserts, fats, eggs, fish, poultry, red meat and dairy products that are lower in cholesterol and saturated fat. The CSI represents a major advance over the old methods of comparing foods based solely on cholesterol or total fat content. Many people stick to foods that they are accustomed to simply because they are unaware of equally tasty lower-fat substitutes. Or they don't know how to tell the sometimes small but still very important differences among these various foods. (Cheeses are a prime example.) The CSI helps solve many of these problems.

PHASE TWO

This phase is characterized by the introduction of many new recipes, designed in particular to gradually help the typical person reduce meat intake from up to a pound a day to no more than 6 to 8 ounces a day. Lunches, and the sandwich in particular, that vehicle for delivering so much meat and cheese into the system, get special attention in this phase. Methods of preparing foods that require less fat are emphasized, as are recipes that use larger amounts of grains, legumes, vegetables and fruits. Numerous, tasty, ethnic dishes are introduced in this phase, including Oriental, Mexican, Mediterranean and Middle Eastern dishes.

PHASE THREE

We often refer to this phase as "a new way of eating." When you reach this phase you will be close to achieving the end-point goals/

objectives outlined earlier. In Phase Three we take a historical approach to the consumption of meat. People have always eaten meat. What they have not done is to eat meat every day, let alone several times a day. Even today, *daily* meat consumption is only possible for the affluent minority of the world's population. It is not to our advantage, in terms of either our health or our resources, to consume large amounts of meat every day.

As President Thomas Jefferson said in a letter to a doctor friend, "I have lived temperately, eating little animal food, and not as an aliment [main course], so much as a condiment for the vegetables which constitute my principal diet."

THE NEW AMERICAN DIET
STEP BY STEP

PHASE I:
SUBSTITUTIONS

This is accomplished by:
- avoiding egg yolks, butterfat, lard and organ meats (liver, heart, brains, kidney, gizzards);
- substituting soft margarine for butter;
- substituting vegetable oils and shortening for lard;
- substituting skim milk and skim milk products for whole milk and whole milk products;
- substituting egg whites for whole eggs;
- trimming fat off meat and skin from chicken;
- choosing commercial food products lower in cholesterol and fat (low-fat cheeses, egg substitutes, soy meat substitutes, frozen yogurt, etc.);
- modifying favorite recipes by using less fat or sugar and vegetable oils instead of butter or lard;
- decreasing use of table salt and using lower sodium salt (Lite Salt)

PHASE II:
NEW RECIPES

This step involves:
- reducing amounts of meat and cheese eaten and replacing them with chicken and fish;
- eating meat, chicken or fish only once a day;
- cutting down on fat; as spreads, in salads, cooking and baking;
- eating more grains, beans, fruits and vegetables;
- making low-fat, low-cholesterol choices when eating out;
- finding new recipes to replace those which cannot be altered;
- using few products containing salt

PHASE III:
A NEW WAY OF
EATING

The final phase means:
- eating meat, cheese, poultry, shellfish, and fish as "condiments" to other foods, rather than as main courses;
- eating more beans and grain products as protein sources;
- using no more than 4-7 teaspoons of fat per day as spreads, salad dressings and in cooking and baking;
- drinking 4-6 glasses of water per day;
- keeping extra meat, regular cheese, chocolate, candy, coconut and richer home-baked or commercially prepared food for special occasions (once a month or less);
- enjoying a wide variety of new food and repertoire of totally new and savory recipes;
- decreasing amount of salt used for cooking

Figure 6. *Summary of the three phases of the New American Diet.*

The total intakes of poultry, shrimp, crab, lobster and meat should not exceed an average of 3 or 4 ounces daily. Happily, however, due to recent discoveries we and others have made, up to 6 ounces of fish, clams, oysters and scallops can be included in the daily diet even during this phase. Fish and shellfish contain a type of fat that actually helps *lower* cholesterol and triglyceride concentrations in the blood (the omega-3 fatty acids).

THE NEW AMERICAN DIET

Whereas emphasis in Phase Two is on modifying the typical lunch, emphasis in Phase Three is on modifying *dinner* with a return to the way people traditionally used meat for most of human history—not as a main course and not at every meal, but instead as a *condiment* to augment or spice up vegetable-, rice-, cereal- and legume-based dishes, much as is found in some of the most appealing Oriental, Indian and Mediterranean cookery.

As we've noted, the current American diet contains about 400 to 500 milligrams of cholesterol per day. This is decreased in Phase One of our diet to 300 to 350 milligrams, to 200 milligrams in Phase Two and to 100 milligrams or lower in Phase Three. Fat content of our diet decreases from 40 percent of total calories in the current, typical U.S. diet to 35 percent in Phase One, to 25 percent in Phase Two and to 20 percent in Phase Three. The goal of only 5 or 6 percent of total calories coming from saturated fats is fully achieved in Phase Three. Carbohydrate intake, with emphasis on the complex variety, gradually increases from about 45 percent of total calories in the typical American diet to 50 percent in Phase One, to 60 percent in Phase Two and to 65 percent in Phase Three.

The dietary fiber content of the New American Diet increases from 15 to 20 grams per day to 45 to 60 grams per day. And though total carbohydrate intake is increased in our diet, the refined sugar content is actually decreased from 20 percent to 10 percent of total calories. Salt intake steadily decreases through the three phases and potassium intake increases. Figure 7 illustrates these changes. Table 1 compares the chemical composition of the present American diet with the New American Diet.

TYPICAL   RECOMMENDED

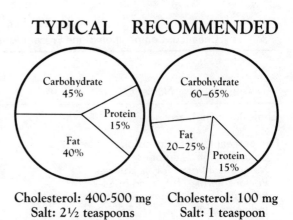

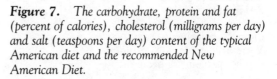

Figure 7. *The carbohydrate, protein and fat (percent of calories), cholesterol (milligrams per day) and salt (teaspoons per day) content of the typical American diet and the recommended New American Diet.*

A Nutritionally Balanced Diet

The New American Diet is nutritionally balanced, offers a wide variety of foods and meets all of the recommended dietary allowances established by the Food and Nutrition

Board of the National Research Council of the National Academy of Sciences. These allowances include those for protein, about which concern is often expressed by people in this country. The protein content of our diet is the same, in fact, in terms of *amount* as that of the current U.S. diet. The *kind* of protein, however, is altered to some extent, with more emphasis on vegetable protein and less on animal protein. People in the United States typically get 68 percent of their protein from animal sources. In our diet, this is altered so that about 44 percent of the protein intake is

from animal sources—still a considerable amount. This is closer to what was eaten in this country in the early 1900s.

Flexibility of the Diet

Gradualness is the key to making *permanent* changes in diet. As we've already noted, we recommend that you proceed at your own pace. We will provide you with goals, information, recipes and with the means of moni-

TABLE 1
Chemical Composition of the Present American Diet and the New American Diet

Nutrient	American Diet		New American Diet (Phase III)	
Cholesterol, mg*/day	400–500		100	
Fat, percent (%) of total calories	40		20	
Saturated fat, % calories		15		5
Monounsaturated fat, % calories		16		8
Polyunsaturated fat, % calories		6		7
P/S value		0.4		1.3
Iodine number		63		99
Vegetable fat, % fat		38		75
Animal fat, % fat		62		25
Protein, % calories	15		15	
Vegetable protein, % protein		32		56
Animal protein, % protein		68		44
Carbohydrate, % calories	45		65	
Starch, % calories		17		40
Sucrose (added to food), % calories		20		10
Fructose, glucose, sucrose, lactose, maltose, % calories (naturally present in foods)		8		15
Dietary fiber, gm*	15–20		45–60	
Sodium, mEq*	200–300		75–100	
Potassium, mEq	60–85		100–140	

* Mg = milligrams; gm = grams; mEq = milliequivalent.

toring your status, all designed to help keep you on the path of progress. The individuality of our diet concept will become evident in other ways, as well, as you read subsequent chapters.

Though we've designed our diet with the family unit foremost in our minds, we recognize that many individuals will want to use this program as well. So will a lot of busy, professional people who don't do a lot of cooking at home or don't have much time to devote to meal preparation. There are many quickies in our New American Diet repertoire. And we will share with you what we've learned about eating out at restaurants and even while on camping trips and the like. It is possible to eat away from home and follow the guidelines of the diet. We'll also have advice for vegetarians, expectant mothers, parents with young children, etc.

Weight Maintenance/ Weight Loss

People are very good at *losing* weight— many have lost hundreds of pounds. The major problem is weight *maintenance,* which few people achieve *after* weight loss. A special chapter will be devoted to the subject of weight loss and weight maintenance.

We believe that the New American Diet provides the best chance for maintaining an ideal body weight once it is achieved—and for maintaining it on a *long-term* basis.

There are a number of advantages to following the New American Diet objectives while losing weight. One, because it is low in fat there is a lot of food—in terms of quantity. Two, it promotes a maximum loss of body fat during weight reduction. This means

there is minimal loss of muscle and water (lean body mass). Three, it does not contain *too much* or *too little* of any one nutrient. Four, it helps one avoid constipation which is often a problem people encounter when losing weight.

We recognize that some individuals will want to lose considerable weight and will need extra encouragement and added motivation to get started. For those people, we will provide a caloric-restricted starter regimen. The purpose of this will be to ensure weight loss from the start while one practices and learns the art of eating a low-fat diet forever. Exercise is an important part of this weight-loss adjunct to our program.

Summary: A Diet for Disease Prevention

Many of you have heard of the concept of defensive driving. The idea behind it is to learn to drive in ways that will help minimize the possibility of your being involved in an accident due to chance or carelessness or the misjudgment of others. The goal is to *prevent* the accident from occurring in the first place. The same concept can and should apply to eating. We call this type of defensive eating "preventive nutrition." The idea here is to learn to eat in ways that will prevent such dietary "accidents" as heart attack, stroke, diabetes, obesity and cancer.

Much is made of the approximately 50,000 people who die on U.S. highways in auto accidents every year. This is proper, but the slaughter on the highways is minor compared to the dietary slaughter we spoke of in Chapter 1 of this section. More than 50 percent of the *entire population* is at serious risk for stroke and coronary heart disease at some point. Up to 20 percent of the general population is or will be hypertensive. More than one in four Americans are destined to die of cancer. And so on.

The New American Diet embraces the concept of preventive nutrition. The earlier in life it is adapted to the better. But it can be started at *any age* after weaning and still deliver significant, measurable benefits. And this is true whether an individual is healthy or already afflicted by one of these diseases. The diet can help halt the onslaught or, in many cases, even reverse some of the damage of disease, but, clearly, its greatest impact is in the *prevention* of disease.

Now is the time to get started. By taking the quiz in the next chapter, you can begin to identify the changes *you* need to make in order to begin reaping the considerable benefits of all the new knowledge we possess with respect to preventive nutrition.

3

HOW DO YOU MEASURE UP TO THE NEW AMERICAN DIET GOALS?

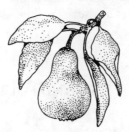

A Quiz to Determine *Your* Need for Change

This quiz was designed to enable you to evaluate your current eating habits and to compare them with the goals of the New American Diet, described in the preceding chapter. By taking this quiz now you will get some idea of what you need to do in order to achieve this way of eating. And by taking this same quiz at various times later on, as you proceed through the program as described in subsequent chapters, you will be able to gauge your progress.

Most of you, eating typical Western world fare, will not score particularly well at the outset. That is to be expected. The disease statistics related to diet that we have been reciting make it evident that most of us have a *lot* of room for making changes in the way we eat. This quiz will help you identify those areas in which you need work. If you fall far short of the goals, don't panic. And don't rush headlong into making changes until you've read the rest of this book. By then you will appreciate the need for *gradual* change. Many of you have spent most of your lives getting into your current eating habits; don't expect to change those overnight. Slow, steady change is the path to *permanent* change.

Directions. For each question in each category below select the answer or answers that *best* describe your eating habits during the last month. The number at the left of each possible answer is the point score. Put your score in the blank after each question. If you checked more than one answer for a question, put the lowest score checked in the blank. For example, with respect to question number 1 under "Meat, Fish and Poultry" below, if you checked bacon, sausage, etc. and also checked wafer-thin lunch meats, then your score is 1. You can compare your score with goal scores at the end of each section. By looking at the goal scores at the end of the "Meat, Fish and Poultry" section, you will see that the goal score is 5, indicating you have a way to go in this category. By looking at the

choice that corresponds under this question with a score of 5 you can see the direction in which you must go. The *higher* the score in each category the closer you are to the goals of the New American Diet. Remember that the goal scores are for the *end-point Phase Three*—so again, don't be alarmed if you fall considerably short of the ideal scores. If your answers are mostly 2 or higher, you're starting out ahead of a great many people. Goal Scores for Phase One and Phase Two will be detailed in subsequent chapters, when you will be asked to retake this quiz.

MEAT, FISH AND POULTRY

1. Which of these have you eaten in the last month?
    1 Bacon, sausage, bologna, pepperoni, regular wieners
    2 Canadian bacon, turkey wieners
    3 Wafer-thin-sliced lunch meats, turkey ham
    4 Soy meat products (such as breakfast links)
    5 None
Score _____

2. Which best describes your typical lunch?
    1 Cheeseburger, typical cheeses, egg salad
    2 Meat (including hamburger), fish or poultry (plain or in a sandwich)
    3 Tuna sandwich, small bits of meat, chicken (in a soup/casserole)

4 Peanut butter sandwich
5 Salad, yogurt, cottage cheese, vegetarian dishes without cheese
Score _____

3. Consider the entrée (main course) at your main meal. How many times a week do you have each of these? (Your number of times per week should add up to 7, for one main meal per day.)
    Beef, lamb, pork, ham, cheese (*Multiply the number of times per week that you have these* _____ *times 2 to get your score* _____ .)
    Veal, wild game (*Multiply the number of times per week that you have these* _____ *times 3 to get your score* _____ .)
    Chicken, turkey, shrimp, crab, lobster

(*Multiply the number of times per week that you have these* _____ *times 4 to get your score* _____.)

Fish, clams, oysters, scallops (fresh/frozen/canned) or Meatless (use grains, beans, vegetables but not egg yolk or typical cheese) (*Multiply the number of times that you have these* _____ *times 5 to get your score* _____.)

Score (total all of your scores for question 3 to get your final score for this question)

_____

4. Estimate the number of *ounces* of meat, regular cheese, fish and poultry you eat in an *average* day. Include *all* meals and snacks. (Remember that there are 16 ounces in a pound. To give some examples to help guide you in your estimate, note that three typical strips of bacon equal 1 ounce; the meat included in a typical sandwich comes to 2 or 3 ounces; a chicken thigh is usually 2 or 3 ounces; a *small* burger patty is about 3 ounces; the average T-bone steak is 8 ounces, 1 slice or a 1-inch cube of cheese equals 1 ounce, etc. Look at labels and pay attention to how much meat and fish weigh when you purchase them.)

   1 Eleven or more ounces per day
   2 Nine to 10 ounces per day
   3 Six to 8 ounces per day
   4 Four to 5 ounces per day
   5 Not more than 1 ounce of regular cheese, 3 ounces of red meat, poultry, shrimp, crab, lobster *or* not more than 6 ounces of fish, clams, oysters, scallops

Score _____

5. Which type of ground beef do you usually eat?

   1 Regular hamburger (30 percent fat)
   2 Lean ground beef (25 percent fat)
   3 Extra lean/ground chuck (20 percent fat)
   4 Super lean/ground round (15 percent fat)
   5 Ground sirloin (10% fat) or eat no ground meat

Score _____

TOTAL SCORE _____ **(Add all of the above scores in this category.)**

Goal Scores for each of the questions above:

Question 1	5
Question 2	4 to 5
Question 3	26 to 30
Question 4	Men/Teens—4; Women/Children—5
Question 5	4 to 5
Total Score	43 to 50

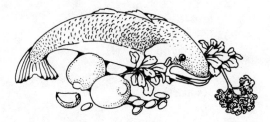

DAIRY PRODUCTS AND EGGS

1. What kind of milk do you *usually* use for drinking or cooking?

  1 Whole milk
  2 Two percent milk
  4 One percent milk, buttermilk
  5 Skim milk, nonfat dry milk or none

Score _____

2. Which toppings do you use?

  1 Sour cream (real or imitation including IMO*), whipped cream
  3 Nondairy toppings such as Cool Whip or Dream Whip
  4 Regular cottage cheese, whole milk yogurt
  5 Low-fat cottage cheese, low-fat yogurt, sweetened or flavored low-fat yogurt

Score _____

3. Which frozen desserts are you most likely to eat at least once a month, if any?

  1 Ice cream
  2 Frozen yogurt (whole milk)
  3 Ice milk, most soft ice cream, Toffutti
  4 Sherbet, low-fat frozen yogurt, ices (sorbet)
  5 None

Score _____

4. What kind of cheese do you use for snacks or in sandwiches?

  1 Cheddar, Swiss, Jack, Brie, feta, American, cream cheese, regular cheese slices or cheese spreads
  2 Part-skim mozzarella, Lappi, light cream cheese or Neufchâtel, part-skim Cheddar (such as Green River, Olympia's Low Fat or Heidi Ann Low-Fat Ched-Style Cheese)
  4 Low-cholesterol "filled" cheese (such as Scandic Mini Chol [Swedish low cholesterol], Hickory Farms Lyte or Cheezola)
  5 Very-low-fat processed cheese (such as Reduced Calories Laughing Cow, Weight Watchers or the Lite-line series of cheeses), or no cheese

Score _____

5. What kind of cheese do you use in cooking (casseroles, vegetables, etc.)?

  1 Cheddar, Swiss, Jack, Brie, feta, American, cream cheese, processed cheese (note: most restaurants use one of these)

* Certain products are listed to provide examples of food items on the market. Often there are other products of similar composition with different trade names.

<u>3</u> Part-skim mozzarella, Lappi, light cream cheese, part-skim cheddar (Green River, Olympia's Low-Fat or Heidi Ann Low-Fat Ched-Style Cheese)

<u>4</u> Low-cholesterol "filled" cheeses (Scandic Mini Chol [Swedish low cholesterol], Hickory Farms Lyte, Cheezola)

<u>5</u> Pot cheese, part-skim Ricotta, low-fat processed cheese (Reduced Calories Laughing Cow, Lite-line, Light n' Lively, Weight Watchers, etc.)

Score _____

6. Check the type and number of "visible" eggs you eat each week.
    <u>1</u> Six or more whole eggs per week
    <u>2</u> Three to five whole eggs per week
    <u>3</u> One to two whole eggs per week
    <u>4</u> One whole egg per month
    <u>5</u> Egg white, egg substitute such as Egg Beaters, Scramblers, Second Nature) or none

Score _____

7. Check the type of eggs usually used in food both commercial and prepared at home (in baked goods, such as cakes and cookies, potato and pasta salads, pancakes, etc.)
    <u>1</u> Whole eggs or mixes containing whole eggs (complete pancake mix, slice-and-bake cookies, etc.)
    <u>3</u> Combination of egg whites, egg substitutes and whole eggs
    <u>5</u> Egg white, egg substitute or none

Score _____

TOTAL SCORE _____ (Add all of the above scores in this category.)

Goal scores for each of the questions above:

Question 1	5
Question 2	5
Question 3	4 to 5
Question 4	4 to 5
Question 5	3 to 5
Question 6	5
Question 7	5
Total Score	31 to 35

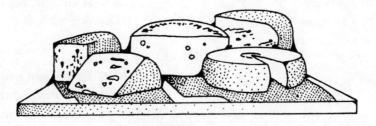

FATS AND OILS

1. What kind of fats are used most often to cook your food (vegetables, meats, etc.)?
   - 1 Butter, shortening (all brands except soft shortening, e.g., Crisco, Food Club, etc.), or lard, bacon grease, chicken fat or eat in restaurants at least 4 times per week
   - 3 Shortening (Crisco or Food Club) or cheap stick margarine (remains hard at room temperature)
   - 4 Tub or soft-stick margarine, vegetable oil
   - 5 None (use nonstick pans or spray)

   Score _____

2. What is your *daily* use of these "visible" fats? (One serving equals *1 teaspoon* (1 pat) of margarine, butter, oil, mayonnaise or Miracle Whip or *2 teaspoons* of imitation or light mayonnaise, salad dressing, peanut butter or diet margarine.) Take all meals and snacks into account.
   - 1 Use 10 servings or more
   - 2 Use 8 to 9 servings
   - 3 Use 6 to 7 servings
   - 4 Use 4 to 5 servings
   - 5 Use 3 servings or less

   Score _____

3. How often do you eat potato chips, corn or tortilla chips, fried chicken, fish sticks, French fries, doughnuts or other fried foods, and croissants and/or Danish pastries?
   - 1 Two or more times *per day*
   - 2 Once *a day*
   - 3 Two to 4 times *per week*
   - 4 Once *a week*
   - 5 Less than twice *a month*

   Score _____

4. What best describes the amount of margarine, peanut butter, mayonnaise or cream cheese that you put on breads, muffins, bagels, etc.?
   - 1 Average (1 or more teaspoons per serving)
   - 2 Lightly spread (can see through it)
   - 4 "Scrape" (can barely see it)
   - 5 None

   Score _____

5. Which kind of salad dressings do you use?
   - 1 Real mayonnaise, Roquefort, blue cheese, Thousand Island, ¾ oil and ¼ vinegar, Ranch Salad Dressing made with sour cream and mayonnaise
   - 2 Miracle Whip
   - 3 Imitation or light mayonnaise, Miracle Whip Light, Italian, Ranch Salad Dressing made with buttermilk and sour cream, IMO or mayonnaise

<u>4</u> French, garlic, ⅓ oil and ⅔ vinegar, Ranch Salad Dressing made with buttermilk and imitation or light mayonnaise or Miracle Whip Light

<u>5</u> Low-calorie dressing, vinegar, lemon juice, Ranch Salad Dressing made with buttermilk and low-fat yogurt or use no salad dressing

Score _____

TOTAL SCORE _____ **(add all of the above scores in this category).**

Goal scores for each of the questions above:

    Question 1   4 to 5

    Question 2   Men/Teens—4; Women/ Children—5

    Question 3   5

    Question 4   4 to 5

    Question 5   4 to 5

Total Score   21 to 25

GRAINS, BEANS, FRUITS AND VEGETABLES

For this part of the quiz, give yourself 5 points for each serving of the following foods you eat each day or per week, as specified. Most people score rather low on this section —which is why we devote a good deal of effort, later in this book, to showing you ways of making grains, beans, fruits and vegetables tasty, exciting parts of your evolving diet.

1. Give yourself 5 points for each serving of fruit eaten *per day*, on the typical day, (1 piece of fruit equals one serving; so does ¾ to 1 cup of real juice—not "fruit-flavored" drinks)

Score _____

2. Give yourself 5 points for each cup of vegetables eaten *per day* (as tossed salad, cooked vegetables, etc.)

Score _____

3. Give yourself 5 points for each cup of legumes eaten *per week* (such as refried beans, split peas, navy beans, lentils, chili, etc.)

Score _____

4. Give yourself 5 points for each small baked potato, ½ cup of potatoes, macaroni or other pasta and ⅓ cup rice eaten *per day*

Score _____

5. Give yourself 5 points for each of the following eaten *per day* (remember sandwiches): 1 slice bread, 1 corn tortilla, 1 muffin, ½ flour tortilla, ½ bagel, ½ cup cooked cereal, 1 cup dry cereal, one 4-inch pancake.

Score _____

6. Give yourself 5 points for each of the following: 5 low-fat crackers, 3 cups lightly buttered popcorn, ½ cup baked corn chips, pretzels (10 small rings) *per day*.

Score _____

7. We believe it's important to eat from each food group regularly. Therefore, *subtract 5 points* for each question 1 through 5 that received a zero.

Total subtracted _____

TOTAL SCORE _____ (Add scores for 1 through 6 above and subtract the score for 7 to get total score.)

Goal scores for each of the questions above. Separate scores are provided in this category for Men/Teens and Women/Children because of differences in calories needed to maintain weight. Older men and women need fewer calories and should therefore score toward the lower end of their appropriate ranges.

	Men/Teens	Women/Children
Question 1	22 to 25	14 to 16
Question 2	18 to 22	13 to 16
Question 3	20 to 25	11 to 15
Question 4	20 to 35	13 to 18
Question 5	39 to 43	29 to 32
Question 6	10	5
Question 7	0	0
Total score	129 to 160	85 to 102

SWEETS AND SNACKS

1. How often do you eat dessert or baked goods such as sweet rolls, doughnuts, cookies, cakes, etc.?
  <u>1</u> Three or more times *per day*
  <u>2</u> Two times *per day*
  <u>3</u> One time *per day*
  <u>4</u> Four to 6 times *per week*
  <u>5</u> Three or 4 times *per week* or less

Score _____

2. How often do you eat candy?
  <u>1</u> Every day
  <u>2</u> Four to 6 times a week
  <u>3</u> Two to 3 times a week
  <u>4</u> Once a week
  <u>5</u> Less than once every two weeks or none

Score _____

3. How much soda pop (not diet soda) or fruit-flavored drinks do you drink *daily*?

    <u>1</u> Four cups or more (1 quart)

    <u>2</u> Three cups (24 ounces)

    <u>3</u> Two cups (16 ounces)

    <u>4</u> One Cup (8 ounces)

    <u>5</u> None

Score _____

4. When you eat cakes, cookies or other baked goods, do you:

    <u>1</u> Eat commercial or homemade from a recipe using the full amount of sweetener called for in the recipe once a day or more often?

    <u>2</u> Eat commercial or homemade baked goods 3 to 6 times a week?

    <u>3</u> Make baked goods using ¾ of the sweetener called for *or* eat commercial baked goods twice a week or less?

    <u>5</u> Make baked goods using ½ or less of the sweetener called for *or* eat commercial baked goods less than once a week?

Score _____

5. Which of the following are you most likely to select as a dessert choice?

    <u>1</u> Croissants, pie, cheesecake, carrot cake

    <u>2</u> Regular cake, cupcakes, cookies

    <u>3</u> Combination of regular and low-fat desserts

    <u>5</u> Low-fat cookies (such as fig bars and ginger snaps), angel food cake, low-fat muffins, desserts from low-fat cookbooks or none

Score _____

6. Which snack items are you most likely to eat in an average week?

    <u>1</u> Potato chips, corn or tortilla chips, chocolate, nuts, party/snack crackers (most are high-fat variety), doughnuts, French fries, peanut butter

    <u>3</u> Combination of higher- and lower-fat snacks

    <u>4</u> Lightly buttered popcorn, low-fat crackers (such as soda or graham crackers), baked corn chips

    <u>5</u> Fruit or *no snacks*

Score _____

TOTAL SCORE _____ **(Add all of the above scores in this category.)**

Goal scores for each of the questions above:

Question 1	5
Question 2	5
Question 3	5
Question 4	5
Question 5	5
Question 6	4 to 5
Total Score	29 to 30

SALT

1. Which kind of "salt" do you normally
   use?
   - 1 Regular salt, sea salt, flavoring salts
       (such as garlic salt), regular soy
       sauce
   - 3 Combination of regular and reduced
       sodium salts
   - 4 Lite Salt, lower-sodium soy sauce,
       reduced-sodium flavoring salts
   - 5 Salt substitute (100 percent
       potassium chloride)or none

   Score _____

2. Do you add salt to your food at the table?
   - 1 Always
   - 2 Frequently
   - 4 Occasionally
   - 5 Never

   Score _____

3. Which type of salt and how much do you
   use in cooking potatoes, rice, pasta,
   vegetables, meat, casseroles and soups?
   - 1 Regular salt (typical amount) and/or
       eat in restaurants 4 or more times
       a week
   - 2 Regular salt (½ typical amount) or
       Lite Salt (typical amount)
   - 4 Lite Salt (½ typical amount)
   - 5 Salt substitute or no salt used

   Score _____

4. What type of cereals do you use?
   - 1 Typical dry cereals (sweetened or
       unsweetened) and/or cereals
       cooked with regular salt (typical
       amount)
   - 3 Combination of typical dry cereals
       and salt-free dry cereals (Shredded
       Wheat, Puffed Wheat, Puffed
       Rice) and/or cereals cooked with
       regular salt (½ typical amount) or
       Lite Salt (typical amount)
   - 5 Salt-free dry cereals and/or cereals
       cooked with salt substitute or no
       salt added

   Score _____

5. How often do you use typical canned,
   bottled, or packaged salad dressings,
   cured meats (lunch meat, ham, etc.),
   vegetables, soups (remember chicken
   broth), chili, entrées and sauces
   - 1 Use more than 15 times a week or
       eat out 4 or more times a week
   - 2 Use 10 to 14 times a week
   - 3 Use 6 to 9 times a week
   - 5 Use 0 to 5 times a week

   Score _____

TOTAL SCORE _____ **(Add all of
the above scores in this category.)**

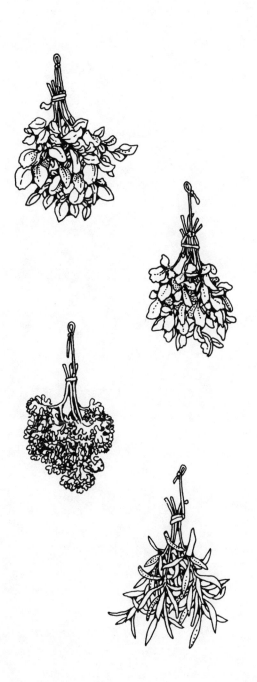

Goal scores for each of the questions
  above:
    Question 1   4 to 5
    Question 2   5
    Question 3   5
    Question 4   5
    Question 5   5

Total Score   24 to 25

The goal scores provided in this chapter are for Phase Three of the New American Diet. The goal scores for Phase One can be found on page 125 and for Phase Two on page 149. The total goal scores for Phase One, Two and Three for Men/Teens and Women/Children are given in table 2.

Total scores less than 141 for Women/Children and 166 for Men/Teens indicate that

TABLE 2

	Women/Children	Men/Teens
Phase I	143–169	166–196
Phase II	194–219	223–260
Phase III	235–267	277–323

you are eating in a manner that puts you nutritionally at maximal risk for the diseases of overconsumption. Scores of 233 or greater for Women/Children and 277 or more for Men/Teens indicate an eating pattern which nutritionally provides maximum protection from the diseases of overconsumption.

Total score for quiz _____

This concludes the quiz. As we've noted, you'll want to take it over again later on. You are ready now to proceed to part 2 and begin working toward the goals of the New American Diet.

PART

2

How to Make
the New American Diet
a *Permanent* Part
of Your Life

1

GETTING THE WHOLE FAMILY INVOLVED— SUCCESS STORIES

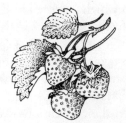

Good News from the Family Heart Study

One of the unique features of the New American Diet is that it is designed for the *whole family*. The choice of food to be eaten is to a significant degree a *learned* activity. Of course, at the most fundamental level, we eat instinctively to survive. But in our present, affluent world there are very few of us who can honestly say that we "eat to live" and leave it at that. Most of us, in order to be more accurate, would have to admit that we "live to eat." This was said nicely by George Bernard Shaw: "There is no love sincerer than the love of food."

Just *how* we eat, *how much* we eat and especially *what* we eat are all learned, for the most part, within the family unit. What we learn, moreover, becomes habit, and the longer we nurture any given habit the more difficult it becomes to change or break that habit. One of the principal goals of our program is to have people learn New American Diet eating habits as early in life as possible —and to do so where it will do the most good, within the family.

By "family" we do not simply mean couples with children. We mean any combination of people within a household including couples without children as well as couples whose children have left home, single parents with children, single people and roommates. We believe that changes in eating habits are best made within the family setting, whatever it may be. It's generally a lot easier for everyone in the family to march to the beat of the same drummer, in terms of food that is eaten, than to have one person attempting to eat something different, as is so often the case for diet programs. The New American Diet is directed toward *every* member of the family.

The dietary program that we have devised is, as we have indicated, based upon decades of research. Recently, as one test of the kind of dietary change we advocate for the Western world as a whole, we conducted a five-year dietary experiment unique in many particulars. Through the Family Heart Study, we sought to determine the extent to which typical families could or would modify their diets toward the New American Diet goals. In this experiment, just as in the program described in this book, the families proceeded at their own rate, incorporating whatever changes they could or wanted to into their daily eating habits.

Five years, of course, is not long enough to assess definitively the impact of dietary change on heart disease or any other disorder. But, as demonstrated in the preceding chapters, we *know* now from decades of research that dietary modification in the prescribed directions *will* result in the significant prevention and amelioration of many diseases. The ultimate goal of the Family Heart Study, then, was not to determine whether the suggested dietary changes would be beneficial— we already knew they would be—but, rather, to see whether *typical* families could, especially as units, incorporate the proposed changes, or at least some of them, into their *permanent* eating behavior or life-styles.

It is of great importance in analyzing the results of this study to realize that the families that participated did not *volunteer* to be part of the project. Instead, the families were selected *at random* and were then *asked* to participate. The idea was to find a cross section of the United States consisting of *typical* fam-

ilies, not those that were, as a whole, motivated to make changes at the outset. We wanted to see if "ordinary" families, some of whom may not even have heard of the risks of a high-fat diet, could be *encouraged* to make the suggested changes by providing support, feedback and general information about the benefits that could be derived from these changes. Beyond that, it was up to each family to decide whether and to what extent to follow the program.

The study, at this writing, has just been concluded. The amount of data gathered on the 233 participating families and the 170 additional families that acted as "controls" for comparison purposes is massive. Analyses of the data will continue for some time and will be summarized in a series of scientific publications. We do know the answers right now, however, to some of our most important questions. In particular, we know that typical American families *can* make significant changes in their diets, in many cases altering eating habits that had become strongly entrenched over years and even decades.

Not only were many of the families able to make these important changes, but they were also able to stick with them. The drop-out rate in the study was astonishingly low. We say "astonishing" because even in some short-term studies requiring far less rigorous participation (among other things, our study required regular blood drawings), drop-out rates are often 75 percent and even higher. At the end of five years, we still had representatives from 90 *percent* of our families. Members of 50 percent of the families actively participated throughout the entire five years. Only a few families dropped out entirely. Many families indicated their intention of continuing with the program for the rest of their lives.

We are highly encouraged by the results of

this study, not only because of the enthusiasm of the families and of the low drop-out rate but also because backsliding to old eating habits definitely diminished in most cases and stopped entirely in many cases as the program progressed. Often the opposite is true since, in many experiments, enthusiasm is high in the beginning but wanes over a period of time. This program seemed to be self-reinforcing. Perhaps most important of all, this study provides persuasive scientific evidence that permanent, positive dietary change is not only possible but also practical *within large groups of people*. All of this encourages us to believe that the ultimate goal —that of moving the entire country and, indeed, the whole Western world toward a lower-fat, higher-carbohydrate but still highly varied and enjoyable diet—is realistic and attainable.

We don't know yet precisely how far each family progressed, but the families as a whole achieved the Phase One goals. Some families were well into Phase Two and some even went all the way to the end-point Phase Three goals. A number of our colleagues suggest that it isn't necessary to achieve the Phase Three goals you'll find discussed in greater detail later in this book in order to begin to reap health benefits. For example, Dr. Gregory Curfman of the highly regarded Massachusetts General Hospital, where he uses our diet as part of a program for the prevention and rehabilitation of heart attacks, reports that most people find Phase Two of our diet sufficiently effective (and enjoyable).

The data from the Lipid Research Clinic's Primary Prevention Trial of the National Heart, Lung and Blood Institute suggested that benefits are continuous—for every 1 percent lowering of the blood cholesterol level there is a 2 percent decrease in coronary heart disease risk. Our position is simply this: *Any* forward progression toward the goals of any phase of our diet is helpful and desirable, but the *more* goals you can achieve the *greater* the protection against the major diseases and disorders of overconsumption, including obesity.

One final point before we proceed to some illustrative and, we hope, inspiring case histories. It seems likely that you and/or your family will make even more rapid progress than did the families in our study. This shouldn't be surprising since we picked the study families at random. Most of you picked this program—as evidenced by the fact that you have purchased this particular book— and are probably already convinced or are leaning toward the conviction that diet plays not merely a role but a *crucial* role in health and disease. In addition, we have learned a lot from the families who participated in this study, and you are the beneficiaries of much of what we have learned, both with respect to mistakes and successes.

All of this makes our job—and yours— that much easier. We realize that it's still a struggle as is all learning—we have never said and never will say that any significant dietary change is easy—and that is why throughout this book we are going to remind you just *why* the kind of changes we propose are so desirable and beneficial.

Success Stories of Typical Families: "Oh, No, What Have We Got Ourselves Into?"

From time to time, during the course of our five-year study, we asked some of our participants to write down their thoughts and reactions to the changes in their diet they were making or trying to make. Here's what Nona, one of our homemakers, wrote. Shortly after deciding to participate in the study, after the novelty of being part of a unique experiment began to wear off, the family's overall reaction was: "Oh, no. What have we got ourselves into?" After all, the changes this family was being asked to make weren't for a day or a week but for *five years* and, perhaps, if everything worked out, for an entire lifetime.

In the first weeks in particular, Nona recounts, "we felt sudden twinges of guilt every time the words red meat, cheese, desserts, high cholesterol or fat were mentioned. We were sure our [group] leaders had a secret way of knowing all the wrong things we were eating and surely could see every new fat globule accumulating in our bodies by merely studying the statistics they so carefully compiled."

But two years into the study, Nona reported that what she and her family had "gotten themselves into" was "a painless way to change lifelong habits of nutrition that may shorten our lives, cause needless health hazards and add pounds or inches few of us really need."

Shirley, an elementary-school teacher, wrote that even though her family had considered participation in the study as something akin to running a gauntlet, "the results," three years into the study, "are readily apparent and measurable . . . the walls of ignorance have been broken down for us and we have *begun* to delve into the processes of 'good health'. . . . As far as our diet is concerned, fresh fruits, vegetables, pasta, popcorn and rice have at least tripled in consumption while eggs, red meat, butter, milk, deep-fried foods, salty snack foods and sugar have decreased in about the same proportion. . . . Our rewards for following this study are numerous: increased vitality, fewer doctor bills, reduced cost of medication, greater appreciation and knowledge of our bodily functions and, hopefully, a longer lease on life."

Jim, an executive, reported halfway through the study that there had been both negative and positive aspects to participation in the study. The negative ones related to "minimum cooperation from our older children." Teenagers, more than any other group, are resistant to dietary change, partly because of intense peer pressures and preoccupation with the emotional upheavals that often attend this stage of life. We'll discuss this problem in more detail later. On the positive side, however, Jim reported many successful changes in diet, including reduction in salt and beef intake in particular. There was real progress, he added, toward lower-calorie meals that were genuinely filling. "The results thus far," he wrote, "have been outstanding. Family members, including 47-year-old Dad, have had amazingly low blood-pressure readings, and the blood studies indicate that we can have positive hope for continued good health. Both Mom and Dad have lost some weight and this is also encouraging."

Elaine, an account executive, reported that while she had made "some strong personal commitments" toward our goals, her husband had been more resistant. (Husbands tend to follow teenagers in the resistance category, though a great many of them adapt easily to the program and, in a number of cases, actually lead the way.) "Both of us," she added, "have high-stress life-styles and demands. Breakfasts and lunches are eaten outside the home by both of us. Our jobs entail frequent schedule changes in midday, throwing the best-laid plans asunder."

To help those of you in similar situations, we are providing, later in this book, guidelines on how to eat out and follow New

American Diet goals. Even some so-called fast foods are acceptable fare, if you know what to look for. We'll also help you, with recipes and other tips provided later on, do what Elaine did to get her reluctant husband to make beneficial changes in his diet. Elaine wrote: "My solution: be as *sneaky* as possible when I can be in control of the food to be eaten. I have done this by finding new recipes which have been accepted by my husband and not preparing the 'old favorites' he used to prefer." That may seem easier said than done, but a good deal of our research has been devoted to finding or developing just such recipes, as you'll discover. Many of them quickly became "new favorites."

Carolyn, a salesperson, reports that her husband, too, has been somewhat resistant to change, but in this case the couples' two sons have actually helped promote a better diet. "They are very concerned," Carolyn writes, "with the number of eggs we eat and tell their dad he eats far too many. Jason says, 'Dad, don't you know an egg yolk has enough cho- lesterol to choke your arteries!' We have gone from *six dozen* eggs a week to two dozen."

Carolyn reports something many of our families have commented on. After gradually making some of our recommended changes, it is remarkable how some once-favorite foods suddenly lose their appeal. "When we elimi- nated most of the animal fats and quit frying food," Carolyn comments, "the boys started saying Twinkies taste like lard, and we all agree."

Bill and Ginger, both business people, had little trouble recognizing the benefits of the changes we proposed. But for them and their family mere recognition was not enough. "Our family has found that *exercise* provides the necessary mental reinforcement. This is due to the fact that we feel good about our- selves and thereby it enables us to implement our diet-changing habits much easier. Be- cause we feel better—healthier—we become more conscious of our eating habits and desire foods that perpetuate our healthier attitude. In addition, we eat less."

This is a point some other participants in the study made, too. The truth of the matter is that the sort of scientific studies that would definitely prove—or disprove—the assumed benefits of aerobic exercise in the prevention of heart disease and other disorders have not yet been done. Exercise, while not an integral part of our dietary program, has psychological benefits and we believe there may be quanti- fiable *physical* benefits as well. Our exercise recommendations, which are optional, are covered later in this book.

Sometimes adverse health—or the fear of it—is a powerful motivating factor. Both Nancy, a housewife, and her husband, John, an attorney, discovered early in our study that they had cholesterol levels that were high for their ages. Even their six-year-old daughter had a cholesterol level that was high even for an adult. Neither John nor Nancy smoked, and neither was overweight. But there was a history of heart disease in Nancy's family. More important, this family's diet before en- tering the study was heavily laden with fat and cholesterol, featuring meat, bacon, but- ter and, typically, three dozen eggs each week. Only a few months into the study, this family managed to make significant changes in diet with a resulting dramatic drop in cho- lesterol levels. Nancy's cholesterol, for ex- ample, plunged in the first five months from 235 to 197. The family cut way back on eggs and meat very early in the study.

"We don't use butter anymore," Nancy commented. "I used to think margarine would be terrible, and it's not. We haven't used egg substitutes. I've found how to cook without egg yolks. Our diet is still high in calories, but low in cholesterol. We snack more on fresh fruit and homemade cookies." The latter, she adds, are made without egg yolks and with margarine instead of butter.

Let's look now at four more families, each with somewhat different perspectives and problems, and see what their impressions are at the *end* of the five-year study.

"Eating Better for Less"

Dick and Linda both work and have three children in school. Linda was the first to be recruited into the study. She went to a breakfast we organized and says, "I was quite shocked they didn't serve bacon and eggs." Nonetheless, Dick soon entered the program, too, even though he came from a family of "dedicated" meat eaters and states emphatically, "psychologically, I could *never* become a vegetarian." Resistance on that score quickly folded, however, because we always make it very clear we don't expect *anyone* to become vegetarian, unless, of course, he or she really wants to. Our research shows vegetarianism *isn't* necessary. Dick was motivated somewhat by the fact that he is diabetic. This particular study focused on heart disease, but we made it known that the same diet could be beneficial in relation to a number of other diseases, too, including diabetes, a disorder also predisposing to coronary heart disease.

"We made some pretty drastic changes in the first six months," Dick recalls, "and then slowed down but kept going after that."

"We were a fairly typical family," Linda says, "in the sense that each of our main meals centered on a big hunk of meat, fried foods and a lot of cheese. We were also into fast foods because they are quick and easy. They also tend to be very fat."

Equipped with information we provided, however, the family found it "surprisingly easy," Linda recounts, "to go from 2 percent milk to 1 percent, briefly, and then all the way to skim. We also switched with relative ease from butter to margarine. We gave up a lot of the Cheddar and other typical high-fat cheeses and started eating yogurt and some of the low-fat cheeses we learned about in the study. We eliminated eggs completely." The ease with which the family was able to go cold turkey on the eggs was particularly surprising to them since they had always eaten a lot of eggs and had long regarded them as one of the healthiest parts of their diet because of the high-protein content.

Reducing meat intake was more difficult for this family. Denise, a teenager, remembers looking at her sandwiches and asking, "Where's the beef?" long before the politicians did. But both she and Lisa, also a teenager now, found that the ethnic dishes that we emphasize made it much easier to switch to meals with less meat. These dishes, in which meat is used as a garnishment rather than as the main ingredient, can present the illusion of a lot of meat and are often very colorful in appearance and highly flavorful in taste, introducing a lot of new spices. Some families have successfully excited interest in the low-meat cuisine of other lands by encouraging their younger children to dress up in the type of clothing worn in the countries whose food is being introduced into their diets.

Lisa noted that some of her schoolmates, aware of her participation in our study, "thought we were a little weird at first." Others, however, wanted to learn more.

Overall, the family has managed to cut down substantially on its meat intake, although this took some time. "Now," Dick says, "we use meat more in the way it is recommended and have completely meatless main meals one or two days a week."

Scott, the eldest child in the family, was most resistant. Sometimes this sort of isolated resistance throws the whole family off. But it didn't in this case (or in most). We've learned that adolescents have more trouble than anyone in making significant changes in diet. Some, of course, have less difficulty. But if there is resistance, our advice to parents is: don't overreact. That can be the worst thing you do. The best approach is to pass on to your teenagers the reasons why you are interested in changing your diet—but always in a matter-of-fact rather than preachy or know-it-all tone. Then let the kids make up their own minds.

It's definitely more of a challenge with teenagers—and it can be a bit more work, too, because the families that have been most successful in getting their older children into the program have been those that have made acceptable food alternatives available as often as possible, especially in the snack category. You'll find a number of good snack recipes in the third part of this book. Another tactic is to give your teenagers more responsibility. Let them take turns preparing meals, asking only that they stay within the recommended guidelines. Not all will spark to this, but some will accept the challenge, especially if it gives them the opportunity to prepare their favorite "exotic" foods, such as Mexican, Chinese, etc.

As for Lisa and Denise, they both say that after five years in this program they believe they will stick with major parts of it now and later in life. And even those teenagers who

resist now are in many cases likely to remember some of what they learned in a family concerned about diet and will return to that learning later in life when they are more settled, have children of their own or are faced with health or weight problems.

Linda observes that following the dietary goals requires a lot of changes in the way food is prepared. But, gradually, she says, "the old standbys have been replaced by new ones." Though Linda had no sign of heart disease herself, her father had open-heart surgery and her mother died of a heart attack. That was motivating; so was the prospect that the diet would help out in the weight department. "That's definitely one of the big pluses of this diet," Linda reports. "You can maintain your weight if it's right to begin with or you can lose some gradually—which is the best way of keeping it off permanently. I didn't have a big problem in this area, but I have steadily lost weight each year. One very important thing I learned from all this is just how poor a concept most people have of dieting and diet in general, with all that overemphasis on protein and so little on complex carbohydrates, which so many continue to think are fattening. People mistakenly think dieting is cutting out breads and pastas. We learned just the opposite in this program."

Both Dick and Linda have enjoyed substantial drops in their cholesterol levels.

"The whole thing just makes so much sense," Linda says. "The gradual approach with the right information and the right feedback is the key. I definitely consider this a lifetime program."

Dick adds, "Another nice aspect of all this is that we now eat *better* for *far less* than we did before. Our budget has improved considerably."

Linda agrees, noting that "We spend less

on food for our entire family than many couples I know." Major savings have been realized, in particular, from the cutback on meat, eggs and butter.

"I Never Felt Hungry on This Diet"

Dan and Susan had their first two children while participating in our study. This was both good and bad. On the plus side, the children have been raised on our diet from day one—and the results, Susan reports, have been remarkable. Foods so many still think are "necessary," "can't-live-without" items are real turnoffs for these young children. They find salt, especially in the quantities used by most Americans, intolerable. And "They're actually repulsed by the thought of eating meat," Dan adds. "The kids won't even touch the best steak."

Pregnancy, however, can be a difficult time for Mom, as Susan found out. Susan hadn't been too keen on getting into the study in the first place. Here's a case where the husband led the way. But both Dan and Susan adapted quickly once they found out they could proceed at their own rate. Dan, as we'll see, found out early in the study that he had a particularly pressing need for this diet, and the couple soon became enthusiastic about the program, progressing far more rapidly than they thought they would. After the first year they had already escalated into Phase Three. But then about a year and a half into the program Susan got pregnant.

"Suddenly," she recalls, "my taste for beans and the like went out the window. I started eating more meat, which means Dan did, too." This isn't unusual. The important thing is not to feel like you've failed because of some temporary backsliding, even if that backsliding persists for some months. This is not, unlike so many diets, an all-or-nothing program. Pregnancy—and some illnesses, such as influenza—can have dramatic effects on appetite and taste perception. It's better sometimes to let your body—rather than your mind—dictate to you. Your taste for the "right" foods will come back, as Susan found out. "After the baby was born," she remembers, "we got back on the program real fast." The same thing happened during the second pregnancy.

Before getting into the study, Dan and Susan were on a very high-fat diet. "I'd always been taught," Susan says, "that a high-protein diet was the healthiest. That means a lot of meat." Both lunch and dinner featured meat, often accompanied by other fatty foods. The couple ate out a lot, too, "and not usually at class establishments," Dan says. "We ate a lot of hamburgers."

At the beginning of the study, Dan learned via some of our blood tests that he had extremely high cholesterol concentrations in his blood. "My readings were as high as 326" milligrams of cholesterol per 100 milliliters of blood, he recalls. "That and the fact that my dad had died of heart disease—blocked arteries—at the age of 49 and that several other relatives on both sides of the family had also had heart disease got me real motivated." Dan was trying to get a job with the fire department and was high on the list of applicants, having done well on all the tests except, as it turned out, one. He was shocked when someone from the department said, "You didn't tell us you have heart disease." The fire department physical exam had also revealed his dangerously high cholesterol levels. "After that," he says, "you'd be surprised how easy it was for us to move right into Phase Three of the diet."

Dan is the sort of person who seems to have an inherited tendency to develop very high cholesterol concentrations in his blood. That doesn't mean however, that altering his diet won't help him. He just has to work at it a bit harder than some of us. When he follows the diet and doesn't eat out in excess, his blood cholesterol levels fall significantly. In the third year of the study he got it down to 210 milligrams per 100 milliliters. It still fluctuates, but it has been under 240 a good deal of the time since the study began, he notes. His blood triglyceride levels had also been high, and those have also come down substantially.

"And now that I'm eating sensibly for the first time in my life," Dan observes, "I've also finally been able to lose some weight"—about 30 pounds. "The best part of it is, I never felt hungry on this diet. I started losing weight right from the beginning without even thinking about it."

The family has meat now in no more than one meal a day and then usually in reduced amounts. "By the end of the first year," Susan says, "we were already spending about $30 a month less on meat. We'd also been buying about six pounds of Cheddar cheese—the fattest kind—per month. By the end of the first year that had stopped, too. We'd gone to quite a bit less cheese and to lower-fat types. Many taste very good. People just don't know about them." (We provide you with a guide to cheeses later on.) They cut back on the beef and added more fish and poultry. Getting more complex carbohydrates into their diet in the form of breads, pastas and legumes was more difficult.

"Taste was a problem for us here," Susan explains. "But part of the solution is spices. Where we had maybe used only a dozen spices, if that, in our food before, we were soon using maybe *thirty* this program introduced us to. That really helped a lot. And before long we were buying grains we'd never even heard of before. Eventually we found this diet could actually bring *more* variety and *more* excitement into our eating habits, not less."

Susan says she feels better *mentally*, too, since altering her diet. Dan says he definitely feels better physically. "It's a new habit with us," Susan concludes. "A habit I think we'll definitely keep for the rest of our lives."

Both parents say they are particularly gratified that their two children started life on the New American Diet, obviously the ideal time to begin.

"Guess What, Mom, We Had Sugar and Meat!"

Bette and Jim both teach school. Both have been involved in coaching athletics and were more sophisticated than average about nutrition before entering the study. One of the most interesting observations they have made is that their two daughters, though only two years apart in age, have considerably different tastes. Jocelyn was only one and a half when the study began, while Jessica was three and a half. Today Jocelyn loves vegetables, while Jessica, who got a later start on the New American Diet, is more resistant to the leafy stuff.

Both children, though, have adapted to major parts of the diet, so much so that when they visited their grandmother, they found the food served them so novel that they felt compelled to phone home with the news: "Guess what, Mom, we had sugar and meat!" It was as if they had landed on some other planet. Even now, at ages seven and nine, they have candy only at Halloween and don't miss it the rest of the year. Bette recalls giving Jocelyn a sucker when she was two and a half. "She didn't even know what it was or what to do with it."

Both Bette and Jim are very health-conscious and were even before they joined our study. Among other things, Bette runs marathons. Still, both found room for improvement in their diets. Bette found she was consuming far more fat in the form of cheese than was healthy and has cut back substantially on that. For Jim, the challenge was salt. "I'd always salted my food very heavily. I also consumed more sugar and white bread than I should have." Gradually he was able to sit down at the table without making sure the salt shaker was both in sight and within reach. Before long it was off the table entirely. Bette says she adds far less salt to foods she prepares and when she does she uses Lite Salt. Jim has also cut back on sugar and now eats whole wheat bread.

The family as a whole was very successful in reducing the fat content of its diet. Jim's blood cholesterol had been in the 190 range (which was much better than average to begin with) before the study began. Several months into the study it was closer to 160 and has remained there. Bette's was 168 at the outset and is now closer to 135.

This family, too, says it is on the New American Diet "for life."

Weight Problem and a Reluctant Husband

Hennie, fifty-nine, and Keith, sixty-three, were one of the older couples participating in our study. Hennie notes that "With a home-ec background and a weight problem I just naturally had an interest in nutrition, and so when we were asked to participate in this research I knew it would be beneficial."

Keith says, "I was included, too, but I didn't know it in the beginning." It was a matter of the wife preparing the food and the husband having to go along with what was placed in front of him. "We've always eaten our meals together," Hennie points out. "We'd always snacked together and we'd gotten fat together." They were committed to meat and often to large servings of it—seven nights a week.

Hennie was never really obese, but she was persistently overweight. "I'd been battling overeating for years—adding pounds and not being able to stop it. I'd tried all kinds of different diets and organizations, including some of the best known. Still, I couldn't get it under control. I worried a lot about it, went to a psychologist, even a minister. I kept a journal hoping that would help me. By the time we got into this program I'd given up on there being any panacea."

With her background in nutritional studies, Hennie says our program struck her as the probable best way of getting control of her eating habits—in a gradual, unforced manner that could take root and hold on. A series of classes we gave, about habits being the problem and not diet per se, gave her a new perspective on her problem. "I stopped counting calories so much and started examining the ways I *felt* about snacking. That, and learning what other people felt about some of the same aspects of eating, was very useful to me. I finally was able not only to stop gaining but was able to lose some weight and to get much better control over my own eating patterns. This has persisted."

Hennie found other aspects of the program helpful to her in this challenge, too. We emphasize exercise for those so inclined, and Hennie continued running regularly and had even climbed our most notorious local volcano—Mount St. Helens—before it erupted. She found our demonstration on carbohydrates and fats helpful, too, as did many of the other families. Later on, we'll be telling you about "the fats of life" and showing you how much fat is in a typical diet, how much fat needs to be removed and how to replace the fat with grains and beans. A "vital part" of the program, Hennie adds, are those demonstrations that show graphically how our diet differs from the standard diet and how substitutions and trade-offs can be made that take much of the pain out of the transition to better, healthier eating habits. You'll have benefit of the same, and additional, material in subsequent chapters.

Well, that was the weight problem. What about "the husband problem"? As we noted earlier, Keith was pretty much stuck with eating what his wife ate, since she prepared all the meals. "I'll admit I wasn't the most eager participant," Keith says. "I rather resented being dragged into this. But I attended the sessions at which the program was discussed. And since I have a background in organic chemistry, I appreciate a good experiment and finally got into the spirit of things in that light."

In fact, it wasn't long before the initially reluctant husband was doing some experimenting of his own. And by the time the study was over, Keith had not only started participating in the food preparation but was also eagerly setting about to find ways to improve on some of our recipes—not by adding fat to them but by adding spices and altering the taste of some of them. Now he has a large folder full of recipes gathered from many different sources—recipes that largely or entirely meet the standards of our program.

"Now," Keith says, "when she cooks, I eat what she prepares and vice versa." Sometimes they work together in the kitchen. In addition, they now have *two* vegetable gardens and an herb garden.

"I have to say, he's become a very good cook in his retirement," Hennie acknowledges. "And I really enjoy having someone work with me in the kitchen."

Hennie and Keith have cut back sharply on their meat intake and now consume a lot more beans, rice and pasta. "We find what we eat now much more varied and much more satisfying than before," Hennie comments. "You can make foods so interesting with herbs. Healthy foods can be made entirely satisfying. You don't need all those rich foods. And another thing: This diet actually takes a lot of the guilt out of eating. We find that with minor alterations we can eat many of the foods we had always thought were bad for us but just couldn't resist." (Finding ways of making favorite foods "respectable" is one of our specialties, as you'll see.)

Asked if they will continue with the diet, Hennie nods in the affirmative, and Keith replies by brandishing his overflowing folder of recipes, announcing, "There's probably only one recipe in this entire file that isn't up to par."

Our goal has been to inspire you, so we have only given you success stories. Naturally there were families who did not or were not able to make considerable changes in their eating habits. The most common reason given was that they had too many other conflicting priorities. Other reasons given for not making changes included family stresses, lack of interest and support within the family, difficulty in acquiring a taste for lower-fat/higher-carbohydrate fare, and simply *not wanting* to make changes.

All of this points up the need to recognize that changing lifelong habits takes conscious effort and requires good communications within each family unit. And any major change requires time and patience.

Since the study ended, a number of families have told us they wished they had been in a position to make *more* changes during the study. We have assured them, and assure you, as well, that, once you have the needed information and have acquired some of the basic skills, you *can* make further changes *anytime*. You are not constrained to any particular timetable, as you will see.

2

BASICS: UNDERSTAND THE GOALS, PREPARE PROPERLY, PROCEED GRADUALLY

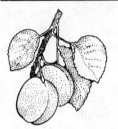

No Deadlines

Remember: This is a program without deadlines. We point you in the right direction but don't prescribe the rate of progress. In other words we don't put you on a rigid diet, but instead propose that you gradually incorporate new eating habits into your life-style. Further, we do not expect you to acquire these new eating habits at any set rate or even in any set order.

Some Guidelines Instead

We don't impose deadlines, but we do provide guidelines. As we discuss the various phases of the program, we'll let you know what many other people have accomplished —or failed to accomplish—in various time periods. We'll also give you the means of monitoring your progress. You will still be encouraged to proceed at a rate that best suits you and your family. We expect some backsliding and take this into account in our guidelines. Nobody is perfect.

Gradualism is the key to our program. You need to make changes slowly and give yourself time to practice and to acclimatize to new ways of cooking and eating. It may take you months to become really comfortable with many of our recommendations; and it's likely to take years to make the major changes we propose and have them become *permanent, natural* aspects of your eating habits. We're not promoting a short-term diet but, rather, a fundamental change in eating life-style— for everyone.

Some people think they can simply make the decision to eat differently and everything will take care of itself. After all, they reason, we understand how good these dietary changes will be in terms of the health benefits now and in the future. Unfortunately, this still doesn't mean "everything will take care of itself." A decision to change isn't enough. *Practice* is also vital. And practice means making mistakes, backsliding, trial and error. But mostly it means pressing on through thick and thin, trying out the recipes we'll provide, continually sampling our suggestions until you find what works best for *you*.

As we begin to introduce you to the first phase of the program we'll share various tips and suggestions with you that will help make things go more smoothly. We'll give you some information on what changes most families seem to find easiest to make in the beginning, how to make choices available to the family that will be well received, how to sneak some new dishes in as side dishes before trying to make them center attractions, the importance of not repeating new foods or new ways of preparing foods too soon, and so on.

We'll also be stressing the importance of making sure everyone gets his or her fill. Remember, our standard program is *not* a calorie-restricted diet. This, too, helps ensure long-term success, for here is a diet that allows you to eat enough to have a feeling of fullness. As you begin to achieve our goals, you'll be eating lower-fat foods and more complex carbohydrates and fiber. The net result may be that you will eventually feel like you are eating as much or even more than before but you'll actually be reducing calories. We'll have a chapter later on weight control and weight maintenance. We'll include in that chapter a special, calorie-restricted diet for those who wish to lose weight. No one *has* to go on this calorie-restricted diet, but we

include it for those who want to shed some pounds before or while getting into our standard program. The loss of weight at the outset may help motivate some individuals.

First Things First

We're as tempted as you are to launch right into the New American Diet program. But before we do that we want you to read the next three preparatory chapters carefully. These contain important, basic information, much of it the product of recent and ongoing research, you need to know in order to make the best use of our program. This information is related to the major components of diet, especially fats, cholesterol and carbohydrates.

The main purpose of our diet is to reduce foods rich in cholesterol and saturated and total fats and replace them with carbohydrates, especially complex carbohydrates. Once you've read about the individual components of the diet, we'll put you through an exercise designed not only to reveal the sources and amount of fat you eat but also to show you how you can get rid of some of that fat and replace it with carbohydrates without gaining weight. Remember, as explained in the introduction to this book, it's the *how* more than the what that distinguishes our dietary program from the others. We're not content simply to give you goals; we tell you how to get there based on our experiences in the laboratory and in the field, among patients, with families and through our studies of the eating habits of other cultures.

The map to your destination will become more specific in the chapters that follow the more basic information, for then we will enter into the three phases of the program, each keyed, in part, to the recipes you will find in part 3.

3

FATS AND CHOLESTEROL: NOT ALL THE NEWS IS BAD

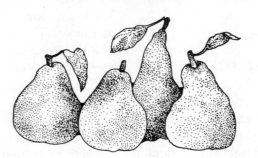

Making the Right Choices

The purpose of this chapter is not to give you a complicated, medical lecture on everything we now know about fats, cholesterol and related substances. That would fill volumes and would do little to change your diet. The purpose of this chapter is to help you understand the need to be more discriminating in your choice of fat- and cholesterol-containing foods. We want you to be able to make lower-fat choices without a great deal of conscious effort and certainly without having to know the cholesterol and fat content of thousands of foods.

There is presently a great deal of confusion, even among health professionals, as well as the public, about the adverse effects of various fatty foods. There are many reasons for this. Some foods such as chocolate, various hydrogenated vegetable shortenings, palm oil and coconut oil are high in saturated fat but are free of cholesterol. Egg yolk and some shellfish (shrimp, crab and lobster) are high in cholesterol, but low in saturated fat. Other foods such as cheeses and red meats contain high amounts of both cholesterol *and* saturated fat. These considerations, coupled with an increased interest on the part of the public and health professionals in disease prevention through dietary alteration, led us to develop an index, a single number, which would express the effects of various foods in terms of their potential to contribute to elevated blood cholesterol *and* atherosclerosis. This single number we have called the Cholesterol-Saturated Fat Index, or simply the CSI. This number takes into account the varying amounts of both cholesterol and saturated fat in a single food.

But before we explain how the CSI works, let's be sure we're in agreement on the meaning and significance of cholesterol and fats.

Cholesterol

Cholesterol, a special type of fat, is usually very closely associated with the saturated fats of animal origin discussed below. Cholesterol from the diet raises the level of cholesterol in the blood. Cholesterol in the blood, as we demonstrated in part 1, is one of the two chief culprits in the early development of atherosclerosis. It is the substance which more than any other produces the blockage in the arteries. References are often made these days to "good cholesterol" and "bad cholesterol." Actually, what these terms refer to is not cholesterol itself but the substances that contain both fat and protein and which carry cholesterol through the blood. HDL (high-density lipoprotein) is the "good cholesterol." HDL helps carry cholesterol out of the tissues and out of the body. LDL (low-density lipoprotein) is the "bad cholesterol." It carries cholesterol into the cells of the body and often into places we don't want it, depositing it on and in arterial walls where it can accumulate, but only when LDL levels are high. Blood level measurements of HDL and LDL, as well as of cholesterol itself, can be useful in assess-

ing health, and in monitoring dietary progress, as will be explained in more detail later in chapter 12.

Saturated Fats

Saturated fats are the fats that are generally solid at room temperature. (The degree of saturation has to do with the chemical structure of the fat.) These dietary fats, like cholesterol, increase the amount of cholesterol in the blood. They do this in part by increasing the amount of LDL, the chief cholesterol carrier.

Saturated fats include most fats of animal origin such as beef, lamb and pork fat, butter and products made from butterfat (cheese and ice cream). Almost all fish and shellfish are exceptions in that their fat, while being of animal origin, is less saturated and contains a unique group of polyunsaturated fats (the omega-3 fats) that will be discussed shortly.

Though most vegetable oils do not contain much saturated fat, a few do. The highly saturated vegetable oils are coconut oil, cocoa butter (the fat of chocolate) and palm oil. Check labels on commercially prepared foods —especially baked goods—because these fats are often used in large quantities or are the only fat used, and in excess they are as capable of raising blood cholesterol as are the saturated animal fats.

Be aware, too, that when you see "contains no cholesterol" on a label you may still be getting a lot of saturated fat in the product in the form of these saturated vegetable fats. Also be aware that when some vegetable oils, such as soybean or cottonseed oil, undergo a process called hydrogenation they, too, may become largely saturated. In the unhydrogenated state they are *unsaturated*. Examples of foods in which vegetable oils have been hydrogenated to the point where they have become highly saturated are hard shortenings and hard margarines and products made from them. Soft margarines, soft shortenings and peanut butter, however, have been less highly hydrogenated and, therefore, contain less saturated fat and are preferable in limited quantities.

Bear in mind that there is absolutely *no dietary need* for either cholesterol or saturated fat. The body can make—from other nutritional sources—all of the cholesterol and saturated fat it needs. You don't have to supply them through your diet. Thus there is no validity to the oft-expressed idea that "you need *some* animal fat in your diet." You *don't*. But we're not proposing that you get rid of all animal fat entirely, though we do propose a sharp reduction in intake. The fact is that you *could* get along very nicely without *any* cholesterol and little saturated fat in your diet.

Monounsaturated Fats

Monounsaturated fatty acids are found everywhere, in both animal and vegetable fats. The foods that contain this kind of fat in the greatest quantity are olive oil especially and, to some degree, peanut oil. It has generally been believed that monounsaturated oils are "neutral" in terms of their effects on blood cholesterol concentrations, neither raising nor lowering them. Olive oil is very low in saturates and this may be the reason that recent experiments have shown some cholesterol lowering from large amounts of monounsaturates in the diet. But, again, since monounsaturates are readily synthesized

by the body, there is no essential need to add them to your diet. We recommend that you cook and bake with *other* vegetable oils, of the more polyunsaturated variety discussed below, and use olive oil, if you particularly like it, for salad dressings and peanut oil for certain special stir-fried dishes (see recipes in part 3). Like all fats, monounsaturated fats, too, are limited in the New American Diet; they should not be used in excess. They too are a potent source of calories.

Polyunsaturated Fats

The polyunsaturated fats are known as *essential* fatty acids. What this means is that they are *necessary* for a variety of bodily functions and, since the body *cannot* synthesize these particular fats on its own, we must obtain them in our diet. Most vegetable oils (with exceptions noted above), *soft* shortenings and *soft* margarines are good sources of polyunsaturates. (Check labels to be sure.) The most common polyunsaturated fats are soybean, cottonseed, corn, sunflower and safflower. These fats, unlike the more saturated variety, in large amounts *reduce* blood levels of cholesterol and LDL. We do not propose, however, that you consume large quantities of polyunsaturates. They are certainly preferable to saturated fats, but there are good reasons to cut back on all fats. Excessive fat of any kind contributes to weight gain and obesity, and excesses of even polyunsaturated fats have been linked to some diseases in animals (but so far not in humans), including certain forms of cancer. Practically speaking, we recommend that people reduce saturated fat intake considerably and use small amounts of the more polyunsaturated fats.

Fish Oils

Fish oils contain a special class of polyunsaturates. The fat found in fish and shellfish, unlike that found in poultry and red meat, is highly polyunsaturated. These omega-3 fatty acids, have recently been found to be particularly useful in lowering blood triglyceride (fat) and cholesterol levels. They also affect another aspect of body chemistry in ways that help prevent heart attack and strokes: They help prevent blood clots from forming and blocking arteries by making certain cells of the blood that are important in blood clotting, called platelets, less sticky.

Up until very recently it was widely believed that fatty fish and shellfish should be avoided. It was assumed that the fats contained in these fish blocked the arteries as much as those found in beef or pork. Some shellfish, moreover, were known to be far higher in cholesterol than other fish and meat.

What helped lead to the discovery of the importance of omega-3 fatty acids and the roles they play in our bodies was a mystery concerning the Eskimos of Greenland that was unraveled by the Danish scientists Dyerberg and Bang. These people consume enormous amounts of animal fat derived largely from fish, seal meat and whale blubber. Yet, despite this, they have low rates of coronary artery disease and heart attack. A lower rate of heart attacks was subsequently noted in certain fishing villages in Japan—with a higher fish consumption and despite a prevalence of high blood pressure caused by excessive salt intake. In a recent report of a twenty-year study in Holland, men who ate more fish also had less coronary disease.

Those of us doing research in this area had to wonder what was going on. We and some of our colleagues discovered over the past several years that the omega-3 fatty acids found in fish, shellfish and some other marine animals (seals, whales, etc.) are very likely the protective factor. They outperform the other polyunsaturates not only in their ability to reduce the cholesterol concentration in the blood but also in their capacity to reduce the blood triglycerides, those circulating fats that can also contribute to heart disease.

This does not mean that you should start gorging on fish, but it does mean that you can eat more fish and shellfish than would previously have been considered prudent. We have made adjustments from these new findings, some of which have come from our own laboratory, in the diet program to be described. In general, these new findings have permitted us to safely allow more fish, and especially fatty fish like salmon, in the diet. An important point to be made is that the fat content of fish ranges from less than 1 percent to 13 percent. This is very different from the fat content of red meat which ranges from 10 percent to over 30 percent. The highest fat fish is almost as lean as the lowest fat red meat.

Just as you shouldn't begin gorging on salmon or lobster, neither should you start immediately taking the fish-oil supplements and derivatives which are now being sold in pharmacies and health-food stores. Also, there are dangers in taking products like cod-liver oil in tablespoon doses on a daily basis because cod-liver oil in large amounts would contain excessive amounts of vitamins A and D which can accumulate in your body over time and have serious toxic effects. A teaspoon per day of cod-liver oil is quite safe with regard to the level of vitamins A and D and does contain the omega-3 fatty acids as well. However, we do not recommend that people take cod-liver oil. Some fish oil supplements being sold mention the specific omega-3 fatty acids by name or abbreviation, such as EPA for eicosapentaenoic acid or DHA for docosahexaenoic acid. Avoid these, too. The safety and efficacy of these supplements have not been established and they remain experimental as far as general use is concerned. Use the fish themselves; you'll find them much more enjoyable and less expensive. Later on in this book, you'll find guidelines on *how much* fish and shellfish you can eat. We stress, as always, the use of foods, rather than supplements, to prevent the diseases of overconsumption.

What about Lecithin?

While we're talking about food supplements that some have suggested can reduce the risks of cholesterol and saturated fats, something should be said about lecithin. Lecithin is a substance derived from soybeans and is sold in stores everywhere. It is claimed that lecithin is an "emulsifier" that "dissolves" fats and cholesterol, breaks them down and renders them harmless. There is no sound scientific evidence whatever that suggests lecithin supplements have any significant effect upon fat and cholesterol metabolism. Some people who want to eat a lot of eggs try to justify this habit as nutritionally sound, arguing that the lecithin in the yolk of the egg counteracts the cholesterol (which is also in the yolk). This is a myth and a potentially dangerous one.

The reason that lecithin is of no value to the body is that the intestine completely digests it, so that it does not add to the lecithin in the blood. Lecithin in the blood is manufactured by the liver.

The Cholesterol-Saturated Fat Index (CSI) of Foods

Though we can derive some protection against heart disease and other disorders by manipulating the *types* of fat we eat, as suggested above, the greatest benefits come from a substantial reduction in both cholesterol and saturated fat intake. If we don't cut back on those, it won't matter how many monounsaturates, polyunsaturates or fish oils we add to our diets. We'll still wind up in trouble. In order to make it easier for people to select foods that are low in *both* cholesterol and saturated fats, we have devised a Cholesterol-Saturated Fat Index (CSI). The CSI enables you to grasp the contribution of both saturated fat *and* cholesterol in one food compared to another food. The CSI reflects our findings that the amount of saturated fat in the diet is just as important as the amount of cholesterol in terms of dietary control of the cholesterol and LDL in the blood.

Look at the numbers under CSI in table 3. The lower the CSI number, the better the food choice for the prevention of heart disease (and the other disorders we discussed in part 1). Apart from the CSI, you'll notice that the number of calories listed for each food varies widely even though in each case we're talking about equal-sized servings within each food category. This will help you realize how different foods can be in terms of their caloric density, that is, in terms of how many calories are packed into a given amount of food. The denser the calories, the easier it is to put on weight with that food.

To begin to understand better how the CSI works, look, for example, at the entry for shellfish (shrimp, crab, lobster). These have a CSI of 6, which is quite low, on par with poultry and some other fish. If we were rating these shellfish on cholesterol alone, however, as has been done in the past, then we would have ended up with a figure, for comparison purposes, far higher than that of poultry and

even red meats. The reason for this is that some shellfish have cholesterol content as much as *twice* that of poultry and red meats, *but*—and this is an all-important "but" that has been overlooked up until now—the saturated-fat content of shellfish is so extremely low that it turns out to be a better choice than *even the leanest red meats!*

For another instructive example, compare a 3½-ounce portion of cooked fish to a 3½-ounce portion of 20-percent-fat beef (the kind you get in ground chuck or pot roasts).

TABLE 3
The Cholesterol-Saturated Fat Index (CSI) and Calorie Content of Selected Foods

	CSI	Calories
Fish, poultry, red meat (3½ ounces or 100 grams cooked)		
White fish (snapper, perch, sole, cod, halibut, etc.), shellfish (clams, oysters, scallops), water-pack tuna	4	91
Salmon	5	149
Shellfish (shrimp, crab, lobster)	6	104
Poultry, no skin	6	171
Beef, Pork and Lamb:		
10% fat (ground sirloin, flank steak)	9	214
15% fat (ground round)	10	258
20% fat (ground chuck, pot roasts)	13	286
30% fat (ground beef, pork, and lamb steaks, ribs, pork and lamb chops, roasts)	18	381
Cheeses (3½ ounces or 100 grams)		
Low-fat cottage cheese, tofu (bean curd), pot cheese	1	98
Cottage cheese, Lite-line, Lite n' Lively, Weight Watchers, part-skim ricotta, Reduced Calories Laughing Cow	6	139
Imitation mozzarella, Cheezola, Scandic Mini Chol (Swedish low cholesterol), Hickory Farms Lyte, Saffola American*	6	317
Olympia's Low Fat, Green River Part Skim, Kiel-Kase and Heidi Ann (lower-fat Cheddars), part-skim mozzarella, Lappi, Neufchâtel (lower-fat cream cheese), skim-american	12	256
Cheddar, Roquefort, Swiss, Brie, Jack, American, cream cheese, Velveeta, cheese spreads (jars) and most other cheeses	26	386
Eggs		
Whites (3)	0	51
Egg substitute (equivalent to 2 eggs)	<1†	91
Whole (2)	29	163
Fats (¼ cup or 4 tablespoons)		
Peanut butter	5	353
Most vegetable oils	8	530

The CSI for the fish is 4, while that for the beef is more than triple that at 13—quite a difference. And this difference exists even though the amount of cholesterol doesn't differ much between these two foods. The fish serving contains 66 milligrams of cholesterol while the beef contains 96 milligrams. The *big* difference, however, is in saturated fat. The fish has only ⅕ gram of saturated fat while the beef, in the same-sized serving, has more than 8 grams of saturated fat. And look at the difference in calories—286 for the beef

versus 91 for the fish. (As the amounts change so do the CSIs. For example, 7 ounces of 20-percent-fat beef would have a CSI of 26 and contain 572 Calories.)

Now check the different categories of cheeses. Here's a food a lot of people have particular trouble with, erroneously believing either that "all cheeses are about equally good or bad for you" or that "there's no good way to tell the difference between them." You'll see that the CSI clearly shows that there are cheeses available that contain less cholesterol

TABLE 3 (cont.)
The Cholesterol-Saturated Fat Index (CSI) and Calorie Content of Selected Foods

	CSI	Calories
Fats (continued) (¼ cup)		
Mayonnaise	10	431
Soft vegetable margarines	10	432
Hard-stick margarines	15	432
Soft shortenings	16	530
Bacon grease	23	541
Very hydrogenated shortenings	27	530
Butter	37	430
Coconut oil, palm oil, cocoa butter (chocolate)	47	530
Frozen desserts (1 cup)		
Water ices, sorbets	0	245
Sherbet, low-fat frozen yogurt	2	290
Tofutti,‡ 16% fat	4	460
Ice milk	6	214
Ice cream, 10% fat	13	272
Rich ice cream, 16% fat	18	349
Specialty ice cream, 22% fat	34	684
Milk products (1 cup)		
Skim milk (0.1% fat), skim-milk yogurt	<1†	88
1% milk, buttermilk	2	115
2% milk, plain low-fat yogurt	4	144
Whole milk (3.5% fat), whole-milk yogurt	7	159
Liquid nondairy creamers: Mocha Mix, Poly Rich	4	326
Liquid nondairy creamers: store brands, Cereal Blend, Coffee Rich	22	344
Sour cream	37	468
Imitation sour cream (IMO)	43	499

* Cheeses made with skim milk and vegetable oils.
† < = less than.
‡ Made with tofu, soy protein and corn oil.

and saturated fat. (Cheese is such a big problem that we'll have a lot more to say about it later on.)

Look, too, at the difference between the whites of three eggs and two whole eggs—zero versus 29! As we've mentioned before, you can substitute three egg whites for two whole eggs in recipes.

As table 3 makes clear, even the softest vegetable fats contain a considerable amount of saturated fat and should be used in modest amounts despite their high polyunsaturated fat content. The same applies to peanut butter and to mayonnaise.

Look at 1 cup of sherbet or low-fat frozen yogurt with a CSI of 2 versus the same-sized serving of a specialty ice cream with a CSI of 34, again, a *very* substantial difference. One woman, when we first introduced her to the CSI, was ecstatic. "I love sherbet," she said, "and now I can actually feel good about eating it. I'd always thought it probably wasn't much better for me than regular ice cream." Milk may have a low CSI—7 for 1 cup of whole milk, but a quart would have a CSI of 28! Many people, however, use milk in and on many foods throughout the day just as they do margarine and mayonnaise. This use can add up quickly—to excessive levels when one considers the optimal CSI *per day*, which will be discussed shortly.

Even though the primary purpose of the

TABLE 4
The Cholesterol-Saturated Fat Index of the Present American Diet and the New American Diet

	Cholesterol (mg/day)	Saturated Fat (gm/day)	CSI* (per day)
American Diet (40% fat, 14% saturated fat)			
1200 Calories	240	19	31
2000 Calories	400	31	51
2800 Calories	500	44	69
New American Diet—Phase I (35% fat, 10% saturated fat)			
1200 Calories	<180†	13	22
2000 Calories	<300†	22	37
2800 Calories	<350†	31	49
New American Diet—Phase II (25% fat, 8% saturated fat)			
1200 Calories	<120†	11	17
2000 Calories	<200†	18	28
2800 Calories	<220†	25	36
New American Diet—Phase III (20% fat, 5% saturated fat)			
1200 Calories	<60†	7	10
2000 Calories	<100†	11	16
2800 Calories	<140†	16	23

* CSI = 1.01 (gm saturated fat) + 0.05 (mg cholesterol). Gm = grams; mg = milligrams.
† < = less than.

TABLE 5

The Cholesterol-Saturated Fat Index of Sample Intakes at 2000 Calories
for the Present American Diet and the New American Diet (Phase III)

American Diet*	Saturated Fat (gm)‡	Cholesterol (mg)‡	CSI
Breakfast			
1 slice white toast	0.2	0	0.2
1 tsp. soft margarine	0.7	0	0.7
1 cup orange juice	0.0	0	0.0
Lunch			
Sandwich:			
2 slices rye bread	0.0	0	0.0
1 Tbsp. mayonnaise	2.0	10	2.5
2 oz. turkey	0.6	49	3.1
Tomato slices	0.0	0	0.0
2 lettuce leaves	0.0	0	0.0
1 oz. potato chips	2.6	0	2.6
1 large apple	0.0	0	0.0
Dinner			
5 oz. grilled filet mignon	11.6	119	17.7
1 large baked potato	Tr.	0	0.0
¼ cup sour cream	6.4	20	7.5
1 cup lettuce salad	0.0	0	0.0
2 Tbsp. blue cheese dressing	3.2	18	4.1
3" x 3" x 1" piece chocolate fudge cake	7.9	52	10.6
TOTALS	35.2	268	49.0

New American Diet†	Saturated Fat (gm)	Cholesterol (mg)	CSI
Breakfast			
2 slices whole wheat toast	0.2	0	0.2
1 tsp. soft margarine	0.7	0	0.7
1 Tbsp. jam	0.0	0	0.0
½ pink grapefruit	0.0	0	0.0
Snack			
1 Cereal Bran Muffin	0.8	1	0.9
Lunch			
1 cup Navy Bean Soup	0.1	0	0.1
2" x 4" piece Corn Bread	1.1	1	1.2
1 tsp. soft margarine	0.7	0	0.7
9 carrot sticks	Tr.	0	0.0
Celery sticks	Tr.	0	0.0
1 cup fresh strawberries	Tr.	0	0.0
4 gingersnaps	0.7	0	0.7
Dinner			
Stuffed Flank Steak Florentine (3 oz.)	2.8	71	6.4
1 large baked potato	Tr.	0	0.0
¼ cup Mock Sour Cream	0.7	5	1.0
1 cup lettuce salad	0.0	0	0.0
2 Tbsp. Western Salad Dressing	0.6	2	0.7
1 cup broccoli	0.0	0	0.0
3 pieces Whole Wheat French Bread	0.1	0	0.1
3" x 3" piece Cocoa Cake	1.6	0	1.6
Snack:			
3 cups air-popped popcorn	Tr.	0	0.0
1 tsp. soft margarine	0.7	0	0.7
TOTALS	10.8	80	15.0

NOTE: Recipes that are set in italics can be found in part 3.
* 2053 Calories, 14% protein, 44% fat, 41% carbohydrate, 15% saturated fat.
† 1931 Calories, 16% protein, 21% fat, 63% carbohydrate, 5% saturated fat.
‡ Gm = gram; mg = milligram.

77

CSI is to help compare and choose individual foods, it is interesting to compare the total CSI of a "typical" American Diet with the New American Diet. Table 4 shows the tabulated CSI of the American Diet and those of the three phases of the New American Diet. The CSI for Phase One of the New American Diet is the same as those of the U.S. dietary guidelines, the American Heart Association's guidelines for the general public, and the guidelines established at a recent Cholesterol Consensus Conference held at the National Institutes of Health. These numbers represent the optimal desirable CSI for different caloric levels.

We have computed two sample food intakes providing approximately 2000 Calories per day—one representing the American Diet and the other representing Phase Three of the New American Diet (see table 5). The CSI of the New American Diet (Phase Three) is approximately only one-third that of the American Diet (15 versus 49).

You'll be referring back to the CSI many times as you get into our program. It is one of the aids we offer to help make low-cholesterol, low-saturated fat choices not only possible but also frequently pleasant. We find that many people will spontaneously make desirable changes in their diet when they have access to the kind of information—providing a variety of choices—contained in the CSI.

Fats and Cholesterol: Summary Recommendations

Our dietary program is designed to encourage a way of eating in which present levels of fat intake, accounting for 40 percent of total

calories in the American Diet, are reduced to 20 to 25 percent of total calories, and we aim to reduce *saturated* fat gradually from present levels of up to 15 percent down to no more than 5 or 6 percent of total calories (see fig. 8). The program is designed with special emphasis on reduction of saturated fats and cholesterol. But it is well to remember that *all* fats in excess are undesirable. They are all calorically dense, contribute to obesity and probably to some forms of cancer. We do, however, recommend an increase in the consumption of those fish that contain omega-3 fatty acids—within limits to be detailed later in part 2, chapter 9.

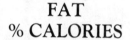

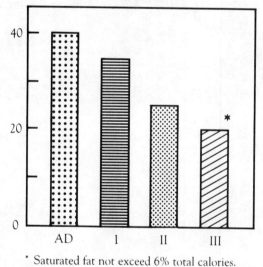

* Saturated fat not exceed 6% total calories.

Figure 8. *The fat content (percent of calories) of the American Diet (AD) compared with the three phases of the New American Diet (I, II, III).*

It is our aim to reduce the typical cholesterol intake of 400 to 500 milligrams daily to 100 milligrams daily—over a period of time (fig. 9). In the course of this, we aim to bring

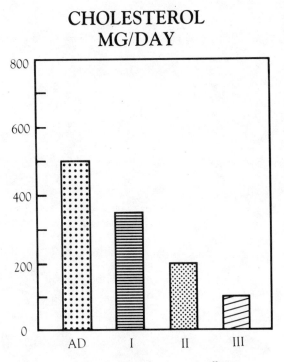

CHOLESTEROL MG/DAY

Figure 9. *The cholesterol content (milligrams per day) of the American Diet (AD) compared with the three phases of the New American Diet (I, II, III).*

blood concentrations of cholesterol down to under 180 milligrams per 100 milliliters of blood. *Any* reduction, of course, will be useful. It has recently been calculated that even a 10 percent reduction in blood cholesterol levels in the United States will eventually save 100,000 lives per year.

If the CSI is used by both consumers and food manufacturers, we think that everyone will be able to reduce the fat in their diets significantly. Though awareness of cholesterol content of foods—and labeling of same by some manufacturers—has helped save lives, we believe that awareness of the CSI of foods may save still more lives and make the choice of foods far more sensible.

Next, let's focus on some basics related to carbohydrates, the foods that will replace some of the excess fat you'll be removing from your diet.

4

CARBOHYDRATES, PROTEIN AND OTHER DIETARY COMPONENTS

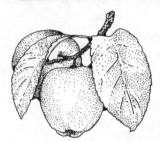

Complex Carbohydrates Are *Not* Fattening

One of the most pervasive—and dangerous —diet myths is that the starchy carbohydrate-rich foods are particularly fattening and/ or that they are somehow nutritionally inferior. Many Americans still associate carbohydrate-containing foods with weight gain; many others regard them as the food of the poor. Protein, meanwhile, is still widely preferred. The notion persists that a diet high in protein and low in carbohydrate provides the best nutrition, the most energy and the least risk of unwanted weight gain. This notion is badly mistaken. Many foods high in protein are also very high in saturated fats and cholesterol, and there is also some evidence that

animal protein itself may, in excess, contribute to some of the diseases our diet helps protect against.

In the New American Diet program the sources, but not the amount, of protein you consume are modified. The amount of fat that you consume is reduced dramatically, especially saturated fat. To replace the calories previously provided by fats, our diet promotes a gradual increase in carbohydrate intake— from 45 percent of total calories (as provided in the standard U.S. diet) to 60 to 65 percent of total calories. Even this is still less carbohydrate than is eaten by many other population groups—particularly those in the non-Western world. Many people consume 75 to 80 percent of their food calories as carbohydrate.

Carbohydrate comes in three general categories: Sugars are carbohydrates made up of one or two simple sugar molecules. Starches are carbohydrates made up of more than ten of these molecules; more complex starches may be made up of several hundred molecules. Fibers are similar to the starches but are not digestible in the human body. The kinds of carbohydrate we encourage you to consume in greater quantities are the starches, especially the more complex starches, and fiber. We recommend *reduced* sugar consumption. Furthermore, most of the starchy foods we suggest such as bread, pasta, rice, other cereals and even potatoes are reasonably good sources of protein themselves. More about protein later.

At present, most Americans eat no more than one food containing significant amounts of complex carbohydrates per meal. The New American Diet goals suggest the consumption of *at least two* such foods per meal. Examples would be to include toast *and* cereal for breakfast, a sandwich *and* bean soup (or a salad with garbanzo or kidney beans in it) for lunch, pasta *and* bread (or rice, corn, potatoes, etc. *and* bread) at dinner. Later in this book, we will be presenting a wide variety of pasta and other recipes containing complex carbohydrates, including many that provide a shift to snacks high in complex carbohydrates such as low-fat cookies, crackers, popcorn, etc. Many of our recipes feature legumes (members of the bean family) and other vegetables. Ultimately, the New American Diet goals suggest getting 3 to 5 cups of legumes into your diet *per week* and 2 to 4 cups of vegetables into your diet *per day*. Review fig. 5 on page 34.

A diet high in complex carbohydrates is just the opposite of fattening. The greater bulk of a high-carbohydrate diet (due in large part to the presence of abundant fiber) en-

ables you to feel full with fewer calories. Fiber absorbs water and becomes even bulkier. And while high carbohydrate foods in general are less expensive than protein, calorie per calorie, they are of no less nutritional value. In fact, foods rich in complex carbohydrates are often good sources of protein (derived from plant rather than animal sources); and these foods are superior to animal protein in that they contain no cholesterol at all, are very low in fat, contribute many vitamins, min-

FEAR OF BREAD
OR
DOES BREAD REALLY MAKE ME FAT?

	Calories	Slices of Bread
MORNING COFFEE BREAK		
Candy bar (1½ oz.)	210	3
ALONG WITH LUNCH		
12 oz. pop/Kool-Ade	144	2
1 oz. bag potato chips	161	2½
PREDINNER		
1 glass wine (6 oz.)	148	2
10 Triscuits	134	2
1 oz. cheese	112	1½
DESSERT		
¾ cup ice cream OR	197	3
3 oatmeal cookies		
DAILY "EXTRAS" TOTAL	1106	16

Figure 10. *Snacks and "extras" a person might consume on a typical day and the caloric equivalent in slices of bread.*

erals and fiber and are good sources of long-lasting energy.

Next time somebody tells you bread—or pasta or potatoes—are fattening, tell him/her about figure 10. This is something developed by one of the Family Heart Study dietitians to show that it would take *sixteen slices of whole wheat bread*—quite a stack!—just to equal, calorically, the snacks somebody might easily consume in a typical day.

Those daily snacks add up to 1106 Calories —equal to sixteen slices or one loaf of bread. And, if you think about it, many of you will have to admit it is very easy to consume even greater quantities of snacks and extras than those listed in figure 10. Yet, people who routinely eat these very high-fat, very high-calorie foods would be horrified if we suggested they sit down and eat a loaf of bread instead.

The choice is not to eat either all of the snacks or all of the bread. Instead, there's a happy medium between those extremes, and one of the goals of this program is to help you find that place for yourself. Another important point is that we have found very tasty ways to include complex carbohydrates in the diet, not as dry bread, but in the form of delicious recipes containing grains, beans and vegetables.

Fiber: Do You Eat Enough?

Fiber is another very important carbohydrate we encourage you to get more of; there's a lot of it in most of the complex carbohydrate foods we recommend. Our goal is to get you to increase your intake from 15 to 20 grams to *45 to 60 grams* of dietary fiber per day. Dietary fiber is only found in plants; it is a term that encompasses a wide variety of car-bohydrates that are believed to be indigestible. These carbohydrates go by such names as cellulose, lignin and pectin. Good sources of fiber include whole grains and cereals, vegetables and fruits. As suggested in part 1, fiber plays an important role in the prevention of a variety of the diseases of over- and undercon-sumption that concern us here. It helps prevent obesity by inducing a feeling of satiety (fullness) through added dietary bulk. It helps prevent certain cancers, diverticulosis, constipation, and several other disorders previously discussed by, among other things, promoting more rapid transit of stool through the system. There is some evidence that certain types of fiber may help lower cholesterol levels but this remains inconslusive. Nonetheless, a diet high in fiber—because it will naturally be low in fat and cholesterol—is an integral part of the diet we use to treat our patients with elevated cholesterol levels. Nearly everyone can benefit from increased fiber intake.

Our fiber goals are also to be achieved very *gradually*. But, in fact, if you know what to eat, getting 45 grams of fiber per day in your diet is not so difficult as it might seem to those who are only getting a fraction of that at present. Some people associate fiber with things like celery and tossed green salads. These do contain fiber, but, because they have such a high water content, they are far from the most concentrated sources. You'd have to eat three good-sized salads or five stalks of celery to get just 5 grams of dietary fiber, but you could get the same amount from just *1/3 of a cup* of cooked beans, peas or lentils. And whereas it would take 4 cups of white rice to provide 5 grams of fiber, you can get the same amount from just 1¾ cups of brown rice or 1 bowl of whole-grain cereal. Two slices of whole wheat bread will give you 5 grams of fiber, but it takes six and a half slices of white bread to deliver that same amount.

Most Americans eat no more than 15 to 20 grams of dietary fiber per day. Figure 11 will help you figure out ways to increase your intake to 45 grams or more.

Later on, we'll introduce you to a number of tasty recipes which have a high fiber content.

Sorting Out and Cutting Back on the Sugars

So far we've been talking about the kinds of carbohydrates we'll be encouraging you to eat *more* of in the course of our diet program. People often assume that we will insist that *all* refined sugars be discontinued in diet. This isn't true. We're realists. Furthermore, the scientific evidence does not suggest this is even necessary. Studies have shown that substantial health benefits can result if people in the Western world will, on average, cut their intake of refined sugar *in half*. Here in the United States the average American gets a rather astonishing 20 percent of his or her total calories from refined sugars. Our goal is to cut this to 10 percent of total calories—not all at once but over a period of time.

In general, we suggest that increasingly you satisfy your cravings for sweets by eating more fruit—three to four pieces a day. Use sugar to sweeten very sour fruits but use much less than recipes normally call for; use sugar to sweeten food made from whole grains (muffins, quick breads, etc.) but, again, use less than what the typical recipe stipulates. (Work toward reducing the amount of sugar called for in most recipes by half.) Be very

FIBER: DO YOU EAT ENOUGH?

Americans currently eat 15 to 20 grams of dietary fiber per day. The goal is 45–60 grams. Here's an example of how to obtain 45 grams of dietary fiber in a day.

4 slices whole wheat bread	10
2 cups brown rice, bulgur, *or*	
1 large baked potato with skin	5–15
1 large serving whole-grain cereal	5
1–2 large servings fruit	5–10
1–2 servings cooked vegetable	5–10
⅓ cup cooked beans, peas, lentils	5
Total	35–55

THE AMOUNT OF EACH FOOD SHOWN BELOW CONTAINS 5 GRAMS OF DIETARY FIBER

2 slices whole wheat bread

6½ slices white bread

1 large serving whole-grain cereal

⅓ cup cooked beans, peas, lentils

3 tablespoons raw bran

1¾ cups cooked brown rice

4 cups cooked white rice

3 servings tossed green salad

5 stalks celery

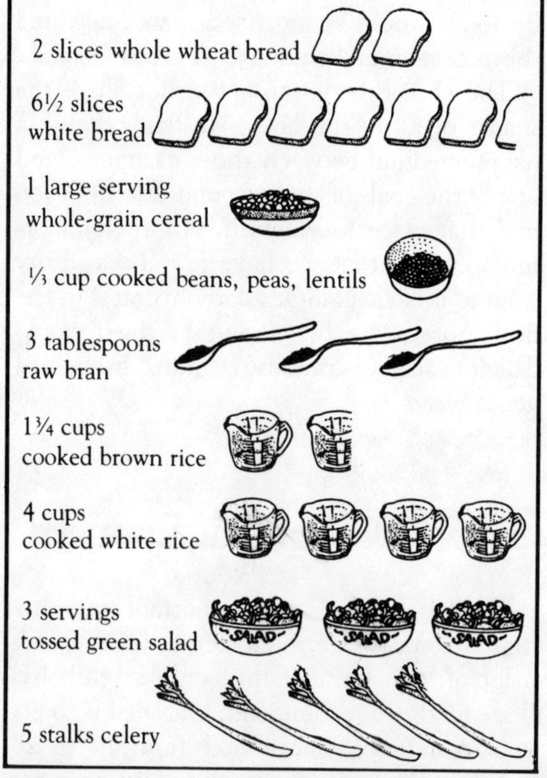

Figure 11. *Amounts of selected foods that contain 5 grams of dietary fiber and an example of how to obtain 45 grams of dietary fiber in a day.*

selective in drinking sweetened "water" whether it is in coffee, tea, juice or soda pop. Make lightly sweetened treats a special rather than a usual event. The ultimate goal is to have pop or candy or dessert in small servings and no more than three times a week. (We'll be more specific about some of this later on.)

What we want to stress now, in this general discussion of carbohydrates, is that a good deal of the sugar you consume is not added by you at the table or in your cooking but is already in food when you buy it. In fact, in the United States, we now get about *half* of our total sugar from packaged foods. (In 1909 we got only one-fourth of our sugar in these foods.) The typical American now consumes about 20–30 teaspoons of sugar *per day*. That adds up to more than *100 pounds per year*. Much of that sugar, as we've noted, comes "hidden" in a wide variety of foods—some obvious and some you probably would never suspect—that you eat all of the time.

If you check labels carefully you'll discover that even the following foods—the type you don't normally think of as "sweet" or "sweetened"—sometimes come with a lot of sugar added: frozen pizza, wieners, boxed rice mixes, bouillon cubes, breads, flavored snack chips, dry-roasted nuts, pickles and relishes, bacon, soy sauce, beef jerky, canned and dry soups, salad dressings and mixes, dry gravy mix, spaghetti sauce, some spice blends, beer, wine, hard liquor (see discussion of alcohol later in this chapter), lunch meat, stewed tomatoes, processed cheese spreads, mayonnaise, some peanut butter, ketchup, crackers, etc.

Some ketchups and salad dressings are actually around 30 percent sugar. Jell-O is more than 80 percent sugar. Some of the prepared mixes used for coating and baking meat and chicken are more than 50 percent sugar

(about the same as a Hershey bar!). Some nondairy creamers are more than 65 percent sugar. "Sugar-frosted" dry cereals are usually 60 to 80 percent sugar and should thus be classified not as cereal but as *candy*. Even some "natural" cereals of the kind "health-food"–oriented individuals might buy are 20 percent or more sugar. Some canned vegetables are 10 percent sugar.

A 12-ounce can of soda pop contains 7 to 8 teaspoons of sugar. A ½ cup portion of ice cream contains 3 to 6 teaspoons; popular candy bars usually weigh between 1 and 5 ounces and contain 3 to *15* teaspoons of sugar; a typical piece of chocolate cake may contain 12 to 15 teaspoons; a level tablespoon of jam contains 3 teaspoons (so does honey and marmalade in the same quantities): a piece of apple pie contains 6 teaspoons; a cup of cocoa or chocolate milk contains 3 teaspoons; a cup of fruit-flavored yogurt contains 6 teaspoons; a 2-inch frosted brownie contains 4; an iced sweet roll contains 7; an iced doughnut contains 4 and so on.

Hidden sugars are everywhere. You have to become adept at reading labels. And beware of claims that "natural" sugars or sweeteners are better for you than what, by implication, are the "unnatural" sugars. Many food manufacturers/processors claim that sucrose—the white sugar you most likely add to foods at the table—is the "bad" sugar. In reality, however, sucrose is as natural as the fructose and glucose found in honey, fruit, vegetables. Sucrose is as much a product of nature as are these other sugars—and the differences, in terms of effects in the body, are small to nonexistent. Honey will put pounds on you and predispose you to tooth decay just as fast as white sugar. (In fact, the stickier, gooier kind of sugar foods, such as caramels, fruit leather, etc., are, recent studies and common sense reveal, *more likely* than white sugar to cause dental cavities.)

Also don't be gulled into believing you're doing yourself a favor if you give up white sugar but then replace it with brown sugar or turbinado sugar which is a coarse light brown crystal. These are often suggested as an improvement over white sugar with no scientific justification. All of the following are various forms of sugar you will find listed on food labels—and you should cut back on *all* of them: brown sugar, corn syrup, dextrose, glucose, honey, lactose, maple sugar, sorghum syrup, turbinado sugar, caramel, dextrin, fructose, grape sugar, invert sugar, maltose, molasses, white sugar.

Look for these sugars among the ingredients listed on product labels. Or, on cereal boxes, for example, look for the type and amount of sugar that has been added to the product, under "carbohydrate information." There are more and more products on the market with *no sugar added.*

Excessive sugar intake is definitely implicated in dental caries. The evidence linking the same excess to diabetes, high blood pressure, heart disease and weight gain is, from a scientific standpoint, still not conclusive. *Some* of the evidence, however, does implicate sugar in these disorders. Certainly sugar is one of the most calorically dense foods you can consume and could therefore be expected to contribute to weight gain which is related to those diseases. There are 16 Calories in every teaspoon of sugar, compared with 1 Calorie in a teaspoon of vegetables, 4 Calories in a teaspoon of rice, 5 Calories in a teaspoon of fish and 9½ Calories in a teaspoon of hamburger. Only alcohol (35 Calories) and fat (45 Calories) deliver more calories per teaspoon.

Before we leave the sugars, a few words about artificial sweeteners: These are products which *do* provide people with more choices. Keep in mind, however, that people in this country have continued to become heavier while consuming millions of pounds of artificial sweeteners. There is no need to use any of these products in order to achieve the goals of the New American Diet. However, for some people artificial sweeteners may play a role in helping decrease sugar intake while continuing to satisfy a sweet tooth. Even so, these products should be consumed with limited frequency and quantity.

Carbohydrates: Summary Recommendations

In summary, the New American Diet goals are to increase the intake of carbohydrate gradually from 45 to 65 percent of calories and dietary fiber from 15 to 20 grams to 45 to 60 grams (fig. 12). This will be accomplished by increasing the intake of whole grains, beans, fruits and vegetables. Refined sugar is to be decreased from 20 to 10 percent of calories. Sugar is used to sweeten sour fruits and whole grain products.

Alcohol: Moderation Is Vital

Alcohol has a high caloric content; it also has many well-known adverse social, psychological and physical effects which argue for its restricted use.

Recently, there has been a great deal of confusion over the relationship of alcohol consumption and factors related to heart dis-

CARBOHYDRATE
% CALORIES

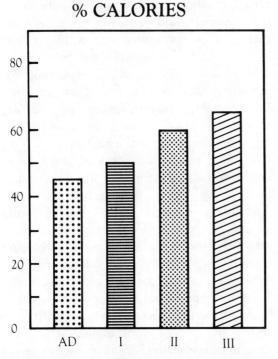

Figure 12.   *The carbohydrate content (percent of calories) of the American Diet (AD) compared with the three phases of the New American Diet (I, II, III).*

ease. There have been findings that alcohol can increase the concentration of HDL in the blood. Since HDL helps carry cholesterol safely out of the system, some drinkers have been encouraged to drink even more, claiming that booze is "good for the heart." This is both wishful and dangerous thinking. The findings related to HDL and alcohol are too scant, contradictory and complex to lend themselves to such simplistic conclusions. Even if alcoholics, as a group, could be shown to have high HDL levels, they would *still* be alcoholics, subject to serious liver disease and all of the other ailments to which this affliction contributes. But, in fact, *some* alcoholics

have been shown to have *low* HDL levels. They also sometimes have elevated triglycerides which, along with cholesterol, contribute to heart disease. Alcohol also raises blood pressure.

It is not possible to give *definitive* or absolute advice on how much one can safely drink. Apart from individual variations, we still have much to learn about the effects of alcohol consumption. In general, however, most of us would be well-advised to restrict ourselves to no more than two or three drinks or less per week.

Those with weight problems should be especially wary of alcohol which, as pointed out above, is packed with calories. Four drinks per day (of the sort people commonly consume) contribute more than *550 Calories.* And when you reflect on the startling fact that, on the average, adults in the United States get up to 8 *percent* of *all* their calories from alcohol, you can begin to understand one of the reasons why so many of us are overweight and have alcohol-related health problems.

One thing is certain: The best scientific evidence to date does *not* provide a green light for alcohol consumption. On the contrary, the best evidence suggests that those who drink are least likely to enjoy better overall health.

Coffee and Tea

You will be relieved to hear that scientific studies have shown little association between coffee drinking and heart disease or other disorders. People who drink too much coffee or strong tea, however, often experience "coffee nerves." They become jittery. It is better to consume coffee and tea in moderation—perhaps 3 cups a day or less. Whether you choose to drink decaffeinated, regular or no coffee or strong tea at all is a matter of personal choice. Tea can be prepared light and still be a good beverage.

Protein: Modifying the Source

Much of what we discuss in this book has focused on fats and carbohydrates. Protein intake undergoes far less modification in our program because the best research findings indicate that we in the Western world are consuming just about the right amount of protein. However, there is scientific evidence suggesting that protein, in too large quantities, can cause deterioration of kidney function over time. The body needs no more than 0.45 gram protein per pound body weight. The actual minimum requirement is 0.16 gram protein per pound body weight. So tripling that amount to 0.48 gram per pound fulfills all the possible protein needs of healthy people. This amount of protein translates to about 10 to 12 percent of the total calories as protein. The New American Diet at 15 percent of calories supplies enough protein but does not provide too much protein.

Any problem with the prevailing pattern of protein consumption does not have to do so much with quantity as with the type or source of protein. Presently, a great percentage of our protein comes from animal sources (eggs, meat, cheese and other high-fat dairy products). Unfortunately, these same foods are also very high in fat and cholesterol.

In the New American Diet program protein intake is maintained at 15 percent of total calories, but a shift is encouraged in the source of those protein calories. Most Americans and others in the developed nations of the Western world get about 68 percent of their protein from animal sources. In our diet program the goal is to reduce this figure gradually to about 44 percent; the remaining 56 percent is then dervied from *plant* protein, i.e., vegetable protein. This amount is similar to what people in the United States were eating at the beginning of the century.

The shift here is not enormous, and no one need worry about getting ample amino acids, the building blocks of protein, from this diet. And though adequate human data are still lacking, there is evidence, in the animal work, that such animal proteins as casein (found in milk) have cholesterol-elevating effects, while such vegetable proteins as those found in soybeans have the opposite, a cholesterol-lowering effect. There is, in addition, both some experimental animal data and some human epidemiological findings suggesting that those of us in the Western world may be at increased risk of developing some cancers due partly to an overconsumption of some animal proteins. Of course, as previously noted, it is often difficult to separate the effects of protein from the fats that are so often present in the same foods, but on balance it appears we might all benefit from a moderate reduction in our consumption of animal protein.

Salt: Cut Your Intake in Half

Though salt is not one of the dietary macronutrients like the fats, carbohydrates and proteins discussed above, it has become such a major "accessory" to the standard diet of the

Western world that it deserves some special mention in this chapter. Americans eat many times the amount of salt that the body needs. The part of the salt molecule that is harmful is the sodium component. Salt intake varies considerably from one person to another, of course, but, in general, we advise people to cut their intake *by at least half.* Reduced salt intake is vital both in the prevention and the treatment of high blood pressure.

Reduction, as usual, takes place gradually. We'll show you how to do this step by step as you proceed through the three phases of our diet. Emphasis is placed on reduction of salt both in the home (at the table and in the kitchen) and in prepared/processed foods. Fortunately, food manufacturers are beginning to market products with reduced or no salt added. Low-salt breakfast cereals and soups are now available in most supermarkets. So are no salt added whole (canned) tomatoes, tomato sauce, juice and various canned vegetables. Lite Salt and various spice combinations that can be used in place of salt are also widely available.

The typical adult in the United States consumes *10 pounds* of salt a year. Forty percent of that typically comes from the saltshaker. Thirty percent is already in processed foods when you purchase them. Another 20 percent is in breads, grains, cereals. Only 10 percent of the salt you eat is naturally occurring in foods, and this amount of salt is not harmful.

Obviously, the first place to start cutting back is in the salt *you* add to food. Many of our patients and test families have expressed surprise over how easy it can be to reduce salt intake. There is some withdrawl discomfort but usually it is of short duration. Many of the people we work with comment on how difficult and distasteful it is to eat foods with the "standard" amounts of salt in them once the salt habits have been changed. Frequently, they express horror at the mere idea of adding salt to foods they haven't even tasted—something many of them used to do without a second thought. The more salt we eat, the more we want; fortunately, this works the other way as well. The less salt you eat, the less you'll want it. Salt is definitely one craving that can be licked.

Now that we've covered the basic food components separately, let's go on to the next chapter and see how we can arrive at a new and better relationship between two of these —the fats and carbohydrates.

5

FAT OUT/ CARBOHYDRATE IN

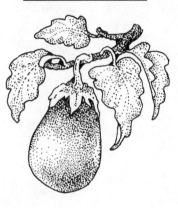

The Astonishing "Fats of Life"

The typical woman of the Western world consumes about 5000 pounds of fat in her lifetime; the typical Western world man puts away even more—about 7000 pounds. Some Americans will consume twice those quantities or even more in their lifetimes. Sympathize for a moment with your body as it struggles to cope with those *tons* of fat. How do we arrive at these dishearteningly huge sums? Well, as the following exercise will demonstrate, we do it a molecule or a teaspoon of fat at a time, day in and day out.

We'll show you in this chapter where all that fat comes form, how much of it is "invisible," how it relentlessly adds up to those figures cited above, how we can get rid of some of it and how we can replace it with other foods, especially with complex carbohydrates. It's this replacement—achieved in a *phased* program—that is at the heart of the New American Diet. This demonstration was developed by two members of the Family Heart Study staff for use in our family study. We found that it was one of the most effective presentations made during the five years of the study.

Typical Daily Fat Intake

Before we get into substituting carbohydrate for fat, let's take a close look at the sources and amount of fat in our diet. This example (see fig. 13) is for a typical man, but

SAMPLE INTAKE FOR
TYPICAL AMERICAN MALE

	Teaspoons of Fat	Lower Fat Alternatives
BREAKFAST		
1 poached egg	1	
2 strips bacon	1½	
1 slice toast	0	
1 tsp. soft margarine	1	
2 tsp. jam	0	
1 cup orange juice	0	
SNACK		
1 cup coffee	0	
1 doughnut	2	
LUNCH		
Sandwich		
2 slices rye bread	0	
2 oz. turkey	½	
1 Tbsp. real mayonnaise	2	
Tomatoes and lettuce	0	
1-oz. bag chips	2½	
1 apple	0	
Water	0	

	Teaspoons of Fat	Lower Fat Alternatives
SNACK		
8 snack crackers	1	
12 oz. soda pop	0	
DINNER		
Cheeseburger:		
1 hamburger bun	0	
4 oz. ground beef (25% fat)	5	
1 oz. Cheddar cheese	2	
1 Tbsp. real mayonnaise	2	
French fries (average order)	3	
2 Tbsp. catsup	0	
Tossed salad	0	
1 Tbsp. blue cheese dressing	1½	
¾ cup ice cream	2	
Water	0	
SNACK		
1 slice toast	0	
1 Tbsp. peanut butter (spread thin)	1½	
1 glass 2% milk, 8 oz.	1	
Miscellaneous (bread, fruit, etc.)	1	
Total	30½ tsp. fat*	

* The objective is to have no more than 20 teaspoons of fat. To keep calories constant, replace with bread, grains and potatoes (11 teaspoons of fat is equal in calories to 7 slices of bread).

Nutrient Composition

Energy (Calories)	3100
Protein (% Calories)	14
Fat (% Calories)	44
Carbohydrate (% Calories)	42
Cholesterol (mg)	572

Figure 13. *Example of a typical intake of fat for the typical American male—for one day.*

the average woman can be instructed by it equally as well. You'll note that from breakfast alone our man consumed 3½ teaspoons of fat—and he's restricting himself to just one egg instead of the two or more many men—and women—eat on a daily basis. And he's using margarine instead of butter, and a con-

servative amount at that. If you'll look now at figure 14, you can see what this breakfast looks like. Those shaded squares and rectangles represent the fat: Each square is the equivalent of a teaspoon of pure fat; each rectangle is half a teaspoon.

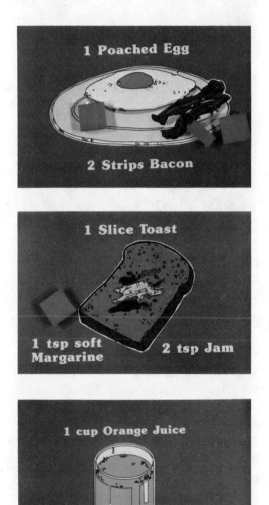

Figure 14. *Breakfast.*

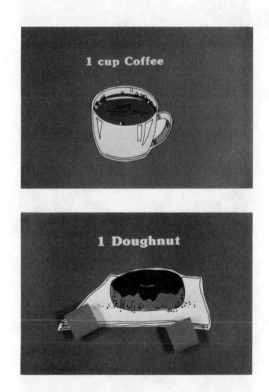

Figure 15. *Morning snack.*

Now, somewhere between breakfast and lunch, there's often some sort of snack, right? In this case, it's a cup of coffee and a doughnut. There go 2 more teaspoons of fat down the hatch (see fig. 15). Well, you're thinking, what's one doughnut? And he didn't even put cream in his coffee.

Next move down figure 13 to lunch. Five more teaspoons of fat. Figure 16 shows you what lunch looks like. For many of you, this

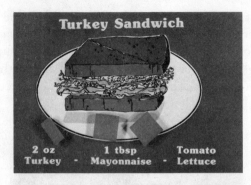

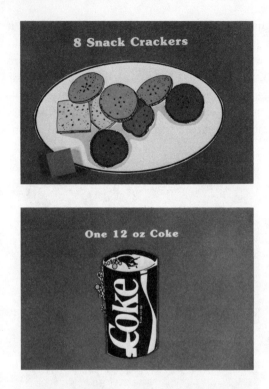

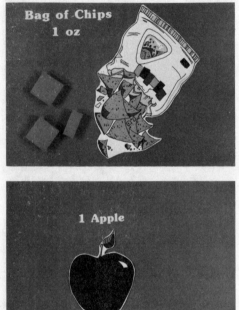

Figure 16. *Lunch.*

Figure 17. *Afternoon snack.*

may seem like a rather Spartan lunch. Many men would eat *two* full sandwiches at lunch. And if you use, say, 2 ounces of bologna instead of 2 ounces of turkey, the meat component of your sandwich would total 3 teaspoons of fat, not ½ teaspoon, as in the case of 2 ounces of turkey. Add a couple ounces of cheese and you'd add another 4 teaspoons of fat. Furthermore, this guy is drink-

ing *water* with his sandwich, not a glass of milk (which, even if only 2 percent fat would add another 1 teaspoon of fat—2 teaspoons if whole milk). A milk shake would add 3 or more teaspoons of fat.

Late in the afternoon, our man has another snack (fig. 17) consisting of 8 snack crackers and a 12-ounce can of soda pop. This contributes 1 more teaspoon of fat to his daily intake.

Move farther down figure 13 now to dinner (visualized in Fig. 18). Dinner contains *15½ teaspoons* of fat, quite a whopping amount. But examine the individual ingredients of dinner in terms of fat content, and see how you compare. This guy is having a cheeseburger as his main dish. Hamburgers and cheeseburgers are not the lowest fat foods around, by any means, but there are hamburgers and there are *hamburgers*. How many

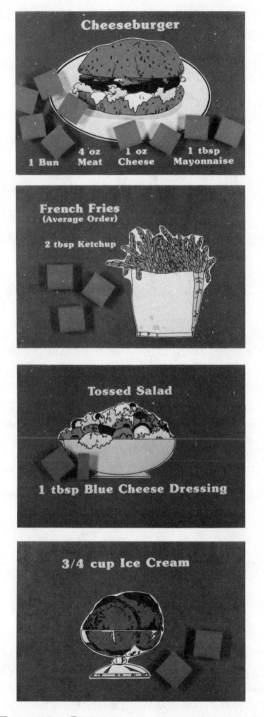

Figure 18. Dinner.

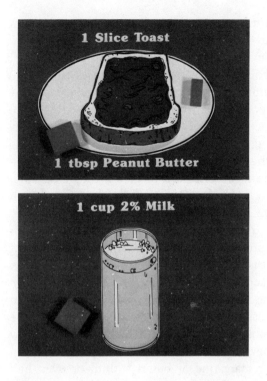

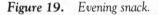

Figure 19. Evening snack.

of you eat the type that have *two* or even *three* layers of meat and/or cheese? The one our maybe-not-so-typical man is eating in this example has just one 4-ounce patty in it and 1 ounce of Cheddar cheese. Again, there's no milk shake or milk with this dinner, although there is ¾ cup of store-brand (as opposed to the even higher-fat gourmet-style) ice cream for dessert.

Later, there's a bedtime snack (figure 19) consisting of a thin spread of peanut butter on a slice of toast and a glass of 2 percent milk, 8 oz. This adds another 2½ teaspoons of fat.

Add one more teaspoon of fat from miscellaneous sources in this day's food intake (bread, fruit, etc.; almost everything contains a little fat), and we arrive at a total of 30½ *teaspoons of fat.* That's equivalent in amount to 1¼ sticks of margarine, the amount consumed by a typical man eating 3100 Calories. For women eating 2000 Calories this would amount to ⅔ of a stick of margarine. The food listed in figure 13 comes to 3100 Calories. Of that, *44 percent* is from fat, amounting to 1373 Calories. This is the way of eating that has contributed significantly to the diseases we discussed in part 1 and, especially, to the *half million* heart attacks suffered each year by those living in the United States.

And yet, if you look at this list of foods carefully, you'll probably have to admit that it isn't much different from your daily fare. In fact, you may have to concede that your *own* fat intake is sometimes even greater. You can easily visualize what 1¼ sticks of margarine look like. It's quite a blob, and, yet, how many times have you put a heap of sour cream or margarine or butter a third or even half that same size on a single baked potato? Or how many times have you put one, two or more ladles of thick cheese dressing on your lunch and dinner salads? It's shocking how fast the fat can add up.

What this exercise should also make clear to you is the "invisible" nature of most dietary fat. Too many of us think of fat in terms of the butter or margarine, salad dressings, or other fats we put on our foods, forgetting or not realizing that many foods, including lean-looking meats and dry, crisp crackers or our favorite cheeses already come with fat galore concealed inside them. Fats directly added at the table constitute only about one-fourth of our total fat intake. The remaining three-fourths is of the "invisible" variety. Little wonder that those hidden molecules of fat can add up so quickly and unexpectedly—from ounces to pounds to *tons* over the days, weeks, months, years. See figure 20 for the sources of fat in the typical diet.

SOURCES OF FAT

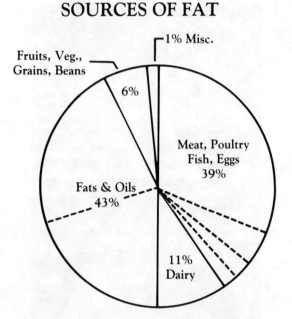

Figure 20. *The sources of dietary fat for people in the United States. Thirty-nine percent of dietary fat is from red meats (30%), poultry (5%), eggs (3%) and fish (1%) as per the broken lines dividing that segment of the circle. Eleven percent is from dairy products. Forty-three percent is directly from fats and oils, 21.5 percent being from visible fats (spreads and dressings) and 21.5 percent from fat used in cooking and baking. Six percent is from fruits, vegetables, grains and beans and 1 percent is from miscellaneous sources.*

Getting the Fat Out and the Carbohydrate In

One of the mistakes many people commit when confronted with the kind of information discussed above is to start cutting back radically on fat without giving any thought to what they are going to replace it with—and, unless you're on a weight-reducing program, you're going to want to replace it with some-

thing. The something that works best in terms of disease prevention, overall good health, energy and weight control is complex carbohydrate.

In our demonstrations we often challenge groups to get rid of at least 11 teaspoons of the fat found in the food listed in figure 13. We put that amount of fat, amounting to 495 Calories, alongside seven slices of whole wheat bread, representing an equivalent amount of complex carbohydrates (also 495 Calories). We then ask people what would happen if they were to eat the diet with the fat in it, and also eat seven slices of bread. The correct answer, of course, is that they would gain weight. Next we ask them what would happen if they take the 11 teaspoons of fat out and replace them with the seven slices of bread. *Weight maintenance* is the correct answer.

Yet most people in this country try not to eat bread, potatoes, and pasta. When they *do* eat them, they add them on, instead of using them to replace dietary fat. It's in this way that these carbohydrate foods erroneously come to be regarded as fattening. What we are suggesting is substituting the carbohydrates for the fats. And *that* we assure you, is *not* fattening.

Let's look again at the daily fare we just examined and see how we might remove at least 11 teaspoons of fat and replace it with high-carbohydrate, low-fat foods of equal calories (fig. 21). A reduction of 11 teaspoons of fat reduces the percentage of calories we get from fat from 44 percent to about 30 percent, still shy of our ultimate goal of 20 percent but within the guidelines for Phase One of the New American Diet, a strong first step in the right direction.

When we do this exercise live, that is, before groups of parents, patients, teenagers, medical students and others, we ask our au-

diences what they would be willing to give up or "trade" for lower-fat foods. The exchange is typically lively, with a good deal of disagreement. The fact that people *do* disagree on what constitutes an acceptable change in diet helps show why so many diets with rigid regimens and meal plans fail. A successful diet program has to provide *many* choices for acceptable change. Thus, what you see in figure 21 is just *one* possible way of getting rid of at least 11 teaspoons of fat. You can figure out many other ways to do this yourself when you get into the three phases of our diet. But even now you can look at figure 21 and, using common sense, come up with a variety of different ways of cutting back on the fat.

In the example provided here the choice is to get rid of the two strips of bacon at breakfast and replace them with a cup of oatmeal and a cup of skim milk. That eliminates 1½ teaspoons of fat. We're on our way. Not only have we reduced some of the fat from our diet but we've replaced it with a filling food—oatmeal, which is also an excellent source of complex carbohydrate and fiber.

Next we go to the midmorning snack. Here the choice is to replace the doughnut with a bran muffin. And there we've eliminated another teaspoon of fat. If you'd opt for a bagel instead of a bran muffin as a replacement for that doughnut, you'd get rid of 2 teaspoons of fat. And you'd be adding some more complex carbohydrate and fiber.

At lunch you could eliminate another teaspoon of fat with minimal discomfort by replacing the real mayonnaise on your sandwich with a light or imitation mayonnaise, many of which are satisfying substitutes. But the choice in this example is to replace that 1-ounce bag of potato chips with 1½ cups of lentil soup, which contains no fat, resulting in a sizable elimination of 2½ more teaspoons of fat.

For your afternoon snack, you can trade those eight snack crackers for *3 cups* of popcorn prepared in an "air popper" which does not use any oil. If you eat it plain you will eliminate another teaspoon of fat. You may decide, however, to put 1 teaspoon of melted margarine on the popcorn. You don't get rid of fat in that case but at least you make a good trade, substituting the low-saturated fat in the margarine for the highly saturated fat in the crackers.

At dinner, if you want to stick to a hamburger, you might try switching to 10- or 15-percent-fat ground beef instead of the 25 percent variety. This would net you a savings of 2 or 3 more teaspoons of fat, or you could go even further and have red snapper or chicken instead of the hamburger. Either of those choices would reduce total fat intake for this day by *four* teaspoons of fat. In the example in figure 21, however, the choice is to keep the hamburger but get rid of the Ched-

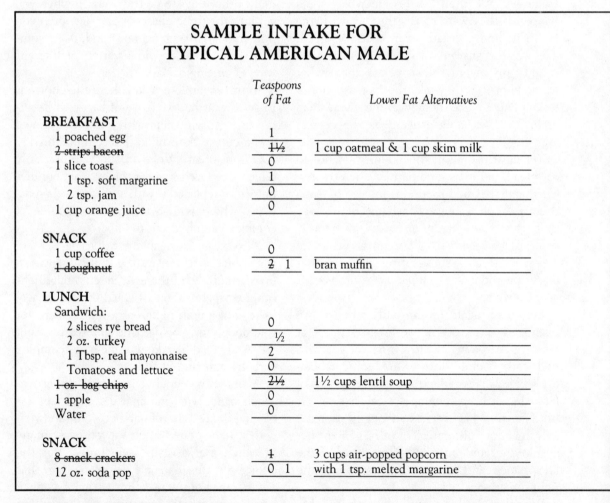

SAMPLE INTAKE FOR TYPICAL AMERICAN MALE

	Teaspoons of Fat	Lower Fat Alternatives
BREAKFAST		
1 poached egg	1	
2 strips bacon	1½	1 cup oatmeal & 1 cup skim milk
1 slice toast	0	
1 tsp. soft margarine	1	
2 tsp. jam	0	
1 cup orange juice	0	
SNACK		
1 cup coffee	0	
1 doughnut	2 1	bran muffin
LUNCH		
Sandwich:		
2 slices rye bread	0	
2 oz. turkey	½	
1 Tbsp. real mayonnaise	2	
Tomatoes and lettuce	0	
1 oz. bag chips	2½	1½ cups lentil soup
1 apple	0	
Water	0	
SNACK		
8 snack crackers	1	3 cups air-popped popcorn
12 oz. soda pop	0 1	with 1 tsp. melted margarine

Figure 21. Example of typical intake for an American man as it might appear after some of the fat had been removed and replaced with carbohydrate.

dar cheese, eliminating 2 teaspoons of fat. Instead of the French fries, a large baked potato is substituted, getting rid of 3 teaspoons of fat. The ketchup is deleted and Mock Sour Cream is selected for the baked potato, *adding* ¼ teaspoon of fat. But by trading blue cheese dressing for our Western Salad Dressing (see recipe, part 3), another 1¼ teaspoons of fat are eliminated. The choice here is to keep the ice cream but if you are willing to substitute low-fat frozen yogurt for the ice cream, you would eliminate another 1½ teaspoons of fat. (Make sure, though, that the frozen yogurt is not made from whole milk or cream!) If you switch to sorbet in place of the ice cream, you'll get rid of 2 teaspoons of fat.

The after-dinner snack is left as it was in the example, but if you choose to drink skim milk instead of 2 percent milk, you'd get rid of another teaspoon of fat. By going to 1 percent milk you can get rid of ½ a teaspoon of fat.

DINNER

Cheeseburger:

1 hamburger bun	0	
4 oz. ground beef (25% fat)	5	
~~1 oz. Cheddar cheese~~	~~2~~	
1 Tbsp. real mayonnaise	2	
~~French fries (average order)~~	~~3~~	large baked potato
~~2 Tbsp. catsup~~	~~0~~ ¼	¼ cup Mock Sour Cream
Tossed salad	0	
~~1 Tbsp. blue cheese dressing~~	~~1½~~ ¼	2 Tbsp. Western Salad Dressing
¾ cup ice cream	2	
Water	0	

SNACK

1 slice toast	0	
1 Tbsp. peanut butter (spread thin)	1½	
1 glass 2% milk, 8 oz.	1	
Miscellaneous (bread, fruit, etc.)	1	
Total	~~30½~~ tsp. fat*	
	19½	

* The objective is to have no more than 20 teaspoons of fat. To keep calories constant, replace the fat with bread, grains and potatoes (11 teaspoons of fat is equal in calories to 7 slices of bread).

Nutrient Composition

Energy (Calories)	3100
Protein (% Calories)	14
Fat (% Calories)	44
Carbohydrate (% Calories)	42
Cholesterol (mg)	572

In the example in figure 21, you eliminate 11 teaspoons of fat. By studying this figure you can easily find many ways of retaining some of your favorite foods here while still getting rid of 11 teaspoons, amounting to 495 Calories. In fact, you can probably find ways of getting rid of 14 to 15 teaspoons without too much pain. This will become much easier when you have more information on substitutions and trade-offs, replacing fat with complex carbohyrate and other low-fat food choices—which will be provided when we get to the three phases of the diet. There you'll learn how to make comparisons for quick and easy substitutions.

This chapter should have demonstrated to you that: (1) you are probably eating far more fat—especially "invisible" fat—than you had imagined; (2) there are *many* ways to reduce dietary fat; and (3) the best substitution for fat is complex carbohydrate, which can be found in a wide variety of delicious foods.

To return now to what we stated at the beginning of this chapter, if you were to reduce your fat intake by just one-third (we hope you'll eventually reduce it by even more), that would take quite a load off your body, at least 1667 pounds less fat to be processed over a lifetime for the typical woman and at least 2333 pounds for the typical man. That can make a big difference in your health, and help to keep you in trim form at the same time.

6

THE THREE PHASES OF THE NEW AMERICAN DIET

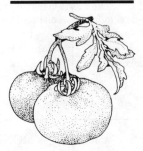

Substitutions/New Recipes/ A New Way of Eating

The three phases of the New American Diet are summarized in table 6, which is on page 104. Phase One concentrates on *substitutions* of foods, especially of lower-fat foods for higher-fat varieties. In Phase Two, we begin to introduce *new recipes*, especially ethnic recipes, such as Chinese, Mexican and Italian, that more closely achieve the goals of our diet. In Phase Three, you will assume what is in many respects *a new way of eating*.

You Determine Your Rate of Progress

Although we continually stress that you must proceed at your own rate, we will, nonetheless, give you some introductory guidelines here on what some others have achieved in a given period of time. Figure 22 shows you what some fairly typical families did during the first year in our program. Don't be discouraged, however, if you and your family don't make all the same changes in the same period of time. There are no deadlines in this program. Actually, when you first look at figure 22 you may think this is quite a bit to accomplish in a single year. But if you consider the changes *a month at a time* they won't seem nearly so challenging. Don't take on everything at once, but instead proceed gradually. What you want to do is to become comfortable with a *few* changes at a time, then add others. The idea is to keep accumulating new eating habits, keep practicing them and keep building toward the larger goals.

Some people find it more convenient to set small goals for themselves *each week* and then to assess their success at the end of each

A YEAR OF CHANGES

MONTH 1 Become aware of how much and how often you eat eggs, liver, red meats and high-fat dairy products (cheese, ice cream, whole milk). Eat and cook with cheeses lower in fat and/or cholesterol (Lite-line, Reduced Calories Laughing Cow, mozzarella, Light n' Lively, "filled" or other part-skim milk cheeses *).	**MONTH 4** Switch to a lower-fat milk (try mixing your current milk with a lower-fat one). Use sherbet, frozen yogurt or ices in place of ice cream. Popcorn is a great snack: (air-popped or with 1 Tbsp. oil per batch).
MONTH 2 Eat breakfasts of whole-grain cereals, toast and muffins more often. Limit whole eggs, bacon or sausage: no more than once a month. Replace one whole egg with two egg whites or ¼ cup egg substitute when making cakes, muffins, waffles, hotcakes, etc.	**MONTH 5** Replace high-fat snack crackers with lower-fat varieties (RyKrisp, soda, ak-mak, graham, Bremner, etc. *). Each week, eat several "meatless" lunches (containing no cheese, eggs, meat, fish or poultry). Try soup, bean burritos, low-fat cottage cheese, bean salad, etc.
MONTH 3 Serve chicken and fish more often in place of red meats. Try a new recipe (but no frying). Limit deep-fat-fried foods (French fries, onion rings, doughnuts, etc.). Replace butter with margarine.	**MONTH 6** Make "mock sour cream" for dips or baked potatoes: mix 1 cup low-fat cottage cheese, 1 tsp. fresh lemon juice and 2 Tbsp. buttermilk until smooth in blender. Prepare legume dishes (lentil or split pea soup, chili, baked beans) with little or no meat.

Figure 22. *A year of changes with suggestions month by month.*

weekly period. If success is lacking or minimal, again, don't be discouraged. Instead, set the same or similar goals for the next week and get to those goals before taking on a lot of new ones. And if you get stuck on some particular goal and just can't seem to achieve it, *set it aside* and work on other things. You can return to the areas that give you particular problems when you've made more progress in other areas. For example, if cutting back on bacon is not working for you, concentrate on eggs instead. Though most people find the three phases of our diet the natural way to proceed, we do *not* insist on any particular order. *Any* of the changes we prescribe, in whatever order, are going to benefit you.

The Weekly Contract

For those who like weekly goals (they could as easily be monthly), the following "contract" is often helpful. Each week or month, take out a new sheet of paper and write down these questions/statements with your answers and goals:

1. This week I am going to work on the following goal or goals (be as specific as possible, e.g., "cut back to no more than three eggs," "reduce the amount of sugar I add to my food by at least one-fourth," etc.).

2. What specifically will I do to achieve this goal? (You might, for example, commit

MONTH 7 Eat two grain products at every meal (bread, cereal, rice, bulgur, tortillas, pasta, etc.).

Have larger servings of grains or potatoes with smaller servings of meat.

Use low-fat plain yogurt (with vanilla and a little sugar) to replace whipped dessert toppings.

MONTH 10 Use ¼ less fat (oil, margarine, shortening) than recipe calls for in cooking and baking.

Use fish or poultry at least 3 times a week for your main meal.

Switch to low-calorie salad dressings and imitation mayonnaise.

MONTH 8 Make your own corn chips by scraping margarine on thin corn tortillas, cut into wedges and bake on cookie sheets for 8–10 minutes at 350°.

When baking, use ⅓ less sugar than recipe calls for. Use part whole wheat flour in recipes calling for all-purpose flour.

Eat fruit 2–3 times a day.

MONTH 11 Eat vegetables at least twice each day.

Try one new way to prepare vegetables each week.

Use beans (garbanzo, 3-bean, etc.) on a tossed salad.

Buy only ground beef with no more than 10–15% fat content.

MONTH 9 Switch to Lite Salt*and use half the amount of salt a recipe calls for in baking or cooking.

Try Kikkoman Lite Soy Sauce.*

Try dessert recipes that have no more than ¼ cup fat (oil, margarine, shortening).

MONTH 12 If you have meat, fish, cheese or poultry for lunch, eat a meatless dinner.

Dine out at ethnic restaurants or places that offer lower-fat choices.

Occasionally, for special celebrations, ignore all suggestions and enjoy!

* Certain products are listed to provide examples of food items on the market which are acceptable choices. Often there are other products of similar composition with different trade names which are also acceptable for use.

yourself to buying less of certain foods you want to cut back on during your weekly shopping, or you might state that on certain days of this particular week or month you are going to eat meatless sandwiches, or that you will try lower-fat cheeses in certain foods or on certain days, or that you will bake your next batch of cookies using reduced amounts of fat and sugar, specifying exactly how much you will reduce these ingredients, and so on.)

3. If I am successful this week in reaching my goal, I plan to reward myself in the following way. (Do something nice for yourself, but don't resort to dietary rewards that undo all the good you've done yourself by making de-

sirable changes. Obviously if you "reward" yourself with a steak just because you reduced your egg intake by three eggs you're going to end up taking two steps backward for every one step forward. For many, just accomplishing a desired goal is adequate reward. But when you feel you've made some really significant progress, treat yourself to a movie, new clothes, time with a friend, or do something else to commemorate the event; this sort of positive reinforcement will help make the progress stick. Use the same psychology on spouses and children.)

4. Estimate your overall success in reaching this goal for this coming week. In other

TABLE 6
Summary of the Three Phases of the New American Diet

Phase I: Substitutions	This is accomplished by:	
	Avoiding egg yolks, butterfat, lard and organ meats (liver, heart, brains, kidney, gizzards)	Trimming fat off meat and skin from chicken
	Substituting soft margarine for butter	Choosing commercial food products lower in cholesterol and fat (low-fat cheeses, egg substitutes, soy meat substitutes, frozen yogurt, etc.)
	Substituting vegetable oils and shortening for lard	
	Substituting skim milk and skim-milk products for whole milk and whole-milk products	Modifying favorite recipes by using less fat or sugar and vegetable oils instead of butter or lard;
	Substituting egg whites for whole eggs	Decreasing use of table salt and using lower sodium salt (Lite Salt)
Phase II: New recipes	This step involves:	
	Reducing amounts of meat and cheese eaten and replacing them with chicken and fish	Eating more grains, beans, fruits and vegetables;
	Eating meat, chicken or fish only once a day	When eating out, make low-fat, low-cholesterol choices;
	Cutting down on fat; as spreads, in salads, cooking and baking	Finding new recipes to replace those which cannot be altered;
		Using few products containing salt
Phase III: A new way of eating	The final phase means:	
	Eating meat, cheese, poultry, shellfish and fish as condiments to other foods, rather than as main courses	Drinking 4–6 glasses of water per day;
	Eating more beans and grain products as protein sources	Keeping extra meat, regular cheese, chocolate, candy, coconut and richer home-baked or commercially prepared food for special occasions (once a month or less)
	Using no more than 4–7 teaspoons of fat per day as spreads, salad dressings and in cooking and baking	Enjoying a wide variety of new food and repertoire of totally new and savory recipes
		Decreasing amount of salt used for cooking

words, guess whether you will be anywhere from zero to 100 percent successful. If you estimate it's less than 60 percent, redefine your goal—either you have chosen too much to do or you don't really want to do it.

5. When the week is over, note what your *actual* success was in accomplishing what you set out to do (e.g., 10 percent successful, 60 percent successful, 100 percent successful).

The *Six* Food Groups

The Four Basic Food Groups largely describes the current standard American diet which we have associated with so many chronic, degenerative diseases. "Six Food Groups" best describes the New American Diet. Both systems deal with the same foods, of course, but the difference is in the group-

SIX FOOD GROUPS—THE NEW AMERICAN DIET

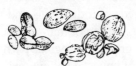

Beans, Nuts, Seeds: Eat 3–5 cups of beans per week (kidney, pinto, lentils, refried, chili, etc.). Use nuts and seeds to spice up grains, beans and vegetables.

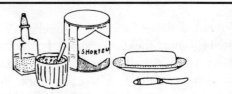

Fats: Use sparingly (4–7 tsp. per day). Think of using half the fat as spreads, mayonnaise or salad dressing and half in cooking and baking (vegetable oils, margarine, shortening).

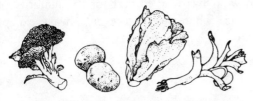

Vegetables: Eat 2–4 cups per day.

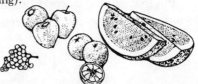

Fruits: Each 3–5 pieces per day—fresh fruit is preferable to juice.

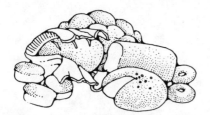

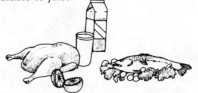

Whole Grains and Potatoes: Eat 2–5 servings at each meal; choose snacks from this group (bread, rice, popcorn, cereals, flour, oats, etc.)

NOTE: Fewer servings are suitable for women and children. The greater number of servings is appropriate for men and teens.

Low-Fat Animal Products: Eat one of the following, aiming for a daily average of *either* 6 oz. of fish, clams, oysters or scallops *or* 3–4 oz. of poultry, shrimp, crab, lobster or lean meat *or* 1–2 oz. of lower-fat cheese. Use low-fat dairy products as desired (skim milk, low-fat yogurt, etc.)

Figure 23. Six Food Groups which represent the New American Diet. Emphasis is placed on the consumption of whole grains, vegetables and fruits. Only one of the six groups contains low-fat animal fats in contrast to the Four Basic Food Groups of the current American Diet in which two groups contain animal products.

ings and interrelationships of the foods and the relative *quantities* in which they are consumed. Emphasis in the new system is on eating more from the vegetable kingdom and using fats and low-fat animal products in moderation.

Figure 23 shows the Six Food Groups of the New American Diet: beans, nuts, seeds; veg-etables; whole grains and potatoes; fats; fruits; low-fat animal products. The recommendations related to each of these are *ultimate* goals. We don't expect you to achieve these from the outset. But figure 23 will help you to understand the directions in which it is desirable for you and your family to go.

Important

Read *all three* of the following chapters before beginning the diet program. It is not necessary to achieve all of the goals of Phase One before proceeding to Phase Two and Phase Three, but it *is* necessary for you to grasp our overall objectives in detail before starting. You may decide to skip around within the program, choosing goals from different phases, and that's fine if it works best for you. But in order to make an informed decision on such matters you first need to know what the whole program entails. From our experience with hundreds of individuals and families followed over a period of many years, we believe the phases provide a logical path of progression. *Most* of you, we believe, will find it easiest to move through the phases as outlined precisely because they are *not* arbitrary but, instead, are based on years of experience and on what has worked best for the majority of others. There are, however, always exceptions.

7

PHASE ONE OF THE NEW AMERICAN DIET: SUBSTITUTIONS

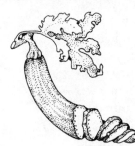

Keep Your Favorite Recipes —But Alter Them

Phase One. This is where you begin to cut back on the cholesterol, fat, salt and sugar in your diet. Substitutions are the key. Cold turkey is okay, if you're talking about the bird—which provides one of the lower-fat meat choices—but not if you're talking about the practical approach. If you tried to cut cholesterol, fat, salt and sugar entirely out of your diet, life would be pretty grim. Chances are you would throw in the towel in a week and return to your typical eating patterns. When we suggest that you eliminate a food or cut back on it, we give you something else to take

its place, usually something similar in taste or texture, but always something with *less* fat, salt and sugar. That is what substitutions are all about.

If you are like most of the individuals and families we counsel, you are probably eating whole eggs, typical high-fat cheeses and meats, salt, sugar, ice cream, butter, etc. on a frequent, daily basis. These foods have become habits with you; you like what you eat. But habits and "likes," as we've already seen, can be changed. You can get rid of or alter old habits and even acquire new ones.

The best way to begin is *not* by throwing out your favorite recipes. *Keep* those recipes, but *change* them so that the fat, salt and sugar contents are gradually reduced over time. A great many recipes can be modified in a variety of ways without drastically altering taste and texture. These gradual modifications will make it much easier for you and family members to change your old habits. As one homemaker in our Family Heart Study put it: "You've got to learn to be a little sneaky, especially in the beginning. You don't tell your teenage son, for example, that you made his favorite cookies *without* egg yolks—not until *after* he tells you how good they are."

Another key to success in Phase One is the *availability* of substitutes. Many of us would readily eat foods with less salt, fat and sugar if they were within easy reach. So if you buy or prepare food for yourself or your family, constantly be alert to the availability factor. Snacks are a particularly big problem here. If you are the person who prepares the meals at your home, you have more than average control over what your family eats. But while you may be quite successful in gradually introducing favorite recipes with lower fat, salt and sugar content, you may still have to contend with a lot of snacking on high-fat, high-salt, high-sugar foods. So, in this chapter, we'll provide you with some tasty, alternative snacks to have on hand to help ease the pangs of withdrawal.

Let's look now at some of the foods to start working on.

Eggs

"Oh, no, how can we live without eggs?" That was the anguished reaction—quite typical—of one woman whose husband announced they were to be part of our study to see to what extent "ordinary" families could decrease the fat content of their food. Eggs are "near and dear" to the hearts of many Americans. Well, we'll go along with the

"near" part of that. The very high cholesterol content of eggs can certainly get "near" the heart, as we've seen; unfortunately, this "nearness" is anything but "dear."

A single egg yolk, if medium-sized, contains 1 teaspoon of fat. Well, that's not so bad, you may be thinking, since that's the same amount of fat you'd get in 1 cup of 2 percent milk. True, but contained in that single egg yolk are 240 milligrams of cholesterol.

SOURCES OF CHOLESTEROL

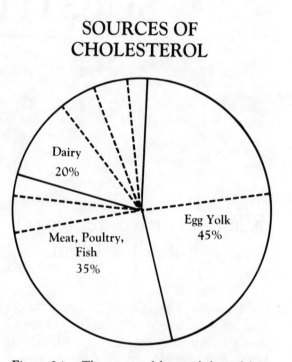

Figure 24. *The sources of dietary cholesterol for people in the United States. Forty-five percent of the dietary cholesterol is derived from egg yolk, with half of that being from visible eggs (2 to 3 eggs per week) and half from eggs used in food preparation (the broken line in the egg yolk segment). Thirty-five percent of the cholesterol is from red meats (28%), poultry (4½%) and fish (2½%). Twenty percent is from dairy products: 9 percent from milk, 5 percent from cheese, 4 percent from butter and 2 percent from ice cream.*

To help you understand how much egg yolk contributes to the typical daily intake of 400 to 500 milligrams of cholesterol, look at figure 24. You can see that 45 percent of dietary cholesterol comes from egg yolk. One-half of that is from visible eggs (two to three per week) and one-half is from invisible egg yolk in foods. So if you think it's okay to put one egg in a batch of pancakes because you only eat two of them, or that it's okay to put one egg in a cake because you only eat one piece and so forth, you are not getting an accurate picture. These little fractions of egg yolk add up to 90 to 113 milligrams of cholesterol each day. When one considers that the goal in Phase Three is to eat 100 milligrams of cholesterol a day, it becomes very clear why we suggest that egg yolk consumption be reduced.

Mercifully, Mother Nature didn't put *any* cholesterol in the whites of eggs. But you can see that just *two* egg yolks a day, *by themselves,* provide nearly 500 milligrams of cholesterol! Short of eating liver or brains, you'd be hard pressed to find a more potent source of cholesterol in your diet than eggs. So one of the most logical, initial substitutions is to *replace egg yolks with egg whites.* You'll be surprised at how successfully most recipes calling for egg yolks can be completed without them. When yolks are called for, use one and a half or two egg *whites* in place of each whole egg specified. This works well in cakes, cookies, pancakes, waffles, in potato salads, etc. You'll get additional ideas when you study the sample meal plans for Phase One later in this chapter —and when you use the many recipes provided in part 3.

There are egg substitutes, both homemade (see recipe section) and commercial, you'll want to be aware of, as well, If you do not like the idea of throwing away all those egg yolks, you might consider buying powdered egg whites. (And it may interest you to know that it is okay to feed the egg yolks you would otherwise discard to your dogs and cats, as they do not get atherosclerosis; unlike humans these natural carnivores excrete the cholesterol). Some commercial egg substitutes are Egg Beaters from Fleischmann's, a frozen product; Second Nature from Avoset Food Corporation, a refrigerated product; and Scramblers from Morning Star Farms, a frozen product. These consist almost entirely of egg whites, with a little fat added to emulsify them. You will find these products available in your local supermarket.

Butter

Butter is another obvious place to make substitutions. This food is loaded with both cholesterol and saturated fat. You can do yourself a big favor by switching to a *soft* margarine. Many people have already made this substitution. Use any tub or soft-stick margarine that suits your taste and budget. We stress *soft* because this ensures that the margarine is made from highly unsaturated fat. If the product gets very soft at room temperature, it is okay. If in doubt, check labels. Some margarines *do* contain animal fat and these should be avoided. A P/S value of 1.0 or greater is desirable, if you are checking labels. (This is the ratio of the amount of polyunsatured to saturated fat.)

By switching from butter to margarine, you'll be going a long way toward cutting the saturated fat and cholesterol content of your diet. One tablespoon of butter has 34 milligrams of cholesterol and 7.5 grams of saturated fat (CSI of 9.3). One tablespoon of typical soft margarine contains *no* cholesterol and only 2.4 grams of saturated fat (CSI of 2.4). Remember, the lower the CSI, the more desirable the food.

Of course, many people have a taste for butter, and some family members may rebel when you try to make the switch. Thus, once again, do not do a 100 percent switch if you fear resistance or are resisting yourself. The best place to start is to put soft margarine in the foods you prepare in place of butter, when the latter is called for in recipes. You may wish to add Butter Buds to keep the butter flavor. Butter Buds, a relatively new product, is widely available. It is essentially "butter" with the fat removed. It can be dissolved in oil, margarine and water and is used to give a butter flavor to foods without adding any fat. You can still put butter on the table if it is customarily found there in your home. You will still be moving distinctly ahead, and you can tackle the butter-on-the-table problem later on.

Another thing you may want to do if butter is really important to you is to use *small* amounts of butter in your recipes for a while, to help make the transition to margarine more palatable in your cooking. Butter used in this fashion thus becomes a *flavoring.* In other words, if 2 tablespoons of butter are called for in a given recipe, you could make 1 or 1½ of those margarine and the remainder butter. As time goes by, you can use more and more margarine, until you're using practically no butter at all. However, by using soft margarine and Butter Buds, we feel that you really should have no difficulty deleting butter from your cooking. Experiment with different brands of margarine, using those that become very soft at room temperature. Different oils and different processing can impart different

flavors. You'll find some you like better than others.

Shortening and Lard

This category is relatively easy. When lard or shortening is called for in a recipe, simply substitute vegetable oils or soft vegetable shortenings. It is generally difficult to tell from the labels, however, which shortenings are made from vegetable oils that have not been highly hydrogenated. Two that we can recommend are Crisco and Food Club. Again, if for some reason anyone notices that the food tastes different, which isn't too likely (though there *are* a few lard addicts, believe it or not, with very keen lard sensors), then do the same thing you did with butter. Use the lard in gradually reduced quantities as flavoring.

Many people are confused about which vegetable oils are the best. There really isn't very much difference among them, although olive oil and peanut oil are a little less unsaturated than soybean, corn, cottonseed, safflower and sunflower oils. Use these oils for special flavoring in salad dressings or for stir frying. Coconut oil and palm oil are vegetable in origin but they are very saturated and should *not* be used.

Peanut Butter

This is a product many Americans profess not to be able to live without. Peanut butter contains no cholesterol, but it *is* about half fat (as are all nuts). The fat in peanut butter is less saturated than animal fat, but if you eat a lot of it you'll still end up getting too much saturated fat. Some peanut butter lovers will need to cut back a little. Use it in a sandwich at lunch (in place of meat or cheese) but stop using it as a snack, except, perhaps, on infrequent occasions. See snack section, later in this chapter, for substitutes.

Some of you may have questions about the "natural" peanut butters versus those which have been partially hydrogenated (hardened). The typical "hydrogenated" peanut butters on the market really are not very hydrogenated and are still very unsaturated. They are okay to use. You may wish to base your selection not so much on this issue as on whether the peanut butter has salt and/or sugar added to it, as most brands do.

Mayonnaise and Miracle Whip

Mayonnaise and Miracle Whip are each a little better than *two-thirds* fat. Many people put 1, 2 or even more tablespoons of one of these into a single sandwich! That's a whopping dose of fat. Fortunately, this is one food you may be able to stop using in one fell swoop. If so, you will be way ahead. There are excellent substitutions available. These have far less fat, often as much as one-half less. So check labels and start using one of the imitation mayonnaises, Light n' Lively, Light Miracle Whip or light mayonnaise. Most people like the taste of these products, but if there's a problem, add a little of the real stuff to these in the beginning. You'll also want to try our Tangy Salad Dressing (recipe section). It's a combination of low-fat yogurt and one of the imitation or light mayonnaise products. It's great in potato and macaroni salads and even as a sandwich spread. It

should be pointed out that Tangy Salad Dressing is water-based instead of oil-based. So it will soak into pastas and potatoes. To avoid a dry product add the dressing just before serving.

Meats

As we've already explained, meats are major contributors of fat, saturated fat and cholesterol in the typical diet. In Phase One, you'll have enough to do without tackling meat head-on. But you can begin by not eating organ meats (liver, heart, brains, kidney, gizzards, all of which are extremely high in cholesterol). Fortunately, a lot of people don't like these anyway. You can also trim as much of the visible fat off meat as possible. Always remember to remove the skin and visible fat from chicken before cooking. A great deal of cholesterol is in the skin of the chicken and some fat is attached to the skin, as well. (See recipe section for ideas about cooking chicken with the skin removed.) This trimming of fat will help considerably, but be aware that there's still a lot of fat *inside* the strands of meat, fat of the "invisible" variety. So keep in mind that as time goes along you will ultimately want to alter your consumption of meat in other ways as well.

There are products designed specifically to replace meats in the diet. These meat substitutes are made of textured vegetable protein from soybeans. Some people like them, others do not. We do not put heavy emphasis on them. We feel the place for textured vegetable protein is to help decrease the cholesterol and saturated fat by using it to stretch red meat. (See for example, the Beef-and Mushroom Spaghetti Sauce recipe in part 3.)

Meat remains a part of our diet through *all*

three phases, but the amounts of meat are gradually reduced and the way in which meat is used is altered. We do not *insist* on meat, however, if you are vegetarian; see discussion on this topic in chapter 11.

If you are eating meat as a main course at many breakfasts and at nearly every lunch and dinner, you should begin to pay attention to this fact. The mere realization of how much meat is being eaten is often surprising to people. You may want to begin replacing some of the higher-fat meats with chicken and fish. (Look again at the CSI in table 3, pages 74–75, to compare the different meats.) In other words, eat leaner beef, pork and lamb, in particular; eat these meats less often; and eat chicken, turkey and fish more often.

Anywhere from a month to several months into Phase One you may want to try having meatless, cheeseless, eggless breakfasts and many such lunches, opting for cereals, fruits, soups, salads, breads, cottage cheese, bean burritos, etc., instead. Look again at "A Year of Changes" (fig. 22, pages 102–3) to see how some families have altered their meat intake over a period of time.

To replace the meat—and other fats— you'll really be cutting back on in Phase Two, you will concentrate on complex carbohydrates including legumes (beans) and whole grains. So, some months into Phase One, you may want to start serving larger portions of potatoes, for example, while simultaneously serving slightly smaller portions of meat. You can get more complex carbohydrates by eating breads, pasta, rice, tortillas, cereals, etc. We'll concentrate on this more heavily in Phase Two. But to whatever extent you can *begin* introducing more grains, beans, fruits and vegetables into your diet now, while reducing meat intake, the further ahead you will be.

And it is not too early to say a few words about hamburger, which, because of its great taste, is the most popular meat in the United States. Just as in the case of ice cream, there are hamburgers and there are hamburgers. There are the one-meat-patty variety and the three-meat-patty variety. There are those with lettuce and tomato and there are those with lettuce, tomato, cheese, mayonnaise and more cheese and more mayonnaise. If you're a hamburger lover, start moving toward the one-patty burger, and use imitation mayonnaise or other similar products. See our recommendations on cheese below, and work gradually toward using a leaner ground beef. The "regular" type is 30 percent fat. Gradually work toward buying ground chuck (20 percent fat), then ground round (15 percent fat), and finally ground sirloin (10 percent fat or less) or a mixture of these last two. The CSI of regular ground beef is more than twice as high as that of ground sirloin.

Cheese

Cheese is a challenge. But we're going to give you information that will help you find substitutes for high-fat cheese. Most people assume cheese is cheese, all about equally "good" or "bad" in terms of fat and cholesterol. Many people, we know from experience, have the vague feeling that they are eating too much cheese but feel powerless to do anything about it. Many of our patients and people who have participated in our studies tell of buying *pounds* of cheese at a time, consuming it in great quantities. The consumption of high-fat cheeses in this country and in the Western world in general is enormous.

The cheese problem is so big and formidable that we have devoted considerable time to it. We have found that if you make people aware of the risks involved in eating large amounts of cheese, they *want* to change their cheese-eating habits. And if you give them lower-fat, lower-cholesterol alternatives, they *will* change those habits—and quickly in many instances. (Review some of the case histories related earlier in this book.)

There *are* low-fat cheeses, and some of them are quite delicious. The CSI that we have developed is particularly useful in evaluating cheeses. Cheese used to be ranked by its overall fat content, and this worked out fairly well so long as most of the cheeses were made from butter fat. Now, however, there are many cheeses that are being made with skim milk and vegetable oils, especially soybean oil. These cheeses still contain considerable fat but much less saturated fat and very little cholesterol. So the CSI gives us a much better way of comparing cheeses.

Before we begin comparing different types of cheese, however, let us look at how cheese stacks up on the CSI with some other foods. In figure 25 you can see how one of the favor-

ite cheeses in the United States—Cheddar—compares with other "protein" foods. Most people are astonished to see that Cheddar cheese compares unfavorably with even beef or pork that has 25 percent fat.

Now let's turn to figure 26 to compare different types of cheeses, again using the CSI. It will be instantly apparent to you that cheeses are *not* all alike. You may not have heard yet of some of the lower-fat cheeses, but check your supermarket. Almost all of them now stock at least some of these lower-fat choices. You'll have to experiment with some of them to find which you and your family like best. Keep moving toward the lower-fat alternatives, but, again, move slowly, gradually.

If you use *cream cheese* in your cooking or at the table or in snacks, you should immediately try Neufchâtel. The CSI for the latter is lower, and Neufchâtel contains fewer calories. There is no difference in texture or taste. And for you Cheddar lovers, and we know your number is legion, there is no great substitute. Still, try switching to Olympia's Low Fat cheese or to regular Green River Part

CHOLESTEROL-SATURATED FAT INDEX
(3½ OUNCE PORTION)

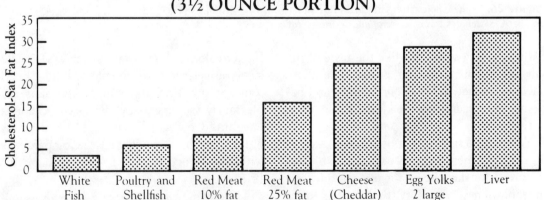

Figure 25. The Cholesterol-Saturated Fat Index (CSI) of 3½ ounces (100 grams) of selected foods compared with cheese (Cheddar). A smaller CSI denotes less cholesterol and saturated fat.

CHOLESTEROL-SATURATED FAT INDEX
OF SELECTED CHEESES (3½-OUNCE PORTION)

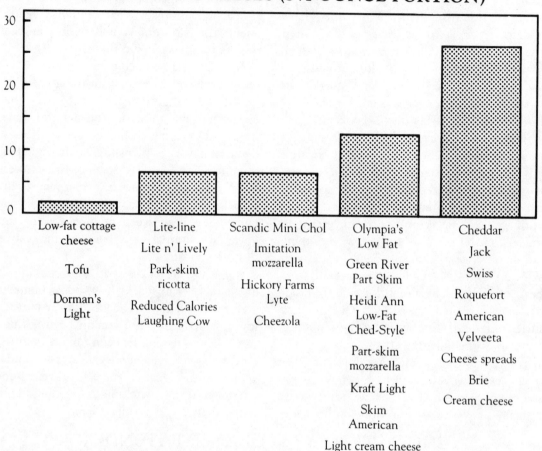

Figure 26. *The Cholesterol-Saturated Fat Index (CSI) of 3½ ounces (100 grams) of selected cheeses. A smaller CSI denotes less cholesterol and saturated fat.*

Skim Cheese (we do not like the taste of the salt-free product). Many people like these cheeses. In fact, most of our families and patients have been delighted with these alternatives.

You may be surprised at how easy it is to go all the way when it comes to picking an easy-to-spread low-fat cheese for use on crackers, in sandwiches, etc. Try Reduced Calories Laughing Cow which comes in wedges contained in a small round box. (There's a higher-calorie, higher-fat variety, so make sure you get the reduced calorie kind.) Even some of our Brie and Camembert fans are pleasantly surprised by Reduced Calories Laughing Cow which contains only 2 grams of fat in each ¾-ounce wedge. Compare this with the 10 or 11 you'll find in an ounce of Brie.

The cheese tips in figure 27 are the same that we give to our patients and others participating in our dietary studies.

CHEESE TIPS

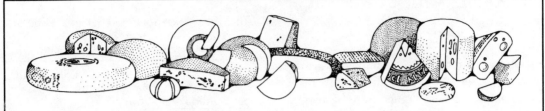

1. Cheddar cheese is the cheese of choice for most people. There are no very low-fat substitutes and there are no substitutes for sharp Cheddar cheese. However, there are somewhat lower-fat choices which make for perfectly good everyday fare—our favorites include (1) *Olympia's Low Fat Cheese*, (2) *Green River Part Skim Cheese* (we do not recommend the salt-free product), (3) *Kraft Light* and (4) *Heidi Ann Low-Fat Ched-Style.*

2. *Part-skim mozzarella* is a good cheese to use in place of Cheddar, Jack or Swiss.

3. *Imitation mozzarella* (made from skim milk and soybean oil) is an even better choice! Would you believe this is the cheese that most pizza places have used in Portland, Oregon, for the last five years? It comes already grated or in blocks.

4. *Scandic Mini Chol*—This cheese has the same total *fat* content as Cheddar and Jack but the fat is *soybean oil* so there is much less cholesterol and saturated fat. This is a white cheese which looks very much like Havarti. It melts beautifully! Look for it in the deli section of the supermarket.

5. *Lite-line* and *Lite n' Lively* are for those who now use cheese slices. We like the Cheddar flavor.

6. For Velveeta lovers, *Cheezola* is the choice. It is another cheese made from skim milk and vegetable oil (usually corn oil). It melts very nicely. This cheese is not widely available. You can order it from Fisher Cheese Company, Dietary Cheese Division, Box 12, Wapakoneta, Ohio 45895.

7. For those who are looking for a snack or a cheese to spread on bagels or low-fat crackers *Reduced Calories Laughing Cow* is a must. Our schoolchildren can trade it for anything so it must be good!

8. The *cream cheese* lovers need to know there is no reason ever to buy cream cheese again. Try *Light cream cheese* or *Neufchâtel*—you can't tell the difference. If you want to go even lower in fat try *part-skim ricotta* (not as smooth in texture but is more flavorful. We like it!). Mixed with herbs or fruits it makes a lovely spread for bagels, etc.

9. For cooking—mix a lower-fat cheese (*imitation mozzarella*) with higher-fat favorites to get the flavor but not the saturated fat and cholesterol.

10. *Low-fat cottage cheese* is an excellent choice for fillings, or can be whipped in the blender for a mock sour cream. *Tofu* (soybean curd) can also be used as a filling, especially when combined with herbs and seasonings.

11. *Parmesan* is a higher-fat cheese, but since it has a strong flavor it can be used in small amounts for flavoring (1 tsp. to 1 Tbsp. per serving).

12. *Brie, Camembert,* and double-cream *Havarti* are superfatted cheese that contain more than twice the fat of Cheddar—use these sparingly, if at all!

13. *For the label readers.* For everyday use consider buying cheeses that contain 6 grams of fat or less per ounce. Cheese made from skim milk and vegetable oil are okay for everyday use even though many contain 6–9 grams of fat per ounce (*Cheezola, Mini Chol, Hickory Farms Lyte*). A *really* low-fat cheese is one that contains 3 grams of fat or less per ounce.

Figure 27. Suggestions for selecting cheeses with lower Cholesterol–Saturated Fat Indexes (CSIs).

Cooking with Lower-Fat Cheeses

There is a tremendous advantage in learning to cook with lower-fat cheeses. In table 7, we have made a comparison of recipes using lower-fat cheeses with similar typical recipes that do not use the lower-fat options. You'll find all of our recipes (designated "lower fat") in the cookbook section (part 3) of this book. Once again, remember that the lower the CSI, the better the food or recipe is for you. Note also how the lower-fat options also provide far fewer calories per serving.

Milk

Do not worry, we are not going to ask you to give up milk. If you presently drink whole milk, try switching first to 2 percent milk. Begin using half-and-half and cream only on special occasions (less than once a month). The CSI for a cup of heavy cream is 73; the CSI for the same quantity of half-and-half is 23; whole milk, which has 3.5 to 4 percent fat content, has a CSI of 7 per cup (which means a CSI of 11 in the typical 12-ounce glass of whole milk). If you drink three glasses of whole milk per day that adds up to a CSI of 33 from milk alone, not counting any that gets used on cereal or in cooking!

This business of fat content in milk is tricky. Some cartons of milk proudly proclaim "3.5 percent fat" in large letters. The unwary consumer may interpret this to mean that there is really very little fat in the milk. After all, 3.5 percent doesn't sound like much. In fact, however, that's about the maximum you'll find in whole milk. Consider that 50 percent of the caloric content of 3.5 percent

TABLE 7
The Cholesterol-Saturated Fat Index (CSI) of Lower-Fat Recipes Compared to Similar Typical Recipes

	CSI	Calories
Super Stuffed Potato (lower-fat), 1 average	2	168
Stuffed potato (typical), 1 average	4	221
Mock Sour Cream (lower-fat), ¼ cup	1	54
Commercial sour cream (typical), ¼ cup	9	117
Ricotta Cheesecake (lower-fat), ½ of 9″ diameter	7	370
Cheesecake (typical), ½ of 9″ diameter	29	647
Cheese Stuffed Manicotti (lower-fat), 3 pieces	6	386
Cheese-stuffed manicotti (typical), 3 pieces	34	699
Spinach Lasagna (lower-fat), 1 (4″ x 4″)serving	8	476
Meatless lasagna (typical), same size	16	527
Lasagna with meat sauce (typical), same size	30	812
Party Carrot Cake (lower-fat), 1 piece (3″ x 3″ x 1″)	2	229
Carrot cake (typical), same size piece	12	539
Spicy Cheese Pizza (lower-fat), ⅜ of 14″ pizza	3	518
Vegetarian pizza (typical), same size	13	695
Pepperoni pizza (typical), same size	21	806
Macaroni Bake (lower-fat), 2 cups	3	427
Macaroni and cheese (typical), 2 cups	12	658

NOTE: Recipes that are underlined can be found in part 3.

milk is fat! And that, as you've just seen, can add up in a day to a lot of saturated fat and cholesterol. By the same token, milk labeled "2 percent fat" also still contains quite a bit of saturated fat and cholesterol, although it is a definite improvement over the 3.5 percent kind.

Almost everybody can easily go from whole milk to 2 percent milk. And people who stop using half-and-half on their cereal for just a few weeks find that it suddenly becomes cloying and much too rich for their taste when they go back and try it again.

Once you feel comfortable with 2 percent milk, give 1 percent a try. Or, if you want to go all out, try skim—which has only ¹⁄₁₀ *of 1 percent* fat in it. Skim milk has a CSI of less than 1 per 12-ounce glass. Don't feel you *have* to get to skim. You'll have made real progress if you get to 1 percent, and even 2 percent is a definite improvement over whole milk.

Buttermilk (without added butter chips or flakes) is another good alternative, particularly in cooking. One cup of buttermilk has a CSI of less than 2. The reason for this low CSI is that buttermilk is made from skim milk and a small amount of added butter fat, usually making it like 1 percent milk.

And what if a recipe flat out insists on cream? Don't be cowed. Try the Mocha Mix in place of cream and then gradually experiment, with other recipes calling for cream, with 2 percent and even 1 percent and skim milk. Many recipes work very well without cream. Be creative and use combinations of skim milk and small amounts of higher-fat choices to suit your tastes at the time. The goal is to think about what you are using every few months, at which time, if you feel you are ready, you can make further changes.

Beware of most commercial nondairy creamers. They are typically made with a very saturated vegetable fat—coconut oil. We've calculated the CSI of a typical store-brand nondairy coffee creamer at 1.4 per tablespoon, which is the same as 1 tablespoon of half-and-half. A tablespoon of Mocha Mix (a nondairy creamer made with soybean oil) and a tablespoon of 2 percent milk each have a CSI of 0.3. Even though 2 percent milk has the same CSI, because it is lower in total fat and calories, it is a better choice for a "creamer" for your coffee. So try to work your way to that.

Getting Adequate Calcium Using Lower-Fat Milk and Dairy Products

Some of the people we advise about dietary matters express concern about getting adequate calcium when changing to a way of eating that very significantly reduces the intake of whole milk and high-fat dairy products. Everybody needs adequate calcium, but it is especially important that *women* get adequate amounts after menopause, for too little calcium may be associated with osteoporosis, a condition in which the bones become thin and brittle and prone to fractures. This is a problem that afflicts women far more than men, in large part because of hormonal differences. Women become particularly prone to osteoporosis as they pass through menopause.

So the calcium question is not one to be taken lightly. The RDA (Recommended Daily Allowance) for calcium is 800 milligrams for both men and women. Calcium is not linked to the fat in milk and other dairy products; thus switching to low-fat dairy products will *not* diminish your calcium intake. You can get all of the calcium you need in 2⅔ cups of *skim* milk daily. If you don't like milk, however, you certainly should not start drinking it just to get calcium. There are many other ways to get it into your diet without drinking milk or taking calcium supplements. Figure 28 provides an example, followed by several *low-fat* calcium sources.

Note that the sample menu for one day in figure 28 provides 801 milligrams of calcium, even though it includes in the way of dairy products only a very small amount of low-fat buttermilk and yogurt. The meal plans for the three phases of the New American Diet you'll

---

MEETING YOUR RECOMMENDED DAILY ALLOWANCE FOR CALCIUM

Meeting your RDA for calcium is especially important if you are a woman past menopause. For an adult woman the recommended intake is 800 mg, for adult men it is also 800 mg.

Two and one-half cups of skim milk will fulfill your requirement, but if you are like many adults you don't drink much milk. You can still meet your recommended intake without supplements. Here's an example:

BREAKFAST:

Whole wheat toast	2 slices	40
Low-fat yogurt	½ cup	207
Berries	½ cup	20

LUNCH:

Romaine lettuce	1 cup	20
Garbanzo beans	¼ cup	45
Ranch Salad Dressing		
(with buttermilk)	2 Tbsp.	30
Whole wheat roll	1	34
Orange	1 medium	55

DINNER:

Meatless chili	1 cup	80
Corn muffins	2	100
Broccoli	1 cup	160
Pineapple	1 cup	10
TOTAL CALCIUM, mg		801

Low-Fat Calcium Sources

Milk Products		Calcium (mg)
Skim Milk, 1 cup		300
Nonfat dry milk, ¼ cup		200
Buttermilk, 1 cup		285
Yogurt, 2%, 1 cup		415
Cottage cheese, 1 cup		150
Ricotta cheese, ¼ cup		160
Parmesan cheese, 1 Tbsp.		75
Mozzarella cheese, 1 oz.		200
Pudding (with skim milk), ½ cup		150

Beans/Grains Products		
Tofu, 3½ oz.		130
Corn tortilla, 1 6″		40
Masa harina, ½ cup dry		70
Soybeans, ½ cup cooked		70
Garbanzo beans, ½ cup		90
Pinto, kidney, etc. beans, ½ cup		35
Muffin, corn bread, 1 average		50

Vegetables/Fruit		
Collard/mustard greens, ½ cup		100
Okra, ½ cup		60
Broccoli, ½ cup		80
Lettuce, 1 cup		20
Rutabagas, 1 cup		65
Green beans, 1 cup		50
Bean sprouts, 1 cup		30
Cabbage, 1 cup		50
Orange, 1 medium		55

Miscellaneous		
Dark molasses, 1 Tbsp.		60
Canned salmon, 3 oz. (with bones)		195
Clams, ½ cup		55
Egg substitute, ¼ cup		30

Figure 28. *Selected low-fat calcium sources and an example of how to obtain 800 milligrams (mg) of dietary calcium in a day.*

find later in this and subsequent chapters contain an average of 800 milligrams of calcium per day.

Ice Cream

Here's an emotional one. How we love our ice cream in this country. Conversations actually revolve around *which* ice cream is the best. People even fight over the issue. And they are willing to stand in long lines to get their favorite brand in cones, cups or large dishes.

It is true, certainly, that ice creams are *not* all alike. The sort of ice creams that create partisan fans to rival those at a Super Bowl game are almost always those with the highest saturated fat and cholesterol content. Unfortunately, almost *all* ice creams contain enough fat and cholesterol to provide, in a single serving, more than is recommended for the entire day. But the gourmet brand ice creams *really* pack a fat wallop. One cup of the typical, store-brand ice cream (10 percent fat content) has a CSI of 13, whereas 1 cup of the richer ice cream (16 percent fat) has a CSI of 18. And when you get into the specialty brands that people line up for, 1 cup has a CSI of about 34! Go back and review the CSI table on pages 74–75, and you'll further understand what a problem ice cream can pose.

We recommend ice cream be eaten on special occasions only, or else, if you don't want to change your ice cream intake, cut back more sharply on your cheese and meat for now. If you are an ice-cream lover, cut back gradually. There are some rich-tasting ice-cream products on the market that have very low CSIs. One of these, currently popular, is Tofutti, which is made from tofu, soy protein

and corn oil. This new product tends to compete with the gourmet ice creams in price but, for some people at least, it also competes favorably with them in terms of taste. Be aware, however, that this low-cholesterol substitute still has quite a bit of fat—and calories—in it. Nonetheless, you're ahead, cup for cup, if you consume Tofutti or some similar product instead of regular ice cream. Check your supermarket. And read the labels.

Other alternatives with very low CSIs are sorbets, low-fat frozen yogurt or sherbet. Some people mistakenly think sherbet is just another ice cream. But while a cup of regular ice cream will have a CSI anywhere from 13 to 34, a cup of sherbet has a remarkably low CSI of 2, as does low-fat frozen yogurt. Sorbets (water ices) have a CSI of 0! Good recipes for Strawberry Ice and Blueberry Ice can be found in part 3.

Sour Cream

A lot of people have the notion that if cream is sour it's good for you. As a matter of fact, 1 cup of sour cream has a CSI of 37, whereas whipping cream, in the same quantity, has a bloodcurdling CSI of 73. However, the whipping cream is 38 percent fat, while the sour cream is made from a 20-percent-fat cream. This still does not mean, of course, that you should eat sour cream with impunity. It, too, has a very high CSI compared with other foods. Eventually, you should stop using sour cream. This includes IMO and other nondairy sour creams. These are made with coconut oil, and 1 cup has a CSI of 43.

Start out by gradually replacing the sour cream called for in recipes with our Mock Sour Cream (recipe in part 3). A cup of this has a CSI of only 4 compared with a CSI of 37 for the real sour cream. Some find yogurt ideal, and it is an excellent choice—provided you use the low-fat or nonfat varieties. Low-fat cottage cheese may prove to be a satisfactory substitute for you.

Snacks

Yes, it *is* possible to snack in a low-fat fashion. Snacking is something most of us will never stop doing, so we might as well not waste time pretending otherwise. A far more productive use of our time will be in developing an assortment of snacks that are low in fat and, when possible, higher in complex carbohydrates.

It's very important to have good snack items on hand. Tasty low-fat snack alternatives can make all the difference during the early, transition phases from a high-fat to a

lower-fat way of eating. Having some of the snacks we suggest below on hand at all times will make it far easier to resist eating a candy bar or having a dish of ice cream, a doughnut or a cheese Danish.

Among the most popular low-fat snacks to have on hand are homemade muffins, Baked Corn Chips and Pita Chips (see recipes in part 3). Always have a variety of fruits and vegetables in the house. Even teenagers can be tempted by these if they are already cleaned and cut and readily available to nibble on. But if it comes down to having to dig a carrot out of the produce bin, wash and scrape it and possibly cut it, or just reach for a Twinkie, the latter is most likely going to win. Vegetables can be made particularly tempting by having an enticing dip on hand to go along with them. (You'll find recipes for various dips in the recipe section, too, including those made with Mock Sour Cream and herbs, yogurt, salsa, bean dip). And do not become fixated on carrots and celery. Those are fine, but you should also try broccoli flowers, zucchini, green pepper rings, cauliflower, raw pea pods and so on.

Unbuttered, unsalted, air-popped popcorn (a little margarine on it is okay) is another snack favorite with many of our families. If you want to add some salt, go ahead, but use a tiny amount of Lite Salt or one of the reduced sodium flavored salts. (See salt discussion later in this chapter.)

Typical snack substitutions are shown in table 8.

Figure 29 shows a more complete list of snack items that meet the New American Diet goals. Recipes for italicized items can be found in part 3.

If you feel the need for a really substantial snack at some point, concentrate on beans. Keep some tortillas or pita (pocket) bread

TABLE 8
Typical Snack Substitutes

Instead Of	Substitute
A doughnut	A raisin-cinnamon bagel or favorite muffin
Ice cream	Low-fat frozen yogurt
Oreos, chocolate chip, and other high-fat cookies	Gingersnaps, graham crackers or fig bars
Commercial chips, nuts, Cheetos	Unbuttered popcorn, *Pita Chips, Baked Corn Chips,** pretzels
Cheddar, Swiss cheese	Reduced Calories Laughing Cow cheese
High-fat crackers like Triscuits, Wheat Thins	Low-fat crackers like ak-mak, RyKrisp, any soda crackers, bread sticks

* Recipes in part 3.

SNACKS FOR THE NEW AMERICAN DIET

FRUIT
Fresh, any
Baked Apple
Fruit salad
Fruit leather

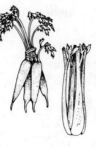

VEGETABLES
Fresh or frozen—any
Super Stuffed Potatoes
Baked yams
Skinny "French Fries"

LOW-FAT COOKIES
Fig bars
Ginger snaps
Graham crackers
Low-Fat Cookies (recipes in part 3)

LOWER-FAT CRACKERS, CHIPS, etc.
ak-mak
Armenian cracker bread
Bremner
Cracottes
Cracklebred
Baked Corn Chips
  (with *Bean Dip* or other dips)
"Gorp" (any combination of Puffed Wheat, rai-
sins, popcorn, pretzels, Wheat or Corn Chex)
Matzoh
Melba toast
Pita Chips
Popcorn, air-popped
Pretzels, unsalted
Rice cakes
RyKrisp
Soda crackers w/unsalted tops

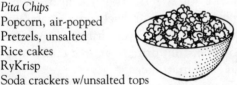

DAIRY PRODUCTS
Lite Ice Milk
Lower-fat cheeses
  Reduced Calories Laughing Cow
  Ricotta cheese
  Low-fat cottage cheese
Low-fat yogurts
Sherbet
Sorbet, water ices

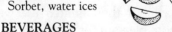

BEVERAGES
Bull Run cocktail (water with lemon juice)
Herbal teas

Hot cocoa (w/skim milk)
Skim milk
Strawberry-Banana Smoothie

BREADS
Bagels
Corn bread
Crumpets
English muffins
French
Italian
Pita bread (pocket bread)
Pumpernickel bread
Raisin bread
Rye
Scandinavian flat breads
Sour dough breads
Tortillas
Whole wheat breads

DIPS, SPREADS
Bean Dip w/Baked Corn Chips
Dill Dip w/fresh vegetables
Hummous w/pita bread
Popeye Spinach Dip w/vegetables, ak-mak or bread
  sticks
Fruit-Nut Sandwich Spread on bagel, English muf-
  fin or graham cracker
Reduced Calories Laughing Cow cheese on bagel,
  or low-fat crackers or any bread
Toast and jam, jelly or honey

CEREALS (with skim milk)
All-Bran
Cheerios
Cornflakes
Grape-Nuts
Puffed Rice, Corn, Wheat
Raisin Bran
Rice Krispies
Shredded Wheat

COMBINATION FOODS
Bean salad
Chili Bean Salad
Egg Salad Sandwich Spread on toast
Lentil Salad
Tabouli
Leftover soups, etc.

Figure 29. *Suggestions for snacks that meet the New American Diet goals.*

121

around and fill it up with beans and salsa or some other low-fat filling, such as Chili Bean Salad, Chowchow or Popeye's Spinach Dip (see recipes, part 3). Keep cans of vegetarian refried or baked beans around for these "heavy" snack moods. You can also make a quick burrito from refried beans and a tortilla.

Chocolate/Sugar/Desserts

We have already dealt with ice cream. Chocolate deserves separate mention as well, since most people dearly love it. Chocolate is the essence of a gourmet dessert or snack. Typical 1½-ounce chocolate candy bars have CSIs of 5 to 8. Some people like to substitute carob for chocolate. A 6-ounce package of carob chips has a CSI of 5 compared with 36 in the same size package of chocolate chips. Our Carob Cookies recipe, which uses carob flour, is very low in fat. When it comes to cooking, cocoa, chocolate extract and Hershey chocolate syrup are better choices than chocolate itself because some of the fat has been removed. If chocolate is really important, in order to indulge occasionally you will want to eat less meat, cheese and high-fat dairy products.

In general, you should aim to cut back on your sugar intake considerably. Sugar, as discussed in chapter 4, provides a lot of calories and very little else. But we appreciate that humans (and bears) will always want to eat some sugar.

Most Americans currently get 20 percent of all their calories from sugar. The typical American now consumes about 100 pounds of sugar a year. Almost all of us could benefit from cutting our sugar intake at least in half. Start working toward that goal by cutting back on the amount of sugar you add to reci-

pes. Work toward a gradual reduction to one-half the amount called for in recipes. If you do this a little at a time nobody will notice the difference. Go as far with each step-by-step reduction as you and your family feel like. Get used to that level and then move on to an even lower level of sugar consumption. Develop the art of *sprinkling* instead of *pouring* sugar. Eventually, you will want to take the sugar bowl off the table.

As we stated in chapter 4, typical Americans are now consuming 20–30 teaspoons of sugar a day. To meet the New American Diet Phase Three goal of 10 percent calories or less from sugar will mean cutting this intake to no more than 14 teaspoons of sugar daily for men and teens and to no more than 10 teaspoons per day for women and younger children. Remember, too, that most of these teaspoons are "hidden" in foods as they come served to you—not added by you. You will want to stage your sugar attack on all fronts. Start eating more fresh fruit and work toward three pieces per day. This will help satisfy your craving for sweets. You will also make real progress if you cut back on the amount of "sweetened" water you drink, in the form of soda pop, fruit drinks, sugared coffee and tea and even fruit juice.

Review the sugar section of chapter 4 for further information on the different types of sugar and the amounts of sugar hidden in different foods, some of which you might never suspect of having a high sugar content. Figure 30 will give you some examples of the amounts of sugar in a variety of foods.

As for sugar substitutes, we feel they are not necessary. But if their limited use will make eating more pleasant for you as you decrease the amount of sugar you eat, then go ahead and use them. But do keep their use to a minimum.

When it comes to desserts, sugar is not the only thing you have to watch out for. Many desserts are loaded with fat, as well. If you usually have dessert with every lunch and dinner, by all means start trying to cut back to once a day. And if you are at the once-a-day level to begin with, try holding the desserts to three or four times a week, or every other day, to begin with. Eat fruit instead of the higher-fat desserts. Or try low-fat or nonfat yogurt with fruit in it. And when you make your own desserts, use recipes that call for no more than ¼ to ½ cup of fat (and then use only vegetable oil, margarine or soft vegetable shortening). You'll find our dessert recipes in part 3. Another tip is to serve desserts when you have fish or meatless main dishes for dinner.

HOW MUCH SUGAR DO YOU EAT?

Americans eat a considerable amount of sugar and other sweeteners such as corn syrup and honey. Average intake is between 20 and 30 teaspoons a day! That's equal to 400–600 empty calories daily. No wonder we recommend cutting down. Meeting the New American Diet goal of 10 percent of calories or less as sugar means for men and teens no more than 14 teaspoons of sugar daily and for women and younger children no more than 10 teaspoons. Use the chart below as your guide to sugar content of foods.

Food and Amount	Teaspoons of Sugar
Candy bar, 2 oz.	6
Life Savers, 3 regular	1
Cake, 2 layer with icing, ¹⁄₁₂ of cake	12–15
Apple pie, ⅙ of 9″ pie	6
Berry, cherry, rhubarb pie, ⅙ of 9″ pie	10–12
Lemon meringue pie, ⅙ of 9″ pie	15
Cookie, 1	1–2
Sweet roll or iced doughnut, 1 ave.	4–7
Muffin, 1 regular	1–2
Ice cream, ½ cup	3–6
Yogurt, sweetened, 8 oz.	6
Soft drink, Kool-Ade, Tang, 12 oz.	7–8
Syrup, jam, jelly, 1 Tbsp.	3
Ketchup, sweet pickle relish, salad dressing, 1 Tbsp.	1

Figure 30. *The sugar content, in teaspoons, of selected foods.*

Salt

Reduction of salt intake begins in Phase One. A high salt (sodium) intake, very common in the Western world, is implicated in the development and aggravation of high blood pressure. (Too little potassium also contributes to this.) We recommend that you first decrease the use of salt at the table. The easiest way to do this is to switch from regular salt to Lite Salt which is available in most grocery stores. Lite Salt is a fifty-fifty mixture of sodium chloride and potassium chloride. Regular salt is entirely made of sodium chloride. By switching to Lite Salt you'll reduce the sodium content of table salt by one-half while also increasing your potassium intake, both of which are desirable.

You also will want to get into the habit of tasting food *before* you add salt to it. Many people reach for the salt shaker the moment food is placed before them, adding salt to already salted foods. Taste first and *then,* if the food tastes very flat, sprinkle on a *little* Lite Salt, taste again, etc. Some people find it works best to not even put the salt shaker on the table. Then, if you really want salt, go get it. After a few weeks or maybe a few months you will suddenly realize that you are no longer making the trip to the cupboard for the salt shaker. You will be surprised how quickly foods that once did not seem salty enough soon seem *too* salty. After a few weeks of a low-salt intake, many people are appalled at how salty some foods that used to seem just right actually are.

After you have succeeded in cutting back on salt at the table, you can begin paying attention to the amount of salt you're using in your *cooking.* You can begin cutting back here, too, gradually aiming at using about half the salt called for in recipes. We will put still more emphasis on salt reduction in Phase Two.

Beverages

The beverage of choice is water. Always serve water at family meals, not just on special occasions. The addition of lemon slices is nice. Begin to cut back on the amount of sweetened water you drink in the form of soda pop, fruit drinks, sugared coffee and tea and even fruit juice. Make cocoa (hot chocolate) using low-fat milk and preferably skim milk. Common sense tells us that we should not drink caffeinated beverages in unlimited quantities. It is a matter of personal choice whether you choose to drink 3 cups or less of decaffeinated or regular coffee or tea per day or drink none. Alcohol should not be an everyday thing. Always offer nonalcoholic choices. We particularly like sparkling apple cider and grape juice. Consider diluting wine, soda pop or fruit juice with salt-free sparkling (soda) water. One such product is Canada Dry Seltzer.

Sample Phase One Meal Plans

The meals in table 9 on pages 126–28, covering a full week, will show you what Phase One of the New American Diet will look like —on the table—once you've essentially achieved the goals of this phase. This is the *end point* of Phase One, not the beginning point. This is the *sort* of pattern you will be working toward in this opening phase.

Review of Goals and Results of Phase One

The meals outlined above—a *sample* of Phase One eating—achieve the basic goals of this part of the diet program:

1. Cholesterol intake is reduced, on average, from 400 to 500 milligrams per day to 300 to 350 milligrams.

2. Fat content of the diet decreases from 40 percent of calories to 35 percent, with much of the reduction in the form of saturated fats.

3. Carbohydrates assume a greater role in the diet, replacing some of the fats. There is a 5 percent increase in calories derived from carbohydrates, especially complex carbohydrates, in Phase One.

In addition, sodium intake is reduced by about 15 percent and potassium intake is increased by about 7 percent, on average, in Phase One.

It is not possible to predict the precise amount by which *blood* levels of cholesterol will be lowered in each individual case as a result of following Phase One of the diet. But, *on average,* there is an expected lowering of up to 6 percent. This means if you have a blood cholesterol level of 260 milligrams in 100 milliliters of blood, it could get as low as 244. It has recently been estimated that for each 1 percent reduction in cholesterol the coronary heart disease risk is decreased by 2 percent. Thus, a 6 percent reduction in blood cholesterol could mean a 12 percent reduction in the risk of coronary heart disease—a significant impact.

How to Tell When You're There

You can help judge your progress toward achievement of Phase One goals by retaking the quiz found on pages 41–51. The following scores correspond with Phase One goals:

MEAT, FISH AND POULTRY

Question 1	2
Question 2	2
Question 3	20 to 21
Question 4	2 (Men/Teens); 3 (Women/Children)
Question 5	2 to 3
Total score	28 to 31

DAIRY PRODUCTS AND EGGS

Question 1	4
Question 2	4
Question 3	3
Question 4	2
Question 5	3
Question 6	4 to 5
Question 7	3 to 5
Total score	23 to 26

FATS AND OILS

Question 1	3 to 4
Question 2	2 (Men/Teens); 3 (Women/Children)
Question 3	3
Question 4	2
Question 5	3 to 4
Total score	13 to 16

GRAINS, BEANS, FRUITS AND VEGETABLES

	Men/Teens	Women/Children
Question 1	15 to 18	10 to 11
Question 2	8 to 12	5 to 8
Question 3	10 to 15	3 to 7
Question 4	5 to 9	3 to 7
Question 5	25 to 30	20 to 25
Question 6	7	4
Question 7	0	0
Total score	70 to 91	45 to 62

SWEETS AND SNACKS

Question 1	3
Question 2	3
Question 3	3
Question 4	3
Question 5	3
Question 6	3
Total Score	18

SALT

Question 1	3
Question 2	4
Question 3	2 to 4
Question 4	3
Question 5	2
Total score	14 to 16

TABLE 9
New American Diet Phase One Meal Plans

	DAY 1	DAY 2	DAY 3	DAY 4	DAY 5	DAY 6	DAY 7
Breakfast	Orange juice, ¾ cup Wheaties, 1 cup Sugar, 1 tsp. 2% milk, ¾ cup Rye toast, 1 slice Soft margarine, 1 tsp.	Pink grapefruit, ½ *Breakfast Volcanos,* 1 svg. with *Mock Hollandaise Sauce,* ¼ cup	Orange juice, ¾ cup Cornflakes, 1 cup 2% milk, 1 cup Sugar, 1 tsp. Whole wheat toast, 1 slice Peanut butter, 1 Tbsp.	Apple juice, ½ cup *Oatmeal Buttermilk Pancakes,* 3 4" Syrup, ¼ cup Soft margarine, 2 tsp.	Grape juice, ½ cup Oatmeal, ½ cup with raisins, ½ Tbsp. 2% milk, ½ cup Blueberry muffin Soft margarine, 1 tsp.	Waffle, with fresh strawberries, ¾ cup Soft margarine, 2 tsp. Syrup, ¼ cup	Breakfast Out: Orange juice, ¾ cup French toast, 2 pieces Syrup, ¼ cup Soft margarine, 2 tsp.
Morning Snack			Bran muffin Soft margarine, 1 tsp.				
Lunch	Tostada: Corn tortilla (fried), 1–6" *Refried Beans,* ¼ cup Ground beef (20% fat), 1 oz. Low-fat cheese, 1½ oz. Lettuce, ¼ cup Chopped tomato, 1 Tbsp. Brownie Apple	In a restaurant: Calzone with mozzarella cheese and Ground beef Lettuce salad, 1 cup French dressing, 2 Tbsp.	Sandwich: Whole wheat bread, 2 slices *Tuna Salad Sandwich Spread,* ⅓ cup Imitation mayonnaise, 2 tsp. Lettuce leaf Carrot sticks Apple Gingersnaps, 3	Chili with beef and beans, 1 cup *Corn Bread,* 1 piece (3" x 3") Soft margarine, 2 tsp. Orange	Hot Dog: Bun Turkey wiener mustard, 2 tsp. Coleslaw, ¾ cup Low-fat fruited yogurt, 6 oz.	Chunky-style vegetable soup, 1½ cups Grilled cheese sandwich: Whole wheat bread, 2 slices Soft margarine, 2 tsp. Cheddar cheese, 1 oz. Lettuce salad, 1 cup Low-cal Italian dressing, 3 Tbsp. Fresh pear	*French Onion Soup,* 1 cup *Chicken Salad with Yogurt-Chive Dressing,* 1 svg.
Afternoon Snack					Soda crackers (unsalted top), 6 Peanut Butter, 2 Tbsp.		

NOTE: Recipes that are in italics can be found in part 3.

TABLE 9—Continued

	DAY 1	DAY 2	DAY 3	DAY 4	DAY 5	DAY 6	DAY 7
Dinner	Portland Fried Chicken, 1½ svg. Corn on the cob, 1 piece Soft margarine, 2 tsp. Tomato, sliced Potato salad, ½ cup Gelatin fruit salad, 1 cup	Veggie quiche ⅙ of 9" pie with no egg yolk and typical crust Sunshine Spinach Salad, 2 cups French bread, 2 pieces (4" diameter) Soft margarine, 2 tsp.	Baked ham, 3 oz. Scalloped Potatoes, 1 svg. Steamed broccoli, ¾ cup with Soft margarine, 1 tsp.	Spaghetti, 1 cup with Marinara Sauce, 1 cup and Ground beef (15% fat), 4 oz. Lettuce salad, 1 cup Low-cal French dressing, 3 Tbsp. French bread, 1 piece (4" diameter) Soft margarine, 2 tsp. Rainbow sherbet, ¾ cup	Special Dinner: Stuffed Flank Steak Florentine, 1 svg. Fluffy white rice, ¾ cup Steamed broccoli, ½ cup, with Soft margarine, 1 tsp. Caraway Dinner Roll Soft margarine, 1 tsp. All Season Shortcake with Strawberries and Yogurt, 1 svg.	Roast Turkey (no skin), 5 oz. Mashed Potatoes, ¾ cup Turkey Gravy, ⅓ cup French-cut green beans, ¾ cup, with Slivered almonds, 1 Tbsp. Homemade biscuits, 2 Strawberry jam, 2 tsp. Apple Loaf Cake, 1 svg.	Lasagna, 3" x 3" (made with 20% fat ground beef, mozzarella and cottage cheeses) Lettuce salad, 1 cup Low-cal French dressing, 3 Tbsp. Sourdough roll, 1 large, with Soft margarine, 2 tsp. Fruit Salad Alaska, 1 svg.
Evening Snack		Vanilla ice milk, ½ cup Oatmeal cookies, 2	Popcorn (air-popped), 2 cups with Soft margarine, 2 tsp. Lemonade or soda pop, 12 oz.				

TABLE 9—Continued

Nutrient Composition	DAY 1	DAY 2	DAY 3	DAY 4	DAY 5	DAY 6	DAY 7	Average	Phase One Goal
Calories	1890	2000	1794	2117	2180	2103	2005	2013	2000*
Protein, % Calories	20	18	17	14	17	16	17	17	15
Fat, % Calories	31	34	28	32	30	32	32	31	35
Carbohydrate, % Calories	49	49	55	54	53	52	51	52	50
Saturated Fat, % Calories	9.2	8.1	7.6	9.8	8.0	7.9	7.2	8.3	10
Polyunsaturated Fat, % Calories	5.0	7.9	9.4	5.4	8.1	8.9	6.3	7.3	8.0
Cholesterol, mg†	258	111	166	155	187	219	320	202	<300‡
CSI	32	24	24	31	29	30	32	29	37
Sodium, mg	2347	3173	2063	2961	2463	3684	2506	2742	2875
Potassium, mg	2889	1767	3121	2282	2785	2438	2212	2499	2535
Calcium, mg	753	1113	850	551	1240	752	697	851	800

* This is a food pattern for people who require 2000 Calories to maintain their weight.
† Mg = milligram.
‡ < = less than.

8

PHASE TWO OF THE NEW AMERICAN DIET: NEW RECIPES

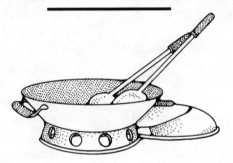

More Bread, Less Meat, Good Grief, What to Eat?

In Phase Two, we continue to cut the fat and reduce meat and cheese intake, but now, instead of just modifying existing recipes—old favorites—we add *new* recipes. In Phase Two, you literally spice up your daily fare by introducing foods from different cultures that taste delicious but are low in cholesterol and high in fiber and other complex carbohydrates. From the Orient come dishes that emphasize fresh vegetables and rice products; from Mexico comes a cuisine that uses tortillas, peppers and beans; from the Mediterranean countries we derive recipes that incorporate pastas and vegetable sauces; and from the Middle Eastern countries we've de-

veloped recipes that employ a variety of wheat products and legume dishes.

Meat is not out, by any means, but in Phase Two we aim to gradually reduce the typical American intake from around a pound or so of meat per day to no more than 6 to 8 ounces per day. Emphasis is placed on lean, well-trimmed meat in order to reduce further the saturated fat content of your diet. The fatter meats, such as bacon, sausage, spareribs, steaks, lunch meats, wieners, etc., should now be used only on rare occasions. The *ultimate* aim of Phase Two is to use meat or regular cheese *no more than once a day.* Work toward eating chicken or fish as the main meal entrée three to five times per week.

Another major goal of Phase Two is modification of the traditional sandwich. By "traditional," we're referring to meat, cheese, butter, mayonnaise, etc. A sandwich does not cease to be a sandwich when you drastically reduce or remove these items. We'll provide you with some instructive and tasty examples of what we mean by a Phase Two sandwich later on in this chapter.

The effort to cut down on fat continues on all fronts in this phase. We'll reemphasize some of the points made in the preceding chapter and add new ones to help you cut back, in particular, on saturated fat and cholesterol.

As we move away from main meals that focus on meat and high-fat dairy products, you will want to acquire, as indicated above, new recipes to replace those which cannot be altered easily to meet Phase Two goals. To replace some of these foods, we will be encouraging the use of recipes that contain larger amounts of grains, legumes, vegetables and fruits.

When you look at our sample meal plans for Phase Two, you will see that we avoid frying foods the way you learned to because this uses too much fat. We have developed the art of "skinny frying" and, as will be obvious when you get to the cookbook section, part 3, we emphasize broiling, baking, steaming, braising and microwaving.

Recipe Modification Continued—Phase Two

Before we proceed to specific guidelines on meats, sandwiches and new recipes, let's expand a bit on what we learned in the preceding chapter—in terms of altering standard recipes so that they contain less fat, salt and sugar. There's almost always room for more

changes. The following section will tell you what to do if you want to alter recipes that do not meet New American Diet goals.

WHAT TO DO IF . . .

The recipe is too high in FAT—
A recipe is too high in fat if it contains more than 1 teaspoon of fat per serving or more than ¼ to ½ cup of fat per recipe. We have successfully reduced the fat in quick breads which had large amounts of fat, but ideally one would choose recipes that contain ½ cup fat or less to start with. The first step is to reduce the fat by one-half and see how you like the finished product. When you decrease the fat in a recipe, you also may need to replace the fat with some liquid such as water, fruit juice or skim milk.

The recipe directions say "sauté"—
Use no more than 1 tablespoon of oil in your skillet.
Use a nonstick pan or a nonstick spray on the skillet.
Steam-cook vegetables or cook in microwave without adding fat.

The recipe calls for whole eggs or egg yolks—
Use one and a half or two egg whites for each whole egg.
Use one egg white and 1 tablespoon egg substitute for each egg.
Use an egg substitute according to package directions.

The recipe calls for butter or lard—
Use a vegetable margarine (soft stick or tub) or a vegetable oil.

The recipe calls for whole milk or cream—
Use canned evaporated skim milk or skim milk.

The recipe calls for creamed soups (chicken, mushroom or celery)—
Use ½ can soup and ½ can skim milk.
Use Homemade "Cream" Soup Mix (It is handiest if prepared ahead and is ready to use. Recipe is in part 3.)

The recipe calls for sour cream—
Substitute low-fat plain yogurt for sour cream in food which is to be heated. (Mix in 1 tablespoon flour for each cup yogurt to avoid separation.) Use Mock Sour Cream (see part 3) for baked potatoes or plain low-fat yogurt with chopped green onions or chives as toppers.

The recipe or meal calls for a high-fat cheese—
Use half the amount of cheese called for.
Substitute a lower-fat cheese (Green River Part Skim, Olympia's Low Fat, part-skim mozzarella).
Try low-fat cottage cheese as a replacement for half the cheese called for in casseroles.

The recipe calls for nuts—
Nuts are almost one-half fat; use them sparingly to add crunch to casseroles and baked products (no more than ¼ to ½ cup per recipe).

The recipe calls for mayonnaise—
Use half the amount or less.
Use low-fat plain yogurt.
Try Tangy Salad Dressing (recipe in part 3).
Use imitation or light mayonnaise or Miracle Whip Light (they have half the fat content).

The recipe calls for salt—
Use half the amount or less.
Use Lite Salt (it has half the sodium).

Use Mrs. Dash (no-sodium dried vegetables and spices which can be used in place of salt as seasoning).

The recipe calls for bouillon or chicken broth—
Dilute the broth (½ water and ½ broth).
Use ½ bouillon cube or half the crystals.

Start paying attention to labels in the supermarket. There are a lot of products now that are unsalted. Look for unsalted canned whole tomatoes and unsalted tomato sauce. If they taste flat to you, remember that you can add Lite Salt to the same level of saltiness as the regular product and only have half the sodium. Compare the sodium content in the dishes in table 10. The recipes can be found in part 3. Obviously you're going to be better off making these with the no salt added

TABLE 10
Comparison of the Sodium Content of Recipes Made with Regular Products and with "No Salt Added" Products

	Regular Canned Tomatoes and/or Tomato Sauce	No Salt Added Canned Tomatoes and/or Tomato Sauce
Marinara Sauce, 1 cup	1056 mg*	41 mg
Eggplant Parmesan, ⅙ recipe	652 mg	146 mg
Hearty Fish Soup, 1 cup	324 mg	117 mg
Rick's Chili, 1 cup	334 mg	189 mg
Country Captain, ¼ recipe	427 mg	65 mg

* Amounts are expressed as milligrams (mg) of sodium.

canned products rather than with the regular canned tomatoes and tomato sauce.

Other products you will find helpful in cutting back on salt (sodium)—
Milder or Lite Soy Sauce from Kikkoman.
Low-salt canned soups.
Unsalted spaghetti sauce from Prego.
Salt-reduced canned tuna (it is packed in water and so is lower is fat).
Salt-free breakfast cereals (Shredded Wheat, Puffed Wheat and Puffed Rice).
Low-salt breakfast cereals (Kellogg's Low Sodium Rice Krispies and Low-Sodium Corn Flakes).
No salt added canned vegetables (now widely available).
Seasonings that contain 75 percent less salt (lemon pepper, garlic salt, chicken seasoning, onion salt and seasoned salt).

Lower-salt and unsalted potato chips (they are *not* lower in fat).

You will find the sodium content of all of the recipes we provide in the nutrient analysis of recipes in the Appendix of this book. By following the guidelines outlined in this section you can meet the Phase Two goal for sodium: *2300 milligrams for women* and 2875 milligrams for men. That is equivalent to 1¼ to 1½ teaspoons of salt for an entire day, counting what is naturally in food as well as what is used in cooking. By now you will *not* be adding salt to foods at the table.

Below are two typical examples of recipe modification in which much of the fat, cholesterol and sodium contents have been reduced. Yet both of these modified recipes are among those we serve to guests. See part 3 for the recipe directions.

Apple Loaf Cake
1 cup oil — (Use ½ cup oil and ½ cup apple juice *or* water)
2 cups sugar
2 eggs — (Use 3 whites or ½ cup egg substitute)
1 teaspoon vanilla
3 cups chopped apples — (Use unpeeled apples)
½ cup chopped nuts — (Use ¼ cup)
3 cups flour — (Use 2 cups white flour and 1 cup whole wheat flour)

¾ teaspoon nutmeg
¾ teaspoon cinnamon
1½ teaspoons baking soda
1 teaspoon salt — (Omit salt)
Whipped topping — (Serve with no topping)

This cake makes 24 servings and, with these changes, each serving contains only 1 teaspoon of fat. The entire cake contains 1400 fewer calories also!

Acapulco Enchiladas
  12 corn tortillas
  3 cups diced, cooked chicken or turkey   (Use white meat)
  ½ cup sliced black olives   (Use ¼ cup)
  ⅓ cup slivered almonds   (Use 2 tablespoons)
  2 cups canned enchilada sauce (mild)
  1 can (8 ounces) tomato sauce   (Use unsalted tomato sauce)
  2 cups sour cream   (Use 2 cups Mock Sour Cream *or* 2 cups
                                                  plain low-fat yogurt
  ¼ cup chopped green onions   (Use ½ cup grated imitation mozzarella
  ¾ cup grated Cheddar cheese   cheese)

Review the preceding chapter to make sure that you have made the major recommended low-fat, low-cholesterol, low-sugar, low-salt substitutions. Then proceed to the following sections where we examine various of the major food groups again, with new recommendations.

Meats and Cheeses

In Phase One, the goals were to trim the fat off meat, to use more fish and poultry and to work toward using lower-fat ground beef. In Phase Two, the primary goal is to eat fish, poultry, meat and cheese no *more than once a day* and to limit the total amount to *no more than 6 to 8 ounces*. Emphasis, more than ever, is on using the fish, poultry and leanest meats more often and the fatter meats less often.

While most people do not eat meat at breakfast, almost everyone eats meat and/or cheese at lunch—often up to 4 ounces or even more. (Two slices of lunch meat make 2 ounces as does one slice of lunch meat and one thin slice of cheese. A small hamburger is 4 ounces.) At dinner it is easy to eat 6 to 12 ounces of meat. A chicken leg and a thigh, for example, is usually about 3 ounces; so is a single half chicken breast. Typical homemade hamburgers contain 6 to 8 ounces of meat

each. Toss in a little cheese on the hamburger or for snacks, say 2 to 3 ounces, and you'll quickly be up to 10 to 18 ounces of meat and cheese in one day. And if, as many do on weekends or vacation, you also have meat for breakfast, say 2 to 4 ounces, your daily total can easily reach 12 to 22 ounces.

Some of you will immediately ask, "If I choose lower-fat meats and cheeses, why can't I eat *more* than six to eight ounces a day?" This is a reasonable question since the CSIs of meats and cheeses do vary considerably. The answer, however, is that the recommendations in Phase Two pertain to the selection of leaner meats and lower-fat cheeses. You can have up to 8 ounces of *those* and still achieve New American Diet goals. If you want to eat the higher-fat meats and cheeses, you will need to limit yourself to 2 to 2½ ounces of those daily to meet the Phase Two goals.

When we say "leaner" we mean those with CSIs of 10 or less per 3½ ounces (see CSI table 3, page 74). This is synonymous with a fat content of 15 percent or less. Some of these include round, flank, sirloin, center muscle of chops, pork tenderloin, as well as ground meat made from these cuts. And when we say low-fat cheeses we mean, for purposes of Phase Two goals, those with CSIs per 3½ ounces of no more than 12. Some of these include lower-fat Cheddars, part-skim and imitation mozzarella, Reduced Calories Laughing Cow, and low-fat cheese slices now available in many supermarkets (look for the diet or low-fat cheese section).

Remember, the goal of no more than 8 ounces (half a pound) of lean meat *and* low-fat cheese per day is just that—an *end-point* goal. It may take you quite awhile to get there. Do not rush it or try to force it. Just keep moving in the recommended direction.

Remodeling the Sandwich

When it comes to meat and cheese, one of the places you are really going to want to work is the sandwich. The sandwich is so central a luncheon and snack feature in the United States and many other Western nations that it deserves special treatment. Many of our patients, Family Heart Study families and individuals, have found it easier at this stage to cut back on meat and cheese more at lunch than at dinner.

Before we go to meatless, cheeseless sandwiches, let's look at some ways you can modify the sandwich and still have it contain *some* of the meat and cheese:

Lunch Meats: Avoid the high-fat varieties, such as bologna, salami, wieners and most other sliced, packaged lunch meats. Better choices are turkey wieners, turkey pastrami, turkey ham and chicken or turkey breasts, thinly sliced. Even lower in fat are the *very thinly sliced,* pressed turkey and other lunch meats. (Use two of these paper-thin slices per sandwich and supplement with lots of vegetables.)

Cheeses: Review the cheese discussion in the above section and in the preceding

chapter and use only those cheeses with the recommended CSI.

Sandwich Spreads: Peanut butter, a popular sandwich spread in the United States, is a good New American Diet choice. We recommend that you use no more than 2 tablespoons for two slices of bread. Omit the margarine. Use jam and jelly, if desired to make more filling for the sandwich. Use imitation mayonnaise or one of the other substitute products discussed in the preceding chapter. If you use margarine on your sandwich develop the art of *scraping* the margarine on, so that you have the thinnest possible layer. Even a sandwich that consists entirely of vegetable filling can be made very tasty by using a good mustard or, if you like it, horseradish.

Breads: Breads made from whole grains are going to be better choices because they contain more fiber and trace nutrients than do the white breads. If you have trouble making the transition from white to dark bread, try making a half-and-half sandwich—with a slice of each kind of bread!

Experiment: If you have always used lots of "everything" in your sandwiches, cut back on one high-fat ingredient at a time. Do not completely eliminate any of the usual ingredients all at once. Add a tasty mustard or horseradish or a greater variety of vegetables as you cut back on the meat and cheese.

For new ideas, look at the sandwich recipes contained in the sample Phase Two meal plan at the end of this chapter or part 3 (cookbook section). These include "Egg" Salad Sandwich Spread, Fruit-Nut Sandwich Spread, Vegetable-Cottage Cheese Sandwich Spread, Falafel with dressings, Chowchow, Baked

Bean Special Sandwich, Pita Pizza, Your Basic Bean Burrito, Pita Bread with Popeye's Spinach Dip or Chili Bean Salad, etc.

Increasing Vegetable/Fruit/ Grain/Bean Intake

As you cut back on the meat, cheese and high-fat dairy products you eat and perhaps begin experimenting with lunches that are entirely meatless and cheeseless on occasion, you are going to arrive eventually at the point where recipe modification alone will not do the job. You will then want to start increasing the amounts of whole grains, fruits, vegetables and legumes (mainly beans of various types) you consume. Review the Six Food Groups of the New American Diet (fig. 23, p. 105). Here is further information to help you when you decide to increase your consumption of foods in each of these categories.

Whole Grains, Breads and Potatoes. As you reduce your fat intake, your goal in Phase Two in general should be to *increase* your intake of grain foods (including breads, pastas, etc.) in the following amounts:

Women and children should eat 1½ to 2½ servings and men and teens 2 to 4 servings of the following *each* day (the quantities specified constitute 1 serving):

1 small baked potato, ½ cup other potatoes, cooked macaroni or pasta or ⅓ cup cooked rice.

AND

Women and children should eat 5 to 5½ servings and men and teens 6 to 7 servings of the following *each* day:

1 slice of bread, 4-inch pancake, 1 corn tortilla, 1 muffin, ½ flour tortilla, ½ bagel, ½ cup cooked cereal, or 1 cup dry cereal.

This may sound like quite a bit, but these amounts add up very quickly. See the example in table 11.

TABLE 11

	Women/Children	Men/Teens
Breakfast	1 slice toast ½ cup oatmeal	2 slices toast 1 cup oatmeal
Lunch	Sandwich— 2 slices of bread	Sandwich— 2 slices of bread
Dinner	Spaghetti— 1 cup French bread— 1 slice	Spaghetti— 1½ cups French bread— 2 slices

Listed below are some of the most commonly used breads, cereals, grains and potatoes. This list will help you get oriented:

Sliced Breads: Whole wheat, rye, pumpernickel, French, Italian, white. We do not suggest that you eat only those breads that are 100 percent whole grain, but you will want to include them because they provide the most fiber and other trace nutrients. We suggest that you use whole or part whole-grain breads in toast and in sandwiches. To add variety to your eating style, use white breads such as a good sourdough French bread with some of your pasta or a tasty raisin-cinnamon bread as a dessert.

Specialty Breads: Dinner rolls, tortillas, pocket (pita) breads, bagels, English muffins, hamburger or wiener buns (try turkey wieners on whole wheat buns or bread for a change), pancakes, waffles, biscuits, muffins.

Breakfast Cereals: Cooked oatmeal, wheat, multigrain cereals, ready-to-eat cereals.

Crackers: Low-fat varieties like ak-mak, Bremner, graham, melba toast, rye, soda (unsalted tops), pretzels, bread sticks, flatbread, rice cakes, etc. Select the low-fat, low-salt varieties.

Grains: Rice, bulgur, barley, buckwheat, cornmeal (polenta), millet, couscous.

Pasta: Spaghetti, macaroni, fettuccine, etc. (Make sure these are *eggless.*)

Potatoes: White or sweet potatoes, yams.

Here are a few breakfast, lunch and dinner suggestions incorporating more breads, cereals, grains and potatoes:

Breakfasts: Our favorites include waffles, oatmeal pancakes, skinny hash browns and, of course, cereals and toast. Modified quick bread recipes like banana and pumpkin are particularly good at breakfast (see part 3 for recipes). Refer to the sample meal plans at the end of this chapter to get an idea about the amount of spreads (margarine and jam) to put on these foods.

Lunches: We like sandwiches, bean soups and popcorn. Soups should be eaten with bread, rolls, muffins if not accompanied by a sandwich.

Dinners: We like potatoes, rice or pasta dishes *and* bread *and,* frequently, beans. Refried beans on tostadas or in Mexican casseroles are also popular. So are baked beans (which go surprisingly well with fish dishes). Hummous makes a nice appetizer.

And try matchstick size strips of tofu (bean curd) in your soups.

You will find many more suggestions later in this chapter when we discuss the kinds of new recipes that will help you to increase your consumption of breads, cereals, grains, and potatoes. The sample Phase Two meal plans, also provided later in this chapter, will give you still other ideas.

Beans, Nuts, Seeds. Here is another of our Six Food Groups that needs more attention when changing to the New American Diet. Some people love beans. Some people don't —or think they don't. Many people have never really given beans a chance. Let's face it, beans have a bad name in some quarters. "They give you gas" is the most common complaint. The truth is, though, that many people can eat fairly large quantities of beans without experiencing this problem. The secret is to *acclimatize* yourself to beans *gradually.* We hear so many people say, "Well, I love beans, they just do not love me." Or, "I wish I could eat them, but I can't." If somebody has not eaten beans for months or even weeks and then sits down to a large plate of them, of course problems will occur. You need to let your system get used to beans slowly by eating small amounts of them frequently, and then you will be able to make them a frequent, easy-to-digest part of your diet. One way to start is to add 2 to 4 tablespoons of garbanzo or kidney beans to green salads several times a week.

It is well worth the effort because legumes (embracing a large number of beans and peas, e.g., split peas and lentils) are among the most nutritious, high-protein, widely available and least expensive foods on the planet. People have eaten legumes—and thrived on them—for millennia. Nearly every culture on the planet makes steady use of them. Mexican and other Latin cultures, of course, are noted for their delicious bean dishes. Oriental cuisine has also made vital use of legumes—especially soybeans, which are pressed, fermented and coagulated to make tofu (bean curd), tempeh (whole-bean tofu) and miso, respectively. (You will find our uses of these foods in part 3.) Europeans, too, rely heavily upon legumes in their cooking, using, especially, garbanzos, split peas and small white beans. In the United States, we favor navy, pinto, lima and kidney beans.

Some have called legumes, with considerable justification, "the perfect food." They contain generous amounts of high-quality protein, lots of fiber, abundant complex carbohydrates and lots of vitamins and minerals. The small amount of fat which they contain is largely polyunsaturated.

There are few foods that can provide the nutritional value of beans *and* the variety of tastes, colors and textures. There are many ways to use beans: as dips, on salads, in a main dish, in soup, in a burrito, as a sandwich filling, even for dessert (see our recipe, part 3, for Pinto Fiesta Cake!). We have bean-spread recipes that work great as sack-lunch items or for snacks. We have even found a way to use beans in lasagna (look for Bean Lasagna in part 3). You will get more ideas when you look at some of our new recipe suggestions later in this chapter.

The goal in Phase Two is to get you to increase your consumption of beans and peas, over a period of time, to the following amounts:

Women/Children—1½ to 2 cups per week
Men/Teens—3 to 4 cups per week

Again, that may seem like a lot of beans, but the examples in table 12 show how easily those quantities can add up in a weekly diet.

TABLE 12

	Cups of Beans per Week	
	Women/ Children	Men/Teens
Appetizers		
Bean Dip with		
Baked Corn Chips	¼	½
Hummous with		
Pita Bread	¼	½
Soups		
Split pea soup	½	¾
Rick's Chili	½	¾
Tossed salad with		
Kidney beans	⅛	¼
Garbanzo beans	⅛	¼
Total (cups of beans)	1¾	3

NOTE: The recipes that are in italics can be found in part 3.

You will want to use nuts and seeds sparingly. They can be used very effectively in small amounts as a means of spicing up grain, bean, salad and other vegetable dishes. If you have never tried them before, you may be delighted by the extent to which a few sunflower seeds, for example, can enliven a tossed green salad. As for peanut butter, it is great for a sandwich spread at lunch (in place of meat or cheese) but not so great as a snack food eaten by spoonfuls.

Vegetables. As we stated in the first part of this book, in 1819, one of our presidents, Thomas Jefferson, wrote to his physician, saying that he had lived temperately, eating little animal food and using it as a condiment "for the vegetables which constitute my principal diet." Jefferson's wisdom about vegetables is echoed in nearly all cultures, from the Chinese to the Tarahumara Indians.

Vegetables are so important to human health because they are potent storehouses of minerals, vitamins and fiber, which in our highly processed foods can often be in short supply. Vegetables, recent research has shown, contain anticancer substances, particularly if they are the green and yellow vegetables with their abundant amounts of carotene and the cruciferous vegetables such as broccoli, cauliflower and cabbage.

The New American Diet is not a vegetarian diet, although we do encourage a significant increase in vegetable consumption. In Phase Two, we suggest that you gradually increase your vegetable intake until you are eating, roughly, the following amounts:

Women/Children—1½ to 2½ cups per day
Men/Teens—2½ to 3½ cups per day

Table 13 shows one way to reach this goal.

TABLE 13

	Women/Children	Men/Teens
Lunch	Salad bar— 1 cup lettuce ½ cup vegetables	Salad bar— 1½ cups lettuce ¾ cup vegetables
Dinner	Broccoli— 1 cup	Broccoli— 1¼ cups
Total	2½ cups	3½ cups

As for the form in which you get your vegetables, fresh, frozen or canned, it is up to you. Keep in mind, though, that most canned vegetables contain a lot of salt. While you will use some of these, look for those that say "no added salt" on the labels. More and more of these are showing up in the supermarket.

(Keep the sodium goals, discussed earlier in this chapter, in mind.)

Vegetables are often used as side dishes, and that is fine, but there are other, more imaginative, ways of using vegetables. Consider these ideas (recipes for italicized items can be found in part 3):

Appetizers: Spicy Stuffed Mushrooms, dips served with raw vegetables as scoopers, vegetables mixed in the dips themselves.

Breakfast or Brunch: Vegetable Frittata, skinny hash brown potatoes (bake or boil potatoes, grate and then cook in skillet with 1 teaspoon to 1 tablespoon vegetable oil).

Lunch or Dinner: Stir-fry dishes, soups of all kinds, *Marinara Sauce* with or without added vegetables on top of pasta, vegetable kabobs, vegetables stuffed in pita bread, *Calzones* or enchiladas, cabbage leaves stuffed with rice and vegetables (*Cabbage Rolls*).

A word of caution about vegetables. If you increase your vegetable intake mainly in the form of salads and at the same time smother them in typical dressings, you are going to defeat yourself. Some people have trouble conceiving of raw vegetables devoid of these dressings. Fortunately, just as there are lower-fat cheeses, so are there many low-fat, low-calorie salad dressings. Some of these are available in grocery stores and you will find recipes for others in part 3 of this book. Figure 31 shows you the CSIs for a variety of salad dressings.

When you eat out, the best way to avoid getting an overdose of fat on your salad is to ask for the dressing on the side. Then you can choose what you want rather than have someone else choose for you. You will get more ideas on how to make vegetables an attractive and tasty part of your daily fare when you study the sample meal plans and new recipes later in this chapter.

Fruit. In Phase Two, we suggest that you work toward eating the following amounts of fruit:

Women/Children—2½ pieces each day
Men/Teens—4 pieces each day
Table 14 shows how to reach this goal.

TABLE 14

	Women/Children	Men/Teens
Breakfast	Blackberries—⅔ cup	Blackberries—1½ cups
Lunch	Orange—1 small	Orange—1 large
Dinner	Apple Crisp*—1 svg.	Apple Crisp*—1½ svgs.
Total (pieces of fruit)	2⅔	4

* Recipe in part 3.

CHOLESTEROL-SATURATED FAT INDEX OF SALAD DRESSINGS (¼ CUP)

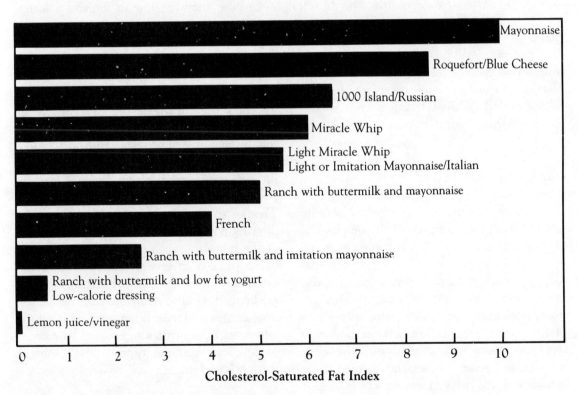

Cholesterol-Saturated Fat Index

Figure 31. The Cholesterol-Saturated Fat Index (CSI) of ¼ cup of selected salad dressings. A smaller CSI denotes less cholesterol and saturated fat.

Making It Work with New (Ethnic) Recipes

The cuisines of many other countries, as we have discussed, come much closer than typical American fare to the style of eating we advocate. We have had considerable success in adapting many of the recipes of other lands to meet the objectives of the New American Diet. It is in Phase Two that you will find it most useful to begin acquainting yourself with these dishes. They will add a great deal of interest and variety to your fare and enable you to make the changes we have been talking about with minimal stress.

There are three groups of ethnic recipes and eating styles we want to introduce to you in Phase Two. Some of you will already be addicted to one or more of these; many of you, however, will have had little experience with any of them, except, perhaps, when eating out. We are going to concentrate here on Mexican fare, Oriental dishes and Middle Eastern/Mediterranean cuisine.

MEXICAN CUISINE

Mexican cuisine, ranging from elaborate feast dishes to the quickest of the quickies, is so versatile that once you become immersed in it you may find yourself "south of the border" several nights each week. It may surprise some of you that we recommend Mexican food as an excellent way of easing into Phase Two of our program. The surprise is due to your familiarity with Americanized versions of Mexican dishes, those accompanied by or smothered in hefty doses of cheese, sour cream, meat, eggs and fat from the deep fryer. This is *not* the way the Mexicans themselves typically eat, except perhaps on an occasional feast day. The Mexican way of eating that we have adapted to our diet conforms more closely to traditional Mexican fare which, we promise you, remains delicious *without* the excesses of fat and cholesterol.

The native Indians of Mexico, who were all agriculturally oriented, improvised a variety of dishes from the avocados, tomatoes, beans, corn, chiles, squash, vanilla and tropical fruit they harvested. Under the influence of the Spanish in the 1500s, the Mexicans added rice, wheat, chicken and dairy products to their diet, giving rise to the cuisine of today, rich in flavor, color, texture and variety.

We warmly endorse the basics of Mexican cooking—corn, beans, rice, chiles and fruit—because they are low in fat and calories, low in cholesterol (or contain none at all), high in fiber, easy to prepare, good sources of protein, vitamins and minerals and are versatile and easy to keep on hand.

Before we get to some recipe suggestions to get you started in Mexican cookery, there are some things you should know about shopping for the makings of Mexican dishes. Outdoor markets are common in Mexico, and fresh produce is displayed in abundance, a feast for the eyes and nose, as well as the mouth. Thanks to modern transportation and the growing popularity of Mexican cuisine, many of the items found in these markets are now being stocked in grocery stores everywhere. Sometimes there is a special section with ingredients for various ethnic cuisines. Even smaller grocery stores often carry a few of the basics, such as tortillas and refried beans.

Here is background information on some of the foods and spices you'll be working with:

Beans
The ones you'll use most frequently are the dried kidney, pinto, red and pink beans.

Black beans are used in the Yucatán, Central and South American cuisine.

Canned Products

Vegetarian refried beans—mashed pinto beans with some spices. If you can't find a vegetarian variety, regular refried beans are acceptable since they contain only a small amount of animal fat. "Spicy" refried beans are also available (Rosarita brand).

Salsa—This is a mixture of tomatoes, chile peppers and spices. It can be mixed with beans to produce that Mex flavor or individually added to any Mexican dish for added zip. Ortega salsa or Picanante hot sauce are good choices.

Enchilada sauce—Choose according to your taste from mild to hot. We have had good success with Rosarita or Old El Paso mild. For a sweeter, milder flavor, mix with tomato sauce.

Taco sauce—This is another variation on seasoned tomatoes and chiles. (Good in homemade chili!)

Tomatillos—Small green tomatoes with distinctive, tart flavor, can be found fresh in some stores or canned.

Chiles

These staples of Mexican cuisine come in a wide variety, ranging from relatively mild types such as the California (Anaheim) green chiles to the superhot jalapeño and Serrano chiles. Experiment with the different types to test your tolerances.

Spices

Cayenne powder—This is ground hot red pepper.

Chili powder—This is a blend of spices. Different brands can range from mild to very hot. Chili powder usually consists of ground dried chiles blended with garlic, oregano and cumin.

Cilantro—This resembles parsley in appearance but not taste. Look for it in the produce section of your grocery store. Cilantro seeds are called coriander and can be found in the spice section of most grocery stores.

Cumin—Aromatic and pungent, this spice is commonly used in Mexican cookery. It is one of the spices used in chili powder.

Tortillas

These are the "breads" of Mexican cuisine. They are flat and round in shape. You can buy them ready-made in many supermarkets. There are some whole wheat versions available in some stores.

Miscellaneous

Masa harina—This is a special corn flour used to make tortillas and tamales.

Polenta—This is a coarse-ground cornmeal that is used in making a tasty side dish of the same name. It is also used in tamale pie.

Corn husks—Dried corn husks are used as wrappings for tamales.

Jicama—With its appealing white, crisp flesh, this turnip-shaped vegetable makes an excellent "dipper."

Now let's look at some ways you can put together irresistible Mexican meals, using recipes (all contained in part 3, the cookbook section). For appetizers try Gazpacho, a cold soup that gives the whole concept of soup a new dimension. Or try our Baked Corn Chips with either Bean Dip or Chowchow. (The leftover bean dip can also be used to make a burrito; just spoon some of it onto a warm flour tortilla, roll it up and you're there.)

For main courses, choose from the following for your opening act: Pollo Tepehuano (pronounced poyo teppawano), a chicken and rice dish from a little town in Durango, Mexico, served with warmed tortillas (either purchased or made by you using any corn tortilla recipe) and Zucchini Mexicali, combining—see recipe for full details—zucchini, carrots, onion, celery, green pepper and tomatoes; or Acapulco Enchiladas topped with our Mock Sour Cream (which has many other uses; see recipe) and served with shredded lettuce, tomato wedges and Refried Beans (either our recipe or the canned variety); or Tamale Pie served with green salad with Western Salad Dressing and Spanish Rice.

For dessert, select one of the following: Strawberry Ice or sherbet, fresh fruit (plain or laced with low-fat vanilla yogurt), or Carob Cookies or Vanilla Pudding with sliced fruit.

Among the other Mexican recipes you will find in part 3 are Chili Bean Salad, Mexican Corn Medley, Creamy Enchiladas, Rick's Chili, Chile Relleno Casserole, No-Meat Enchiladas, Acapulco Bean Casserole, Tostadas, Taco Salad, Your Basic Bean Burrito and Fruited Punch.

ORIENTAL CUISINE

Learning something about Oriental dishes is another excellent way of adding variety to your diet while achieving some more Phase Two goals. Along with the Mexican dishes you have already been introduced to, these Oriental recipes—and others you will find in part 3—are almost certain to become a permanent part of your cooking repertoire. We favor Oriental recipes because they stress a lot of vegetables, little fat, and meat is used more as a condiment or supplement to main dishes than as the centerpiece of the main dish. Again, if you check your local supermarket, you will likely find a section of the store that stocks many of the ingredients of Oriental cooking. But even without such help it is easy to make a number of delicious Oriental meals.

We must caution once again that the kind of Oriental dishes you get in typical Chinese restaurants may not be at all typical of what the Chinese themselves have traditionally eaten. Many of these restaurant dishes have been elaborately sweetened, salted and/or fattened to cater to the American palate. Such foods, if used at all by the Chinese, are reserved for special occasions, feasts and the like. Learn how to eat the *real* Oriental way. Try some of the following recipes (included in part 3); they make learning easy and enjoyable:

Hot and Sour Soup, Cashew Chicken, Oriental Sauce for Fish, Eggplant Szechuan Style, Chinese Salad Rich Style, Steamed Buns (with a savory filling), Moo Shoo Pork (which is often served with thin pancakes called Peking Doilies, available in Chinese groceries), Pepper Steak, Spicy Chicken with Spinach, Chinese Cucumber (or Asparagus) Salad and Stir-Fried Mushrooms and Broccoli.

MIDDLE EASTERN AND MEDITERRANEAN CUISINE

Thoughts of the Mediterranean conjure up images of a landscape full of cypress, pine, walnut, olive, fig and palm trees, and of tomato and grapevines, and of a variety of sun-drenched countries with distinctive cultures and cuisines that have in common a pool of low-fat, high complex carbohydrate staples. From Spain to southern France, Italy and Greece, from Morocco and Northern Africa to the Middle East, the diverse peoples of that region have developed a remarkable eating style based upon fish, grains, lentils, garbanzo beans, fruits, vegetables and fermented dairy products. Olives, figs, almonds, apricots, oranges, garlic, basil, mint, cumin, thyme, oregano, barley, bulgur, onions, leeks, zucchini, cucumber, pasta and fish—and still more pasta and fish. It sounds like the New American Diet!

Little wonder that medical researchers concerned with nutrition have taken such an interest in Middle Eastern and Mediterranean cooking with their high complex carbohydrate and low-fat characteristics. The fats that are used are olive, walnut, sesame and peanut oils. No butter on bread in these parts. No need anyway—the breads are crusty and are most often used to mop up juices on the plate. Lamb and goat meats are included, but not generally as main courses.

Actually, though you may not always realize it, many of our most cherished foods (such as pizza) come from this part of the world. And you do not usually have to go to the specialty markets to find the ingredients for Middle Eastern and Mediterranean recipes. Most of the ingredients you need can be found in our supermarkets and fish markets.

The New American Diet recipes (see part 3) have been heavily influenced by the cuisine of this part of the world. To begin sampling it, try such appetizers as our Great Little Snackers or try a fragrant Hummous (a delicious dip made from garbanzo beans) served with Pita Bread. If the Hummous does not appeal to you, try another dip—our Eggplant Delight. Antipasto is just that—a mixture of

fresh vegetables to be eaten "before the pasta," that is, before the main course.

Soups are the mainstay of the evening meals in Mediterranean lands, though you may want to try them at lunch, as well. Try the Greek Lentil Soup or the fragrant peasant soup from Southern France, Bean and Basil Soup, or its cousin from Italy, the Minestrone Soup. Basil again takes culinary center stage in Zucchini and Basil Soup. For something really different, try our Icy Olive Soup. Salads, to accompany the soups, or to stand by themselves, make plentiful use of legumes, grains and vegetables. Lentil Salad and Tabouli will introduce you to some new ways of using traditional staples. Greek Salad and Cucumber Cumin Salad will introduce you to some new uses of yogurt.

Our cookbook section contains a large number of main dishes using mainly grains and beans or vegetables. Many of them are Mediterranean-inspired. Try the Herbed Lentil Casserole, Romano Rice and Beans, Zucchini Spaghetti Dinner, Falafel (the Middle Eastern version of the "hamburger" made from ground garbanzo beans and spices), Moroccan Vegetable Stew, Cheese Stuffed Manicotti, Spinach Lasagna, Zucchini Pie, Spicy Cheese Pizza and Calzones ("pizzas in a pocket").

To accompany fish and chicken dishes, try "sunny" dishes such as Tomatoes "Provençale," Ratatouille Provençale (a flavorful mixture of tomatoes, eggplant and zucchini), Eggplant Parmesan (capable, we have found, of pleasing even the most ardent eggplant hater), colorful Stuffed Zucchini Boats or Bulgur Pilaf (which can be used in place of rice or potatoes, as a basic staple to add variety to your meals).

For fish, we go to Marseilles, in France, for a version of its famous Bouillabaisse, a simple dish created by the wives of fishermen to make use of unsold fish (and now on the menus of many fancy restaurants). Or try the quick Fish à la Mistral, as swift to prepare as the wind in France for which it is named. For an elegant fish dish try Fillet of Fish Florentine.

If it is chicken you want, you can get it in the Mediterranean mode via our Chicken and Vegetables Provencale or Chicken Italian. For a Lebanese touch, try Lemony Chicken Kabobs. Neither Mediterranean nor New American Diet cuisine offers many dishes using beef, though there are two that use *lean* beef: Pizza Rice Casserole and Stuffed Flank Steak Florentine.

For desserts, people from these lands typically choose fresh fruits, reserving fruit pies, cakes or ice cream for special occasions.

Breakfasts are usually a piece of toast and jam or a gruel. Bread, at any meal, is typically the whole-grain version of the classic French bread. (See our recipe for Whole Wheat French Bread.)

PASTA—MEDITERRANEAN CUISINE CONTINUED

Pasta is such an important and satisfying part of Mediterranean cuisine that we are going to give it its own separate section here. If you do not familiarize yourself with pasta and make it a regular part of your eating fare you are really missing out on one of life's culinary pleasures. Pasta is a simple mixture of wheat flour and water. Pasta has fed large segments of the world population for centuries. Though we think of pasta as uniquely Italian, it was most likely first developed in China and then introduced into Italy by Marco Polo. Asiatic Indians and Arabs were also early consumers of pasta, which rapidly

became an attractive alternative and addition to bread in all regions where wheat was grown. Pasta can be eaten hot or cold and maintains its texture better than most other wheat products when dried. It can be stored in this dried fashion for long periods of time, making it an especially useful staple.

Our studies have convinced us that pasta is one of the most important foods known to mankind—and one of the healthiest. It is a good source of protein, it contains no cholesterol (unless it is made with whole eggs), it is very low in fat of any kind, it is low in calories but is still filling, it is a good source of minerals and vitamins of the B group and of fiber (when whole wheat is used), it is inexpensive, easy to store and its production is "low on the food chain," meaning it does not take much energy to produce it.

One of the nicest things about pasta—from the cook's point of view—is that it qualifies as a "convenience" or even "fast" food. It can be prepared very quickly; if the sauces and toppings that accompany it have been prepared ahead, it can be the workingwoman's, single person's or busy homemaker's lifesaver. And since pasta is so versatile it can be served frequently. It comes in an enormous variety of shapes and flavors and can be served hot or cold, in soups, salads, as main dishes, in casseroles and with an assortment of sauces, as raviolis, etc. (You will find a list of different types of pasta in table 15.)

If you live in a city or town of any size you may have shops that sell freshly made or fresh-frozen pasta—ready to be cooked by you at home in a matter of minutes. You can buy sauces at these places, too, although the ones made with cheese are going to contain more fat than the ones we recommend. Even when you buy your pasta ready-made the price remains surprisingly low. Compare the cost of a pound of fresh pasta to a pound of meat.

Some people are a little leery of approaching a pasta stand for the first time, intimidated by all those strange names. They wonder, when do you order "vermicelli" as opposed to "linguine" or "fettuccine"? The fact is, most of these Italian names merely describe different *widths* and *shapes* of pasta. "Spaghetti," familiar to most Americans, is really no different from "fettuccine" (which is what many call noodles), or the others named above, except in terms of the width of the cut. When you approach the pasta stand you are likely to see big sheets of pasta, often, these days, in different colors. Pasta entrepreneurs keep coming up with new "flavors"—spinach, tomato, herb, even "hot red pepper" and jalapeño pasta. All you have to do is pick your flavor and your width and tell the salesperson how much you want. They will cut it for you, using a special machine, right on the spot.

A word of caution, though, about buying your pasta, rather than making it yourself. Just as bread comes in different nutritional packages, so does pasta; it all depends on what goes into it. Make sure the pasta you buy is not loaded with eggs, fats and refined flour. These precautions apply both to the dried and fresh pastas.

Table 15 will help familiarize you with a variety of pastas.

Now, why don't you try your hand at preparing some pasta dishes at home? If you have a pasta machine you can make a wide variety of pastas (always remember to use three egg whites for every two whole eggs called for in pasta recipes). But if you do not have a pasta machine you can still make many dishes, using dried, fresh or fresh-frozen pastas you buy at the store as starter materials. Other pastas can be made in the home with some other inexpensive special equipment. Even raviolis, those little pasta squares stuffed with

TABLE 15

Name	English Translation	Description
Acini	Acino "grapeseed"	Small spherical pasta resembling rice
Anelli	"Ring"	Ring-shaped, used in soups
Cannelloni	Cannella "straw"; cannelloni can also be flat spheres of pasta rolled around stuffing	Hollow, pipe-shaped, served with a stuffing; cannelloni are large; cannellini are smaller
Cappelletti	Cappelle "hat"	Little, stuffed, hat-shaped dumplings, similar to tortellini
Fettuccine	Fettina "little slice"	Narrow, ribbonlike
Fusilli	"Gun" (the grooved inside of the barrel)	Spaghetti twisted like a corkscrew
Gnocchi	"Gnoccho" is a placid, simple soul	Semolina or potato dumpling served traditionally on Thursdays in Rome and Naples "If it's gnocchi, it must be Thursday"
Lasagna	—	Extra-wide flat noodles with rippled edges
Linguine	"Tongue"	Narrow rods slightly flattened
Macaroni	—	Tubelike, many shapes
Manicotti	Manica "sleeve"	Largest of tubelike pasta; 4" long, served with a stuffing similar to cannelloni

TABLE 15 (Continued)

Name	English Translation	Description
Mostaccioli	"Mustache"	Diagonally cut tubes, about 2" long
Nastrini	Nastro "bow"	In various sizes, also called strichetti
Noodles	—	Flat strips of pasta of various widths
Orzo	"Barley"	Pasta resembling elongated rice, or barley
Ravioli	—	Pasta squares served with a filling
Rigatoni	Rigato "line," "groove"	Large, grooved pasta tubes
Spaghetti	Spago "string"	Long, thin rods
Tagliatelle	Taglione "to cut by hand"	Very narrow noodle type
Tortellini	"Little cakes"	Similar to cappelletti, but twisted specially, from Bologna, Italy
Vermicelli	Verme "worm"	Very thin spaghetti type, often used in soups

cialty stores. These particular raviolis are made with either a fresh chicken or a canned chicken filling. And the sauce that accompanies them is our Marinara Sauce which is low in fat and contains no cholesterol.

After making your pasta debut with raviolis, move on to Cheese Stuffed Manicotti, which is particularly easy to prepare since the manicotti shells do not need to be precooked in our recipe. Rich tasting though this dish is, you will get only 7 grams of fat and 17 milligrams of cholesterol with a CSI of 4—in two pieces.

Then try Pasta Primavera, a wonderful "spring pasta" that combines cooked fresh vegetables with pasta; Four Star Pasta Salad, a beautiful and unusual salad served with a pungent sauce and sometimes combined with shrimp; Alphabet Seafood Salad, one of our personal favorites that includes tuna, black olives, alphabet pastas, onion and a sprightly yogurt/sweet pickle/Dijon mustard dressing; Easy Oven Lasagna, an old favorite prepared an easier way—with *uncooked* noodles (and ground turkey or leanest ground beef); Minestrone Soup (a superb-tasting, very low-fat, no-cholesterol variety). Some of the dressings used in the pasta salad recipes contain yogurt (water-based) instead of mayonnaise (oil-based). These dressings need to be added just before serving so the pasta does not absorb all of the dressing and become too dry.

You'll want to start trying many of our sauces, in addition to those mentioned above. For spaghetti, see our recipes for Tomato-Mushroom Spaghetti Sauce, Beef-Mushroom Spaghetti Sauce, and Turkey-Mushroom Spaghetti Sauce. For other fresh-cooked pasta, be it linguine, fettuccine or whatever cut or shape suits your fancy, see our Clam Sauce for Pasta, our Light Mushroom Sauce for Pasta, and our Marinara Sauce.

delicious fillings that please most family members, aren't particularly difficult to make. And you can make a lot of them at one time and then freeze them just like the Italians do. See our recipe in part 3 for Homemade Raviolis. The only special tools you will need are a ravioli rolling pin and a ravioli cutter, both available in most department or kitchen spe-

Isn't This Going to Be a Lot More Work?

Whenever you change your eating habits, it is likely to mean some extra work—at least in the beginning. Even if it was a *lot* more work, which it isn't, we'd still argue that it is worth the extra effort, given the considerable health benefits and the greater chances of permanently controlling weight that result from this program. The fact is, however, the New American Diet meals are, in many instances, quick and simple to prepare. Once you make the initial effort to replace some of your old standbys with these new recipes, *they* will become your new "old standbys," and you will get many of them on the table with no more effort than you are expending right now. Even our most exotic recipes, though they may take a little time to master in the beginning, have the benefit of bringing new excitement and variety into the kitchen. And there are plenty of nonexotic recipes for those frequent occasions when you want to get something on the table in a matter of minutes.

SOME DINNERS-IN-A-HURRY SUGGESTIONS

—Pizza is a good quickie, provided it is made to low-fat specifications. You can get your crust and sauce ready-made from Appian Way, or you can use purchased sauce and our quick version of Pizza Crust. Serve with green salad.

—Boiled potatoes with low-fat cottage cheese and steamed vegetables.

—Macaroni and cheese from the package (but omit margarine and use skim milk), served with canned soup (Progresso brand lentil is an excellent choice, to cite one example), bread or wheat rolls and fruit.

—Spaghetti with Prego or Ragú brand spaghetti sauce (so long as it is the meatless variety), served with steamed vegetable and/or green salad and bread or rolls.

—Fish à la Mistral served with Bulgur Pilaf, steamed carrots or broccoli and rolls or French bread.

You will find many other quickie ideas in part 3. It is wise to have a number of foods on hand for quick meals when you need them. Frozen fish is an excellent choice. It can be baked, while still frozen, over a bed of onions and tomatoes or other vegetables and liberally seasoned for an elegant quickie.

Canned soups, especially bean soups, are other good choices. You can "customize" these and enrich them to make a main meal by adding potatoes, vegetables, rice, tomato paste or leftover meat. These additions also help make them less salty.

Pasta, as already discussed, is another candidate for a quickie. Pick up some fresh pasta on your way home from work or keep several varieties on hand, frozen or dried. Add Marinara Sauce or some low-fat cheeses, in moderation, along with some vegetables, perhaps even some clams with mushrooms and eggplant. Improvise. It's hard to go very far astray with pasta.

Rice is another staple to have on hand at all times. Mix it with canned beans and/or celery and onions, any leftover vegetables and lots of herbs. Or mix in tofu, a little low-fat cheese, steamed vegetables and various herbs and you will have another tempting, tasty quickie.

If you tire of rice, try Couscous (pronounced coos-coos), the Moroccan pasta you buy in boxes in many supermarkets and can prepare in a matter of minutes. It makes a superb, nutritious base upon which to heap steamed vegetables and small pieces of chicken. Or it can be served by itself with spaghetti sauce. This grain takes only 3 or 4 minutes to cook.

You can also make meals out of a variety of now widely available convenience foods, such as instant tabouli, falafel mixes and veggie-burger mixes (made of cooked, ground and dried beans and grains).

In table 16 are some sample meal plans for Phase Two.

Review of Goals and Results of Phase Two

The meals outlined above—a *sample* of Phase Two eating—achieve the basic goals of Phase Two of the diet program:

1. Cholesterol intake is reduced, on average, from 300 to 350 milligrams at the end of Phase One to approximately 200 milligrams at the end of Phase Two.

2. Fat content of the diet decreases from 35 percent at the end of Phase One to 25 percent at the end of Phase Two, with much of this additional reduction in saturated fats.

3. Carbohydrates assume a still greater role in the diet, further replacing fats. There is another 10 percent increase in calories derived from carbohydrates, especially complex carbohydrates, in Phase Two.

In addition, sodium intake is reduced by another 22 percent, and potassium intake is increased by 58 percent, on average, in Phase Two.

It is not possible, as previously noted, to predict the *exact* amount by which blood levels of cholesterol will be lowered in each individual as a result of following the Phase

Two diet. But, on average, there is an additional expected lowering of up to 7 percent from Phase One. This means that a person who started with 260 milligrams of cholesterol per 100 milliliters of blood could now be at 227. This is a highly significant further reduction. As we stated before, for each 1 percent reduction in cholesterol achieved by the population, there will be a 2 percent decrease in coronary heart disease risk, according to calculations from recent research findings.

How to Tell When You've Achieved Phase Two Goals

You can assess your Phase Two progress by retaking the quiz found on pages 41–51. The following scores correspond with Phase Two goals:

MEAT, FISH AND POULTRY

Question 1	3
Question 2	3
Question 3	22 to 25
Question 4	3 (Men/Teens)
	4 (Women/Children)
Question 5	3 to 4
Total score	34 to 39

DAIRY PRODUCTS AND EGGS

Question 1	4
Question 2	5
Question 3	4
Question 4	4 to 5
Question 5	3 to 4
Question 6	4 to 5
Question 7	5
Total score	29 to 32

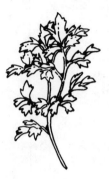

FATS AND OILS

Question 1	3 to 4
Question 2	3 (Men/Teens)
	4 (Women/Children)
Question 3	4
Question 4	4
Question 5	4 to 5
Total score	18 to 21

GRAINS, BEANS, FRUITS AND VEGETABLES

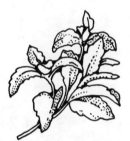

	Men/Teens	Women/Children
Question 1	19 to 21	12 to 13
Question 2	13 to 17	9 to 12
Question 3	16 to 19	8 to 10
Question 4	10 to 19	8 to 12
Question 5	31 to 38	26 to 28
Question 6	9	4 to 5
Question 7	0	0
Total score	98 to 123	67 to 80

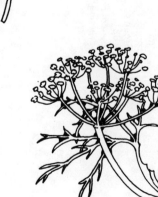

SWEETS AND SNACKS

Question 1	4
Question 2	4
Question 3	4
Question 4	5
Question 5	3 to 5
Question 6	4 to 5
Total score	24 to 27

SALT

Question 1	4
Question 2	5
Question 3	5
Question 4	3
Question 5	3
Total score	20

TABLE 16
New American Diet Phase Two Meal Plans

	DAY 1	DAY 2	DAY 3	DAY 4	DAY 5	DAY 6	DAY 7
Breakfast	Pink grapefruit, ½ Oatmeal, 1 cup Brown sugar, 1 tsp. 1% milk, ¾ cup Orange-date muffins, 2	Cantaloupe, ½ Spanish omelet: Egg substitute, ½ cup Chowchow, ¼ cup English muffin, 1 Strawberry jam, 2 tsp.	Orange juice, ¾ cup *Our Granola*, 1 cup 1% milk, ¾ cup	Strawberries, ½ cup Cream of Wheat, 1 cup Sugar, 2 tsp. 1% milk, ¾ cup Raisin bread toast, 2 slices Soft margarine, 2 tsp.	Fruit cup: Banana slices, ½ cup Orange sections, ½ cup Bran Flakes, 1 cup 1% milk, ¾ cup Whole wheat toast, 2 slices Grape jelly, 2 tsp.	Orange juice, ¾ cup Apple crepes: *Crepes*, 2 Apple pie filling, ½ cup Low-fat plain yogurt, 2 Tbsp.	Waffles, 2 Blackberries, ⅔ cup Blackberry syrup, ¼ cup Soft margarine, 2 tsp.
Morning Snack			Banana, 1				
Lunch	*Thick Crust Pizza* with mozzarella cheese, green peppers, onions, mushrooms, 1½ svgs. Apple *Oatmeal cookies*, 2	*Moroccan Vegetable Stew*, 2 cups Soda crackers (unsalted tops), 6 Green salad, 1 cup Low-cal French dressing, 2 Tbsp.	Stuffed tomato: Tomato, 1 *Alphabet Seafood Salad*, 1 cup Bagel, 1 Reduced Calories Laughing Cow, ¾ oz. Honeydew melon, ½ cup	Lunch in a Cafeteria: Baked potato, 1 large *Mock Sour Cream*, ¼ cup (brought from home) Chives, 1 Tbsp. Three bean salad, ¾ cup French bread, 2 pieces (4" diameter) Soft margarine, 2 tsp. Apricots canned in own juice, ½ cup	*Rick's Chili*, 1½ cups Oyster crackers (unsalted tops), 10 *Skinny "French Fries,"* 1 svg. Fresh green grapes, ½ cup	*Red Root Soup*, 1½ cups Sandwich: Whole wheat bread, 2 slices Turkey salami, 2 oz. Alfalfa sprouts, ¼ cup Mustard, 2 tsp. Tomato, 2 slices Fresh Pear 1% Milk, 1 cup	Sandwich: Whole wheat bread, 2 slices Peanut butter, 2 Tbsp. Vegetable sticks: Carrots, ½ cup Celery, ½ cup Fig bars, 2 Orange

TABLE 16—Continued

	DAY 1	DAY 2	DAY 3	DAY 4	DAY 5	DAY 6	DAY 7
Afternoon Snack		Low-fat raspberry yogurt, 6 oz.					
Dinner	*Orange Baked Chicken,* 4 oz. Steamed rice, 3/4 cup *Stir-Fried Mushrooms and Broccoli,* 1 svg. Dinner roll, 1 Soft margarine, 2 tsp. Fortune cookies, 2 1% milk, 1/2 cup	*Marinated Mushrooms,* 1 svg. Spaghetti, 1 1/2 cups, with Red clam sauce: *Marinara Sauce,* 1 cup Clams, 3 oz. Parmesan cheese, 2 Tbsp. *Ratatouille Provençale,* 1 svg. *Whole Wheat French Bread,* 4 (2" diameter) pieces Soft margarine, 2 tsp. Cherry cobbler, 1/2 cup	*Baked Corn Chips,* 1/2 cup *Guacamole,* 1/4 cup *Acapulco Bean Casserole,* 2 svgs. Lettuce salad, 1 cup Low-cal French dressing, 2 Tbsp. Daiquiri ice, 1/2 cup	*Beef Stroganoff,* 1 cup Noodles (eggless) 1 1/2 cups Spinach salad, 1 cup Low-cal Italian dressing, 2 Tbsp. Steamed broccoli, 3/4 cup Wheatberry roll, 1 Soft margarine, 2 tsp.	*Pepper Steak,* 1 svg. Brown rice, 1 cup Lettuce salad, 1 cup *Red French Salad Dressing,* 2 Tbsp. Whole wheat dinner rolls, 2 Soft margarine, 2 tsp. *Cocoa Cake,* 1 svg.	*Lemony Chicken Kabobs,* 1 1/2 svgs. *Potato Puff,* 1 svg. *Tomatoes "Provençale,"* 1 svg. Baked winter squash, 1/2, with Brown sugar, 1 tsp. *Poppy Seed Cake,* 1 svg.	*Popeye's Spinach Dip,* 1/2 cup with Vegetables: Radishes, Green pepper, Cauliflower, 1/4 cup each *Hearty Fish Soup,* 1 1/2 cups Green salad, 1 cup *Ranch Salad Dressing* made with Imitation mayonnaise, Low-fat yogurt and Buttermilk, 2 Tbsp. *Apple Crisp,* 1 svg. with Plain low-fat yogurt, 2 Tbsp.
Evening Snack				Fresh fruit: Peaches, 1/2 cup Pears, 1/2 cup			

NOTE: Recipes that are in italics can be found in part 3.

151

TABLE 16—Continued

Nutrient Composition	DAY 1	DAY 2	DAY 3	DAY 4	DAY 5	DAY 6	DAY 7	Average	Phase Two Goal
Calories	2128	1928	1908	1992	1985	1732	2020	1946	2000*
Protein, % Calories	17	15	15	17	17	27	13	17	15
Fat, % Calories	24	24	25	29	24	22	33	26	25
Carbohydrate, % Calories	59	61	59	53	59	52	54	57	60
Saturated Fat, % Calories	4.8	5.0	7.9	6.8	4.8	4.7	6.3	5.8	8.0
Polyunsaturated Fat, % Calories	5.9	5.0	5.8	9.2	5.5	6.0	11.2	6.9	8.0
Cholesterol, mg†	96	65	98	100	103	113	83	94	<200‡
CSI	16	14	22	20	16	15	19	17	28
Sodium, mg	1856	2063	2453	2442	2155	2578	2319	2267	2300
Potassium, mg	2280	3835	3994	3440	3809	4969	3811	3734	3900
Calcium, mg	1260	991	887	1087	543	972	888	833	800

* This is a food pattern for people who require 2000 Calories to maintain their weight.
† Mg = milligram.
‡ < = less than.

9

PHASE THREE OF THE NEW AMERICAN DIET: A NEW WAY OF EATING

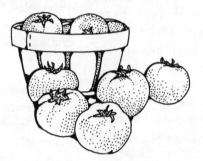

Making the Decision to Put It All Together *Every Day*

When it comes to Phase Three, you are going to need to sit down and do some hard thinking, either alone or in conference with your family. The question you must ask yourself—and answer—is: "Do I (we) want to go all the way?" If you've achieved most or all of the goals of Phase Two, you've made very substantial changes in your eating habits, changes that are likely to have very significant and positive impact on your health. Some decide that Phase Two is far enough. Remember that *any* change in the desired direction is better than no change at all—and no one need feel he or she has failed if the

decision is to stop after Phase Two (or even Phase One).

But there is absolutely no question at all in our minds that by far the *greatest* benefits will be reaped by those who reach our end-point goals, by those who *do* "go all the way." The difference between Phase Two and Phase Three goals isn't really all that great in many respects. But in Phase Three you need to do *daily* what you may, in Phase Two, only be doing several times per week. In Phase Three you have to put it all together each and every day.

In Phase Two you are consuming no more than 6 to 8 ounces of meat, fish, poultry *and* cheese per day. The fat you use is from 5 to 8 teaspoons per day, and the milk and other dairy products you are cooking with and eating are generally made from 1 percent fat or

153

less. In Phase Three you will need to further reduce your meat/poultry/shrimp/crab/lobster intake to a total of 3 to 4 ounces *or* fish/clams/oysters/scallops to 6 ounces per day, to limit the amount of fat used in cooking and eating to 4 to 7 teaspoons per day, and to use, for the most part, dairy products which are made from skim milk.

There are other goals you will want to work toward, but this is the crux of the situation. Can you do it? As you make your decision refer back to the quiz on pages 41–51 for ideas; list those things you could begin to do *now* to make further changes. You may find that you have already gone as far as you want to go. That is okay. You may, however, wish to review the situation periodically, say every six months, since you might be ready to make some more changes later on. Our feeling is that if you have come this far, you *will* most likely find ways to make more changes that bring you closer to the end-point goals, either now or in the future.

By the time you reach Phase Three you will have a different perspective about a lower-fat way of eating. Suddenly, you will find that you are no longer backsliding frequently but instead are being more consistent in your lower-fat eating. In short, you will discover that new habits have indeed been formed. Now, instead of devoting so much of your energy just to trying to stick to eating less fat, you will be looking for new ideas to add variety to your newly established eating patterns.

Another pleasant surprise will be your reduced food bill. And you will derive satisfaction, as well, from the realization that your new way of eating contributes to a lowered risk for a number of diseases that presently limit and make miserable many of our lives. Another benefit is a sparing of our natural resources because this way of eating takes less energy to produce.

Phase Three Goals

The groundwork for Phase Three has all been put in place in Phase Two. The major fine tuning that now must be made is a further reduction in meat and fat, especially saturated fat, along with a concommitant *increase* in complex carbohydrates.

We return now to the Six Food Groups of the New American Diet: the whole grains and potatoes; the beans, nuts and seeds; the vegetables; the fruits; the low-fat animal products and fats. Let's look at each of these and see what you need to do:

Whole Grains and Potatoes. Eat two to five servings at *each meal*. Choose from breads, pastas, potatoes, rice, cereals, etc. This can be achieved, for example, by eating toast and cereal for breakfast, a sandwich and bean soup or Baked Corn Chips for lunch, by large servings of potatoes, pasta or rice and bread for dinner, and by eating popcorn, muffins or bagels as snack foods.

Beans, Nuts, Seeds. By the time you've achieved Phase Three goals you will be eating 3 to 5 cups of cooked legumes (beans, peas) *each* week. This can be done by putting beans on salads, serving a variety of bean soups, putting beans in casseroles, using a number of our Mexican dishes, etc. Continue to use nuts and seeds very sparingly and only to spice up grains, beans and vegetable dishes. Use no more than ¼ to ½ cup of nuts per recipe (unsalted, of course).

Vegetables. Eat 2 to 4 cups *per day*. Have vegetables both at lunch and at dinner in one form or another.

Fruits. Eat three to five pieces of fruit *per day*. Fresh fruit is best, but frozen is fine and so is canned fruit as long as the fruit is canned in its own juice, without syrup added. Or, if canned in syrup, drain and rinse the fruit.

Low-Fat Animal Products. Use skim milk, nonfat yogurt and cheeses. Limit ice cream to once a month and keep the quantity to one scoop or less. Your total of red meat, poultry, shrimp, crab and lobster intake should not exceed 3 to 4 ounces per day. The only exception here is that up to 6 ounces of fish, clams, oysters and scallops may be consumed each day. This is not in addition to other meat and cheese but is *in place of* them. This greater quantity of fish is suggested because of the omega-3 fatty acids they contain which, as previously explained, are substances we and others have discovered help hold down blood cholesterol and triglycerides and help protect against blood clotting.

In a typical Phase Three day (you will find a sample Phase Three meal plan for a full week later in this chapter), meat, poultry and fish will be included in only one meal. Leaner meats are heavily emphasized. The meat that is used in the main dish will, typically, be lean beef, pork or lamb one or two days out of the week. Poultry will be used more often —two or three days out of the week; fish will be used two or three times a week. And one or two days may be entirely meatless and cheeseless. Remember that you need to stick to the lower-fat cheeses (CSIs of 12 or less per 3½ ounces) and that when you have cheese you include it in the meat allotment. Thus, if you have 3 ounces of lower-fat cheese on any given day, you should not have *any* meat at all that day.

Fats. Use very sparingly, no more than 4 to 7 teaspoons *per day*. That's a total, includ-

ing both what is in prepared fo cooking, as well as what is ac the table. Avoid typical fried use our "skinny fried" recipes ir added fat to 2 to 4 teaspoons per day (in the form of margarine, mayonnaise, salad dressing). Use peanut butter as a meal item, not as a snack. Reduce saturated fat very sharply by limiting red meat or regular cheese to twice a week. (These are general recommendations; it's up to you to make these fit the end-point goals more precisely.) Use only skim milk. Limit chocolate, as well as ice cream, to once a month. Use nonfat or low-fat yogurt. Use low-fat cheeses as specified above. Avoid coconut, palm and hydrogenated vegetable oils. By Phase Three *all* butter, lard and drippings should be replaced entirely with vegetable oil or soft margarine.

In order to get cholesterol consumption down to the target goal, you will also, in Phase Three, eliminate egg yolks *entirely*, avoid all organ meats and limit daily meat consumption as previously stipulated and as further described in the discussion below.

There are some goals not included in the Six Food Groups that need to be mentioned. These include salt, sugar and alcohol.

To achieve *salt* goals, you will add *no salt whatever* to any food at the table; will cook with small amounts of Lite Salt or reduced sodium soy sauce, using 50 percent *or less* than quantities called for in recipes; will primarily use no-salt-added canned products or will choose fresh and frozen products with no salt added; will limit regular—salt-added— canned soups, vegetables, salad dressings, sauces or entrées to five or fewer items per week and will use salt-free cereals.

To achieve the *sugar* goals, you will eat baked desserts (modified in fat, cholesterol and salt content, as well as sugar) three to four times a week or less. Candy, preferably the nonchocolate varieties (i.e., gum drops), soda pop and fruit-flavored drinks will be consumed once every two weeks or less.

Alcohol will not be an everyday thing. Two to three drinks *or* fewer *each week* is the Phase Three goal.

Let's concentrate now on the most difficult parts of all this—the further reduction of meat and cheese, attended by an increase in complex carbohydrate intake.

Putting the Lid on Meat and Cheese

An increasing number of people are concerned about their level of meat consumption. Many others, however, are reluctant to confront the issue, believing that the only other choice is to eat no meat at all. We promote the idea that there *is* life in the middle. Even though we suggest people cut back on meat in Phase Two and even more in Phase Three, meat remains a part of the New American Diet.

What we discourage is the use of meat, poultry or shellfish as *the* sole item in the *main* course. They can be used *in* the main course but should not be the centerpiece of it. Otherwise, there would be a very tiny serving on your plate. Meat and cheese in Phase Three are almost always used as condiments in vegetable, grain, bean, pasta dishes. They are used to spice up these dishes, as is common in the Oriental, Mediterranean and Mexican cuisines we introduced you to in Phase Two.

Once again, eat no more than one serving per day of fish, poultry, lean meat *or* low-fat cheese, in these quantities: 6 ounces of fish,

clams, oysters, scallops *or* 3 to 4 ounces of red meat, shrimp, crab, lobster or low-fat cheese. That's the general rule. Once you've got that mastered, work toward getting the red meat and cheese intake down to no more than twice a week. In other words, if you have always eaten a lot of red meat, you might find that in order to comply with this goal you will want to have your 3 or 4 ounces in the form of red meat every day for a while. But gradually you can start having poultry and fish more often. The ultimate goal is to have poultry two or three times a week, fish two or three times a week, red meat once or twice a week and no meat or cheese once or twice a week.

You may, however, after experimenting along these lines, still find that eating lean red meat every day is what you personally want to do. This is still going to be a beneficial choice provided you select the *leanest* meats, stick to the prescribed quantities and avoid cheeses, chocolates, ice cream, etc. In other words, ultimately you have to decide what is important to you and do the best *you* can. Sometimes you can break some of the rules by eating more of one thing and less of another. We'll return to these trade-offs, later in this chapter.

When we talk about lean red meats we're talking about those with CSIs of 10 or less per 3½ ounces. Save the fatter meats, including bacon, sausage, lunch meats, spareribs, etc. for only very special occasions, if at all. These high-fat meats fall into the same category as ice cream, high-fat cheese, chocolate, etc. In Phase Three you should eat only *one* of these foods no more than once a month.

There are a couple of tips that may help you cut down on your meat intake in general:

1. Buy *appropriate* amounts of meat. By purchasing just the right amount for yourself or your family you won't be tempted to over-

consume in order not to waste. For a family of four, a typical example might be: red meat—1 to 2 pounds boneless per week; plus fish—4 to 5 pounds per week; plus poultry—2 to 3 pounds boneless per week (or 5 to 6 pounds if bone is included; this is the equivalent of two whole, average-sized chickens).

2. If there are too many complaints about too little meat and especially of ground beef, which has become an American staple, try making the same dishes with ground turkey or ground sirloin (which has only about 10 percent fat) or try a mixture of ground sirloin and textured vegetable protein, a soybean product that is very low in fat. (An example of such a recipe is Beef-Mushroom Spaghetti Sauce.) Thus everyone can fill up without getting excess amounts of fat and cholesterol.

As for the cheeses, remember to stick to those with CSIs of 12 or less per 3½ ounces on the CSI chart. You can regard 1 ounce of cheese with CSIs of 6 to 12 (per 3½ ounces on the chart) as equal to 1 ounce of lean meat.

Fish Dishes. You don't have to become a fish lover to make it to the end-point goals of Phase Three but it certainly helps. The great thing about fish is that you can eat more of it than you can of any meats and still stay within Phase Three guidelines. You can, in fact, eat almost twice as much fish as you can red meats, cheese or poultry—up to 6 ounces per day. This is a change from our previous recommendations and is based upon new scientific findings related to some of the fats fish contain. We used to recommend only 3 or 4 ounces of fish per day and frowned on the use of shellfish completely since they have substantial amounts of cholesterol. However, by using the CSI, which considers both cholesterol and saturated fat together, we can see

that fish, clams, oysters and scallops have very low CSIs. We now recommend up to 6 ounces of these in one day. Shrimp, lobster and crab can be consumed in the same manner as poultry and red meat—up to 3 to 4 ounces a day.

As we noted earlier in this book, Greenland Eskimos and some others who consume large amounts of fish and marine mammals that contain considerable cholesterol nonetheless have low rates of heart disease. Our research group fed healthy individuals and those with elevated blood levels of cholesterol and triglycerides a pound of salmon a day along with some additional salmon oil. This diet resulted, among the healthy subjects, in a 15 percent *reduction* in levels of total blood cholesterol and LDL (low-density lipoproteins associated with heart disease). VLDL (very low-density lipoproteins) and triglycerides (fat) levels also fell—by 40 to 45 percent. The reductions were even greater in the subjects who started out with elevated levels of cholesterol and other blood lipids.

Well, you may be thinking, if a *pound* of salmon a day was so beneficial, why shouldn't *we* eat more than 6 ounces of fish a day? First of all, most of you wouldn't want to eat a whole pound of fish each day even if we said it was okay to do so. But, beyond that, eating this much would calorically crowd out other foods which we think, overall, are very beneficial, such as the complex carbohydrates. So stick to the guideline of having fish two or three times a week for dinner with the limit of a 6-ounce portion.

Many people want to know *which* fish are particularly good sources of the omega-3 fatty acids, the substances that lower the cholesterol and the triglycerides and decrease blood clotting. Almost all fish contain these fatty acids but among particularly good sources are mackerel, tuna, salmon, bluefish, sardines, herring, shad, butterfish, sablefish, pompano, lake trout and rainbow trout. Remember we said earlier (page 72) that the highest-fat fish is almost as lean as the lowest-fat red meat and the CSI is even better in the fish. The CSI of 3½ ounces of salmon (high-fat fish) is 5 compared to a CSI of 9 for 3½ ounces of 10 percent fat red meat (low-fat meat). Therefore, both lean and fatty fish can be eaten.

Some precautions: As stated earlier we do *not* recommend taking fish oil per se, especially cod-liver oil which, taken in tablespoon quantities, would contain toxic amounts of vitamins A and D. Up to one teaspoon of cod-liver oil, which some of you were given daily as children, will not contain toxic amounts of vitamins A and D and will contain considerable omega-3 fatty acids. However, we do not recommend using it or the new fish-oil supplements that are available. And beware of canned fish packed in vegetable oils. Avoid them. These oils are not generally the kind that are going to provide you with the omega-3 fatty acids (those are in the fish themselves). When you buy canned fish try to get the type that comes packed in water or in fish oil. Or, if you get the fish packed in vegetable oil, drain the oil off and rinse with water. Also be aware that most canned fish also has a lot of salt added. Look for no-salt or low-salt labels. Again, rinsing well with water will help get rid of some of this salt.

Some of the favorite fish dishes of our staff and the families we've worked with include Tandoori Fish, Fillet of Fish Florentine, Salmon Mousse, Sweet 'n' Sour Supper (simple since it uses canned tuna), Bouillabaisse (very French), Lively Lemon Roll-Ups (a lot of children like these "fish wrapped up with broccoli inside"), Hearty Fish Soup (a particular favorite), Sesame Halibut (the comment we often get is: "It doesn't taste like fish!") and Skinny Sole (fillet of sole rolled in cornmeal and fried in a tiny amount of oil and served with ketchup; even dedicated fish-resisters fall for this one).

Our fish dishes range from baked fillet quickies to elegant dishes. We offer a number of sauces, and our fish dishes come in a variety of ethnic accents: Oriental, Hawaiian, Creole, French, etc. See part 3.

Chicken and Turkey Dishes. We put a lot of emphasis on these, too, since the CSIs for turkey and chicken are lower than those for most other meats. Here, too, you'll find that our dishes come in a wide variety of "flavors," including Oriental, Continental, curries and so on. Among our favorite chicken dishes are Basic Stir-Fried Chicken (this becomes one of the new "old favorites" very quickly among most of our families because it is so quick and easy; with the right vegetable combinations —several are suggested in our cookbook section, part 3—it makes a delicious meal that can be repeated frequently). For ethnic variety, try our Cashew Chicken, Far East Chicken, Orange Baked Chicken, Chicken Italian, Parmesan Yogurt Chicken, etc. If you are a turkey fan, you'll want to try Turkey-Vegetable Chowder, Simply Wonderful Turkey Salad, Turkey-Mushroom Spaghetti Sauce and Turkey-Lettuce Stir Fry.

Beef, Pork and Veal Dishes. Where's the beef? We still have it, and, on those occasions when you'll be eating red meats, you'll find the beef in a stir-fried dish, Pepper Steak. You'll also find it in our Pizza Rice Casserole, our Stay-Abed Stew, in our Taco Salad, in our more elegant Stuffed Flank Steak Florentine and so on.

You can find pork in our Moo Shoo Pork recipe and veal in our very French Veal Stew with Dill and Veal Roll-Ups recipes. These are the only recipes we have for pork and veal and there are none for lamb, though we have nothing against them, provided you select *very lean* cuts only and stick to the meat guidelines, in terms of quantities. We've concentrated on beef because it is more popular and is more widely used.

Taking the Lid Off Complex Carbohydrates

So far we've been talking about putting the lid *on* meat and cheese consumption. Now we want you to take the lid *off* those foods that provide complex carbohydrates—which is what you replace the fat with. There is even more emphasis in Phase Three on the consumption of more whole grains and legumes —to replace calories lost from decreasing fat intake. In Phase Two we devoted a great deal of effort to changing the typical Western world lunch—principally by replacing meat with beans, grains and low-fat animal products. In Phase Three, emphasis is placed on remodeling dinner, as well.

As you get into Phase Three you'll find that those dishes which use mainly grains, beans and vegetables will be the mainstay of your eating pattern. It is from main dishes consisting mostly of these foods that you are going to get the bulk—and the energy—to replace the fat you're deleting. These lower-fat grain, bean and vegetable dishes contain many fewer calories than comparable typical recipes (see page 116), as well as being lower in saturated fats and cholesterol. Our recipes are as kind to your waistline as to your arteries.

On days when you choose to have little or no meat or cheese you will find that these dishes will be as tasty and satisfying as dishes heavily laden with meat and cheese used to be. For those who have trouble getting into completely meatless meals, try serving a dish with meat (only very lean meat, of course) as a main course but make sure you have one or more appetizing side dishes consisting of our grain, bean and/or vegetable selections. Gradually, you will start filling up on these side dishes and will eat less of the main entree. After a while, a taste for these side dishes is typically acquired even in resistant cases and quite often becomes sufficiently intense that main meat courses can be entirely eliminated on many days. "Practice makes perfect" even—or perhaps especially—when it comes to eating.

Casseroles are particularly good dishes for weaning off of meat. We have a good selection, ranging from Acapulco Bean Casserole to Broccoli with Rice. Other favorites include Bean Stroganoff, Romano Rice and Beans, Garbanzo Goulash, Moroccan Vegetable Stew, Spinach Lasagna, Creamy Enchiladas, Zucchini Pie, Cauliflower Curry, etc.

Another way to increase carbohydrate intake as well as add tremendous variety to your eating style is to build up your repertoire of vegetable recipes. You'll find many ways of making vegetables exciting accessories to meals in our "Side Dishes" section of part 3, where we concentrate on different ways of preparing vegetables, potatoes, grains and beans to go along with entrées to be selected from other sections of our cookbook. These vegetable side dishes include such offerings as Zucchini Mexicali, Ratatouille Provençale, Skinny "French Fries," Homemade Tatertots, Curried Rice, Refried Beans and so on.

Trade-offs

Earlier in this chapter we spoke of trade-offs. Trade-offs offer a means of getting around some of our guidelines and recommendations. They allow you, for example, to eat red meat more often than we recommend (though not in quantities greater than we recommend) provided you are willing to give up other things, such as your chocolate or dessert quota. Trade-offs, as a concept, constitute our recognition that people have unique tastes and will not follow every one of our guidelines precisely. Ultimately, you have to become the scorekeeper.

The chocolate lover may decide that it's worth giving up extra meat in order to eat more chocolate. The same goes for the person who adores butter. To some, ice cream is far more important than meat and cheese. Or some may want to eat regular cheese but be willing to give up some of the meat, the ice cream and the chocolate. Still others may like eating out a great deal or may have to eat out frequently because of business or travel consideration. Those individuals will need to pay attention to what they are eating on the road and then make up for the difference at home, by eating even more meatless or cheeseless dinners and lunches than we call for.

Trade-offs enable you to be adaptable, provided you use common sense and exert some discipline. They close the door on restrictiveness and open the door to variety, and in the long run, will enable you to go further with the program than you would otherwise do. It takes eight or nine months to begin to get a real feel for trade-offs. Then you can use what you've learned to create your own unique eating style. Be creative and flexible. But don't delude yourself, either. Keep the end-point goals firmly in view so that you can achieve maximum prevention of those diseases of over- (and under-) consumption that still limit the lives and potential of so many of us.

In table 17 are some sample Phase Three meal plans.

Review of Goals and Results of Phase Three

The meals outlined above—a *sample* of Phase Three eating—achieve the *end-point* goals of the New American Diet:

1. Cholesterol intake is reduced, on average, from 200 milligrams at the end of Phase Two to approximately 100 milligrams at the end of Phase Three.

2. Fat content of the diet decreases from 25 percent at the end of Phase Two to 20 percent in Phase Three. Saturated fat, in Phase Three, accounts for only 5 to 6 percent of total caloric intake.

3. Carbohydrates, accounting for approximately 50 percent of total calories in Phase One, and for about 60 percent in Phase Two, account for 65 percent in Phase Three. The dietary fiber content of the diet has increased from about 15 to 20 grams per day, in the typical American Diet, to 45 to 60 grams per day in Phase Three. And though total carbohydrate intake has increased substantially, carbohydrate in the form of added sugar has decreased from 20 percent of calories, in the typical American Diet, to 10 percent of calories in Phase Three.

In addition to the above, sodium intake is reduced by another 13 percent, on average, in Phase Three, arriving at our end-point goal of 1725 milligrams per day for women and 2415 milligrams per day for men. The potassium intake remains little changed from Phase Two.

Protein intake remains constant and abundant at 15 percent but, in Phase Three, the

TABLE 17
New American Diet Phase Three Meal Plans

	DAY 1	DAY 2	DAY 3	DAY 4	DAY 5	DAY 6	DAY 7
Breakfast	Orange juice, 3/4 cup; Applesauce, unsweetened, 1/2 cup; Oatmeal Buttermilk Pancakes, 4; Soft margarine, 2 tsp.; Syrup, 1/4 cup	Cantaloupe, 1/2; Puffed Wheat, 1 cup; Skim milk, 3/4 cup; Whole wheat English muffin, 1; Strawberry preserves, 2 tsp.	Fresh raspberries, 1/2 cup; Shredded Wheat, 1 cup; Skim milk, 3/4 cup; Whole wheat raisin bread, 2 slices; Soft margarine, 2 tsp.	Sliced banana in Plain low-fat yogurt, 6 oz.; Cereal Bran Muffin, 2; Orange marmalade, 1 Tbsp.	Pink grapefruit, 1/2; Skinny hash browns: Shredded potatoes, 1 cup; Vegetable oil, 1 tsp.; Whole wheat toast, 2 slices; Blackberry preserves, 2 tsp.	Honeydew melon, 1/2; Oatmeal, 1 cup; Skim milk, 3/4 cup; Whole wheat English muffin, 1/2; Honey, 2 tsp.	Orange juice, 3/4 cup; German Oven Pancake, 1/2, with Blueberries, 1/2 cup and Peaches, 1/2 cup and Powdered sugar, 1 tsp.
Morning Snack		Cereal Bran Muffin			Whole wheat cinnamon raisin bagel		
Lunch	Greek Lentil Soup, 1 cup; Melba rounds, 6; Reduced Calories Laughing Cow, 3/4 oz.; Green grapes, 1 cup	Burrito: Flour tortilla (8"); Refried Beans, 1/2 cup; Chowchow, 1/2 cup; Plain low-fat yogurt, 2 tsp.	Chili Bean Salad, 1 cup served in Whole wheat pita bread; Potato Leek Soup, 1 cup; Orange	Four Star Pasta Salad, 1 svg.; Corn on the cob, 1 piece; Soft margarine, 2 tsp.; Wheatberry roll; Apple	Salad Bar: Lettuce, 1 cup; Cherry tomatoes, 4; Radishes, 4 slices; Cucumber slices, 1/4 cup; Kidney beans, 1/4 cup; Garbanzo beans, 1/4 cup; Dressing: Vinegar, 3 Tbsp.; Oil, 4 tsp.; Baked Potato with Low-fat cottage cheese, 1/4 cup	Minestrone Soup, 2 cups; Corn Bread, 1 piece (3" x 3"); Fruit cup: Orange sections, 1/4 cup; Banana slices, 1/4 cup; Grapes, 1/4 cup	In Restaurant: Crab Louie: Crab, 3 oz.; Egg white, 1; Lettuce, 1 1/2 cups; Carrot (grated) 1/4 cup; Cucumber, 1/4 cup; Tomato, 1/2; Black olive; Thousand Island Salad Dressing, 1/4 cup (brought from home); Whole wheat rolls, 2

TABLE 17—Continued

	DAY 1	DAY 2	DAY 3	DAY 4	DAY 5	DAY 6	DAY 7
Afternoon Snack		Blueberry frozen yogurt (low-fat), 4 oz. on cone					
Dinner	Cashew Chicken, 1 svg. Steamed rice, 1½ cups Lettuce, 1 cup Red French Salad Dressing, 2 Tbsp. Fresh sliced pineapple, 1¼ cups Hot Fudge Pudding Cake, 1 svg.	Turkey Vegetable Chowder, 2 cups Baked potato Soft margarine, 2 tsp. Carrot-Raisin Salad, ¾ cup Whole wheat dinner rolls, 2	Lively Lemon Roll-Ups, 1 svg. Steamed carrots, ⅔ cup Sunshine Spinach Salad, 2 cups Whole wheat sourdough rolls, 2 Apricot Meringue Bars, 2	Pizza Rice Casserole, 1 svg. Green peas, ⅔ cup Baked squash, ½ Whole Wheat French Bread, 4 pieces (2" diameter)	Parmesan Yogurt Chicken, 1 svg. Fettuccine, 1½ cups Steamed broccoli, 1 cup Whole wheat dinner rolls, 2 Grape ice, ½ cup	Baked Snapper with Spicy Tomato Sauce, 1 svg. Baked potato Soft margarine, 2 tsp. Stuffed Zucchini Boats, 1 svg. Waldorf Salad, 1 svg. Caraway Dinner Rolls, 2 Pinto Fiesta Cake, 1 svg.	Spaghetti, 1½ cups with Marinara Sauce, 1 cup and Parmesan cheese, 2 Tbsp. Lettuce Salad, 1 cup Western Salad Dressing, 2 Tbsp. Steamed green beans, ½ cup Whole Wheat French Bread, 4 pieces (2" diameter) Wine or sparkling grape juice, 6 oz.
Evening Snack	Popcorn (air-popped), 3 cups Soft margarine, 1 tsp.	Banana	"Egg" Salad Sandwich Spread, ¼ cup on Soda crackers (unsalted tops), 6	Graham crackers, 3 Skim milk, 1 cup	Apple Gingersnaps, 2		Popcorn (air-popped), 3 cups with Soft margarine, 1 tsp.

NOTE: Recipes that are in italics can be found in part 3.

TABLE 17—Continued

Nutrient Composition	DAY 1	DAY 2	DAY 3	DAY 4	DAY 5	DAY 6	DAY 7	Average	Phase Three Goal
Calories	2218	1873	2017	1918	2018	1790	1993	1975	2000*
Protein, % Calories	12	15	19	16	16	18	16	16	15
Fat, % Calories	14	16	19	19	19	20	19	18	20
Carbohydrate, % Calories	73	69	63	64	65	62	59	65	65
Saturated Fat, % Calories	3.2	4.3	4.0	4.9	3.8	4.0	4.1	4.0	5.0
Polyunsaturated Fat, % Calories	4.7	4.3	6.7	5.6	7.2	6.7	5.2	5.6	8.0
Cholesterol, mg†	41	57	119	74	70	114	101	82	<100‡
CSI	10	12	15	14	12	14	14	13	16
Sodium, mg	1685	1921	2066	1722	1733	1567	1869	1795	1725
Potassium, mg	3370	4338	3494	4191	3162	4615	3054	3746	3900
Calcium, mg	528	1076	986	1157	549	792	900	855	800

* This is a food pattern for people who require 2000 Calories to maintain their weight.
† Mg = milligram.
‡ < = less than.

end-point goal of attaining about 56 percent of total protein from vegetable sources and 44 percent from animal sources is achieved.

We cannot predict the *exact* amount by which blood levels of cholesterol will be lowered in *each* individual as a result of following the Phase Three diet. But, on average, there is an expected lowering of 16 to 20 percent over baseline measurements related to the standard American diet. This means that a person who started with 260 milligrams of cholesterol per 100 milliliters of blood could now be at 213. This is a very significant reduction. Since each 1 percent reduction in blood levels of cholesterol reduces by 2 percent the risk of coronary heart disease, this drop in cholesterol could mean a decrease of about 35 percent in the risk of coronary heart disease.

How to Tell When You've Achieved Phase Three Goals

You can assess your Phase Three progress by retaking the quiz found on pages 41–51. The following scores correspond with Phase Three goals:

MEAT, FISH AND POULTRY
Question 1   5
Question 2   4 to 5
Question 3   26 to 30
Question 4   4 (Men/Teens)
              5 (Women/Children)
Question 5   4 to 5

Total score   43 to 50

DAIRY PRODUCTS AND EGGS

Question 1 5
Question 2 5
Question 3 4 to 5
Question 4 4 to 5
Question 5 3 to 5
Question 6 5
Question 7 5

Total score 31 to 35

FATS AND OILS

Question 1 4 to 5
Question 2 4 (Men/Teens)
            5 (Women/Children)
Question 3 5
Question 4 4 to 5
Question 5 4 to 5

Total score 21 to 25

GRAINS, BEANS, FRUITS AND VEGETABLES

	Men/Teens	Women/Children
Question 1	22 to 25	14 to 16
Question 2	18 to 22	13 to 16
Question 3	20 to 25	11 to 15
Question 4	20 to 35	13 to 18
Question 5	39 to 43	29 to 32
Question 6	10	5
Question 7	0	0
Total score	129 to 160	85 to 102

SWEETS AND SNACKS

Question 1 5
Question 2 5
Question 3 5
Question 4 5
Question 5 5
Question 6 4 to 5

Total score 29 to 30

SALT

Question 1 4 to 5
Question 2 5
Question 3 5
Question 4 5
Question 5 5

Total score 24 to 25

10

WEIGHT LOSS/WEIGHT MAINTENANCE

REPLACING "YO-YO" DIETING WITH LIFELONG WEIGHT CONTROL

The Real Problem Is Weight *Maintenance*

If you are struggling with weight control, you have no doubt already tried many diets, and you have probably lost weight on most of those diets. People are very good at losing weight; many have lost hundreds of pounds. They are also very good at gaining it all right back. Follow-up studies of a wide variety of popular diets indicate that the failure rate is 90 percent or greater for these weight-loss diets. Most dieters lose weight but fail to keep it off for more than a few months. So then it's back to another diet.

And with each new diet you may have found it more difficult to shed the excess weight. This practice of alternately losing and gaining weight on one diet after another has been called "yo-yo" dieting in some circles and has been labeled "the rhythm method of girth control" by Dr. Jean Mayer, a prominent nutritionist who is president of Tufts University. Whatever you call it, the practice is both ineffective over the long term and, worse, is *dangerous*, as you'll see later on in this chapter. You'll also learn why many diets might actually be fattening in the long run.

Obesity is a problem throughout the Western world, and the greatest nutritional concern of people in the United States is, in a word, calories. Obesity poses very serious medical and psychological perils. While we understand weight loss scientifically—and people can and do lose weight—we still have a very great deal to learn about weight gain and weight maintenance. It is easy, for example, to predict how much weight a person will lose from a particular diet. No matter what one's weight, a pound of fat will ultimately be lost for every 3500 Calories deficit. It is not possible, however, to predict the amount of weight a person will gain. It may, according to current estimates, take anywhere from 500 to 5,000 Calories or more to result in 1 pound of gained weight! The body has as yet a poorly understood mechanism to resist weight gain called "thermogenesis."

The hard facts are these: If you have a persistent weight problem, it's not going to be easy to achieve *and* maintain the lower weight you're aiming for. *We do believe, however, that the New American Diet provides the best chance for maintaining a lower body weight once it is achieved—and for maintaining it on a long-term, possibly permanent, basis.*

And there are a number of advantages to using the New American Diet in your effort to get the weight off in the first place. First, on our diet you can eat *a lot* because what you do eat is so low in fat and high in bulk. The quantity of food you eat in the diet is, at 1000 Calories, about the same in bulk that you'd get in the present American diet at 1600 Calories!

Second, the New American Diet promotes the maximum loss of body fat during weight reduction. This means there is little loss of muscle and water (lean body mass). Our diet reduces fat and spares lean body mass far more than many popular diets. We'll explain later in this chapter why this distinction is so important and why, from a scientific point of view, it makes it easier to resist the insidious yo-yo effect that plagues so many dieters.

Third, the New American Diet does not contain either *too much* or *too little* of any one nutrient. And, fourth, it helps avoid the constipation which is often a problem people encounter while losing weight.

Definitions and Consequences of Obesity

A federal consensus conference, convened by the National Institutes of Health, recently declared that obesity, previously considered by some as merely a nuisance or a psychological disorder, is a *physical disease* with potentially fatal consequences. Dr. William Castelli, director of the famed thirty-six-year-old Framingham Heart Study, declared at the conference: "Obesity is as powerful a risk factor as any that we know, including smoking and high blood pressure." The Framingham data strongly suggest for the first time that obesity is an "independent risk factor" in heart disease and that it can contribute to premature death in otherwise healthy men. (The same probably holds true for women, as well, though the data will have to be further analyzed before this is clearly demonstrated.)

But, in addition to cardiovascular disease, the federal panel of experts found, on the basis of the best available research evidence, that obesity can also contribute significantly to high blood pressure, to cancers of the breast and uterus in women, to cancer of the prostate in men, to cancers of the colon and rectum in both men and women and to the development of so-called Type II (adult-onset) diabetes in susceptible individuals.

The *psychological* problems related to obesity were recognized by the panel—but not as causes but rather as one of the consequences of obesity. In fact, the panel concluded that the "enormous psychological burden" obesity imposes on an individual "may be the gravest effect of obesity."

It was not the purpose of this particular panel to prescribe treatments for obesity (a future panel will address that issue) but, rather, to define obesity and describe its known consequences. The panel found that *any* degree of obesity will increase health risks. It cited the 1983 Metropolitan Life Insurance Company table of "desirable" body weights (for men and women of different heights and frame sizes) in arriving at its definition of obesity. Weight 20 percent or above those cited in table 18 is defined as the sort of obesity that calls for *medical intervention,* according to the panel. And this is so, the panel added, even if the individual is healthy in every other respect. Individuals with diabetes and high blood pressure, high blood fat levels or those who have a family tendency toward such problems require treatment for overweight even earlier.

The type of food eaten to produce the weight gain may contribute more to the health problems than the small excess body weight itself. In addition, many researchers believe that the "desirable" weights cited by Metropolitan may be too high to begin with; these figures have been highly controversial since they appeared in 1983.

Information was presented at the conference that indicates that approximately *34 million Americans* are obese (20 percent or more above the "desirable" weights). More than *11 million* of these are *extremely overweight* and thus are at very high risk of developing one or more of the diseases mentioned above. The risks for these individuals are *several times higher* than for the general population.

The panel recognized that better methods are needed to evaluate obesity and its risks in different individuals. It recommended further investigation of one promising new method developed by Dr. Per Bjorntorp and colleagues at the University of Göteborg in Sweden. This method compares waist and hip measurements. In the Swedish studies, it was found that a potbelly in men may carry with it greater risk of cardiovascular disease than just being generally overweight or carrying the excess poundage elsewhere on the body. The risk for cardiovascular disease seems to increase sharply when a man's waist measurement is the same as or bigger than his hip measurement. The same is true, he adds, for women whose hips are not at least 20 percent larger than their waists.

Methods of determining the composition of your body (fat versus lean body mass) which are much more sophisticated than simply getting on a set of scales are currently being developed in medical centers throughout the world. A practical, at-home way of getting *some* idea of body fatness is to compute your Body Mass Index (BMI). You can do this most easily if you have a pocket calculator handy.

How to calculate your body mass index:

1. Convert your weight from pounds to kilograms by dividing your weight in pounds by 2.2

2. Convert your height from inches to centimeters by multiplying your height in inches by 2.54.

3. Square your height in centimeters by multiplying it times itself.

4. Divide your weight in kilograms by your height in centimeters squared.

5. Multiply the answer by 10,000. This is your Body Mass Index (BMI).

This all sounds terribly complicated but it isn't. Here's an example. Let's say you're a

TABLE 18
1983 Metropolitan Height and Weight Tables for Men and Women
According to Frame, Ages 25–59

Height (In Shoes)†		Weight in Pounds (In Indoor Clothing)*		
		Small Frame	Medium Frame	Large Frame
Feet	Inches			
		MEN		
5	2	128–134	131–141	138–150
5	3	130–136	133–143	140–153
5	4	132–138	135–145	142–156
5	5	134–140	137–148	144–160
5	6	136–142	139–151	146–164
5	7	138–145	142–154	149–168
5	8	140–148	145–157	152–172
5	9	142–151	148–160	155–176
5	10	144–154	151–163	158–180
5	11	146–157	154–166	161–184
6	0	149–160	157–170	164–188
6	1	152–164	160–174	168–192
6	2	155–168	164–178	172–197
6	3	158–172	167–182	176–202
6	4	162–176	171–187	181–207
		WOMEN		
4	10	102–111	109–121	118–131
4	11	103–113	111–123	120–134
5	0	104–115	113–126	122–137
5	1	106–118	115–129	125–140
5	2	108–121	118–132	128–143
5	3	111–124	121–135	131–147
5	4	114–127	124–138	134–151
5	5	117–130	127–141	137–155
5	6	120–133	130–144	140–159
5	7	123–136	133–147	143–163
5	8	126–139	136–150	146–167
5	9	129–142	139–153	149–170
5	10	132–145	142–156	152–173
5	11	135–148	145–159	155–176
6	0	138–151	148–162	158–179

* Indoor clothing weighing 5 pounds for men and 3 pounds for women.
† Shoes with 1-inch heels.
SOURCE OF BASIC DATA: *Build Study,* 1979 (Society of Actuaries and Association of Life Insurance Medical Directors of America, 1980).
Copyright 1983 Metropolitan Life Insurance Company.

woman who is 5 feet 4 inches weighing 137 pounds. This is how to compute your Body Mass Index.

1. Divide 137 pounds by 2.2 which gives us *62.3 kilograms.*

2. Multiply 64 inches by 2.54 which comes to *162.6 centimeters.*

3. Square the height by multiplying 162.6 times 162.6 arriving at *26,439.*

4. Now divide 62.3 by 26,439 to get an answer of *0.0023564.*

5. Multiply 0.0023564 by 10,000 to get the Body Mass Index of *23.6.*

To avoid this calculation we have provided table 19, which gives the body mass index for a variety of heights and weights.

People who are at "desirable" weights will have BMIs of approximately 22.5 or less. (This and subsequent numbers were derived from the Metropolitan tables using the weight of the midpoint of the medium-frame person.) The value of the BMI is that it provides a number which is independent of the differences that occur in height and weight for varying ages and is also independent of the differences in height and weight that occur between males and females at any age. Therefore, *one number* can be used to delineate obesity for everyone of *any age* and *any height*— and this is the Body Mass Index (BMI). As you can see, the woman in our example is a little overweight according to the BMI.

At 10 percent above "desirable" weight the BMI will be about 24.8; at 20 percent above the desirable weight the BMI will be about 27. These numbers will be slightly different for small- and large-framed people.

When we applied this measure of obesity to randomly selected individuals largely representative of the population as a whole we found that the mean (intermediate) BMI measurement for men over age 16 was 24.7; for women over age 16 it was 23.5; for boys ages 6–15 it was 17; and for girls ages 6–15 it was 17.2. The typical man or woman in the United States is somewhat overweight and has a BMI associated with being 8 to 10 percent above "desirable" weight. Individuals in populations noted for a low incidence of obesity, and the diseases related thereto, typically have BMIs *less than 22.*

Some of the Possible Causes of Obesity

Why do people become fat? There are many reasons, of course. Some of the reasons, accounting for individual variability, are genetic and are not well understood scientifically. These differences make it easier for some people to put on excess weight than for others. But there is another factor that is very important. This factor relates to the question of why people in developed nations such as the United States tend toward overweight.

Why, in other words, do we overeat? The answer can probably be found in our not-so-distant past: a mechanism that has helped ensure our survival in times of food shortages is still with us, enduring in our case long beyond its usefulness, now harming rather than helping us. In prehistoric times, in the era of the caveman, and throughout much of our history on this planet and even today, people have been confronted by frequent periods of food *scarcity.* Nature gave us a "thrifty gene" which induced us to eat more than we really needed during times of plenty so that we would store

TABLE 19
Body Mass Index for a Variety of Weights and Heights

Height in Inches

Weight in Pounds	56	57	58	59	60	61	62	63	64	65	66	67	68	69	70	71	72	73	74	75	76	77	78
80	17.9	17.3	16.7	16.2	15.6	15.1	14.6	14.2	13.7	13.3	12.9	12.5	12.2	11.8	11.5	11.2	10.9	10.6	10.3	10.0	9.7	9.5	9.3
85	19.1	18.4	17.8	17.2	16.6	16.1	15.6	15.1	14.6	14.2	13.7	13.3	12.9	12.6	12.2	11.9	11.5	11.2	10.9	10.6	10.4	10.1	9.8
90	20.2	19.5	18.8	18.2	17.6	17.0	16.5	16.0	15.5	15.0	14.5	14.1	13.7	13.3	12.9	12.6	12.2	11.9	11.6	11.3	11.0	10.7	10.4
95	21.3	20.6	19.9	19.2	18.6	18.0	17.4	16.8	16.3	15.8	15.3	14.9	14.5	14.0	13.6	13.3	12.9	12.5	12.2	11.9	11.6	11.3	11.0
100	22.4	21.7	20.9	20.2	19.5	18.9	18.3	17.7	17.2	16.7	16.2	15.7	15.2	14.8	14.4	14.0	13.6	13.2	12.8	12.5	12.2	11.9	11.6
105	23.6	22.7	22.0	21.2	20.5	19.9	19.2	18.6	18.0	17.5	17.0	16.5	16.0	15.5	15.1	14.7	14.3	13.9	13.5	13.1	12.8	12.5	12.1
110	24.7	23.8	23.0	22.2	21.5	20.8	20.1	19.5	18.9	18.3	17.8	17.2	16.7	16.3	15.8	15.4	14.9	14.5	14.1	13.8	13.4	13.1	12.7
115	25.8	24.9	24.1	23.2	22.5	21.7	21.0	20.4	19.8	19.2	18.6	18.0	17.5	17.0	16.5	16.1	15.6	15.2	14.8	14.4	14.0	13.6	13.3
120	26.9	26.0	25.1	24.3	23.5	22.7	22.0	21.3	20.6	20.0	19.4	18.8	18.3	17.7	17.2	16.7	16.3	15.8	15.4	15.0	14.6	14.2	13.9
125	28.0	27.1	26.1	25.3	24.4	23.6	22.9	22.2	21.5	20.8	20.2	19.6	19.0	18.5	17.9	17.4	17.0	16.5	16.1	15.6	15.2	14.8	14.5
130	29.2	28.2	27.2	26.3	25.4	24.6	23.8	23.0	22.3	21.6	21.0	20.4	19.8	19.2	18.7	18.1	17.6	17.2	16.7	16.3	15.8	15.4	15.0
135	30.3	29.2	28.2	27.3	26.4	25.5	24.7	23.9	23.2	22.5	21.8	21.2	20.5	20.0	19.4	18.8	18.3	17.8	17.3	16.9	16.4	16.0	15.6
140	31.4	30.3	29.3	28.3	27.4	26.5	25.6	24.8	24.0	23.3	22.6	21.9	21.3	20.7	20.1	19.5	19.0	18.5	18.0	17.5	17.1	16.6	16.2
145	32.5	31.4	30.3	29.3	28.3	27.4	26.5	25.7	24.9	24.1	23.4	22.7	22.1	21.4	20.8	20.2	19.7	19.1	18.6	18.1	17.7	17.2	16.8
150	33.7	32.5	31.4	30.3	29.3	28.4	27.5	26.6	25.8	25.0	24.2	23.5	22.8	22.2	21.5	20.9	20.4	19.8	19.3	18.8	18.3	17.8	17.3
155	34.8	33.6	32.4	31.3	30.3	29.3	28.4	27.5	26.6	25.8	25.0	24.3	23.6	22.9	22.3	21.6	21.0	20.5	19.9	19.4	18.9	18.4	17.9
160	35.9	34.7	33.5	32.3	31.3	30.3	29.3	28.4	27.5	26.6	25.8	25.1	24.3	23.6	23.0	22.3	21.7	21.1	20.6	20.0	19.5	19.0	18.5
165	37.0	35.7	34.5	33.4	32.2	31.2	30.2	29.3	28.3	27.5	26.7	25.9	25.1	24.4	23.7	23.0	22.4	21.8	21.2	20.6	20.1	19.6	19.1
170	38.1	36.8	35.6	34.4	33.2	32.1	31.1	30.1	29.2	28.3	27.5	26.6	25.9	25.1	24.4	23.7	23.1	22.4	21.8	21.3	20.7	20.2	19.7
175	39.3	37.9	36.6	35.4	34.2	33.1	32.0	31.0	30.1	29.1	28.3	27.4	26.6	25.8	25.1	24.4	23.7	23.1	22.5	21.9	21.3	20.8	20.2
180	40.4	39.0	37.6	36.4	35.2	34.0	32.9	31.9	30.9	30.0	29.1	28.2	27.4	26.6	25.8	25.1	24.4	23.8	23.1	22.5	21.9	21.4	20.8
185	41.5	40.1	38.7	37.4	36.2	35.0	33.9	32.8	31.8	30.8	29.9	29.0	28.2	27.3	26.6	25.8	25.1	24.4	23.8	23.1	22.5	22.0	21.4
190	42.6	41.1	39.7	38.4	37.1	35.9	34.8	33.7	32.6	31.6	30.7	29.8	28.9	28.1	27.3	26.5	25.8	25.1	24.4	23.8	23.1	22.5	22.0
195	43.8	42.2	40.8	39.4	38.1	36.9	35.7	34.6	33.5	32.5	31.5	30.6	29.7	28.8	28.0	27.2	26.5	25.7	25.1	24.4	23.8	23.1	22.6
200	44.9	43.3	41.8	40.4	39.1	37.8	36.6	35.5	34.4	33.3	32.3	31.3	30.4	29.6	28.7	27.9	27.1	26.4	25.7	25.0	24.4	23.7	23.1
205	46.0	44.4	42.9	41.4	40.1	38.8	37.5	36.3	35.2	34.1	33.1	32.1	31.2	30.3	29.4	28.6	27.8	27.1	26.3	25.6	25.0	24.3	23.7
210	47.1	45.5	43.9	42.4	41.0	39.7	38.4	37.2	36.1	35.0	33.9	32.9	32.0	31.0	30.2	29.3	28.5	27.7	27.0	26.3	25.6	24.9	24.3
215	48.2	46.6	45.0	43.5	42.0	40.7	39.4	38.1	36.9	35.8	34.7	33.7	32.7	31.8	30.9	30.0	29.2	28.4	27.6	26.9	26.2	25.5	24.9
220	49.4	47.6	46.0	44.5	43.0	41.6	40.3	39.0	37.8	36.6	35.5	34.5	33.5	32.5	31.6	30.7	29.9	29.0	28.3	27.5	26.8	26.1	25.4
225	50.5	48.7	47.1	45.5	44.0	42.5	41.2	39.9	38.7	37.5	36.3	35.3	34.2	33.3	32.3	31.4	30.5	29.7	28.9	28.1	27.4	26.7	26.0
230	51.6	49.8	48.1	46.5	45.0	43.5	42.1	40.8	39.5	38.3	37.2	36.1	35.0	34.0	33.0	32.1	31.2	30.4	29.6	28.8	28.0	27.3	26.6
235	52.7	50.9	49.2	47.5	45.9	44.4	43.0	41.7	40.4	39.1	38.0	36.8	35.8	34.7	33.7	32.8	31.9	31.0	30.2	29.4	28.6	27.9	27.2
240	53.8	52.0	50.2	48.5	46.9	45.4	43.9	42.5	41.2	40.0	38.8	37.6	36.5	35.5	34.5	33.5	32.6	31.7	30.8	30.0	29.2	28.5	27.8
245	55.0	53.1	51.2	49.5	47.9	46.3	44.8	43.4	42.1	40.8	39.6	38.4	37.3	36.2	35.2	34.2	33.3	32.3	31.5	30.6	29.8	29.1	28.3
250	56.1	54.1	52.3	50.5	48.9	47.3	45.8	44.3	42.9	41.6	40.4	39.2	38.0	36.9	35.9	34.9	33.9	33.0	32.1	31.3	30.5	29.7	28.9
255	57.2	55.2	53.3	51.5	49.8	48.2	46.7	45.2	43.8	42.5	41.2	40.0	38.8	37.7	36.6	35.6	34.6	33.7	32.8	31.9	31.1	30.3	29.5
260	58.3	56.3	54.4	52.6	50.8	49.2	47.6	46.1	44.7	43.3	42.0	40.8	39.6	38.4	37.3	36.3	35.3	34.3	33.4	32.5	31.7	30.9	30.1

excess fat to burn during times of scarcity. The extra fat was important for survival when confronted by injury, disease, famine and other forms of stress.

Little wonder then that, for long periods of time in human history, fat was considered desirable and, indeed, beautiful. Because only the rich and/or the strong had the resources to acquire fat it was considered a status symbol indicative of wealth and power.

Now that the Western world is, in a relative sense, awash in plenty, fat no longer distinguishes the rich and powerful from the poor and weak. Fat is out of fashion but, alas, thanks to that persistent "thrifty gene" it is still far from being out of sight. Modern technology has provided us with a plentiful supply of food, not just seasonally but twelve months out of every year. Our "natural" drive is to eat when food is available and so we do—very often to excess. Technology has also greatly reduced our expenditure of energy. Machines do our work and transport us. Thus, people in our society need less food than in former times. (More about the role of exercise later.)

Another reason people in developed nations tend to be overweight almost certainly has to do with our heavy intake of fat in the diet, accounting for 40 percent of all our calories. In scientific studies, rats permitted to eat as much as they wanted whenever they wanted, became significantly fatter when given high-fat fare than when given low-fat food. The scientific evidence is not quite so conclusive for humans, but it is known that the people of the Western world, where diet is high in fat, are heavier than the people of other countries where low-fat food is more typical. And within the United States itself it has been shown that strict vegetarians weigh 25 pounds less, as a group, than nonvegetarians, as a group. The reason why high-fat diets may promote weight gain is unknown. However, the fat which is eaten is, within a matter of minutes after it is absorbed and transported to the blood, deposited in the fat tissues. On the other hand, carbohydrate and protein in the diet go to the liver and do not directly provide fat for the fat tissues. Of course, excessive calories from carbohydrate and even protein may ultimately be converted to fat by the liver and transported for storage in the fat tissues, but this process requires considerable energy.

What all of this comes down to is that perhaps the most basic cause of a population being overweight is simply the overconsumption of calories over the needs of the body for energy, and particularly of calories derived from fat. This may seem obvious, but, judging by all of the diverse and sometimes contradictory theories that have been put forward over the years, it is not. We would all do well to focus more attention on the obvious: *overeating* and especially overeating *fat*. The role of reduced physical activity is also important in producing obesity. In our culture muscles are used less and less in daily work; thus the need for calories in the midst of an abundant supply is less than in past generations.

Why Some Diets Can Be Dangerous—And Even Fattening (And Why the New American Diet Can Make Long-Term Weight Control Feasible)

The hazards of repeated weight loss and re-peated weight gain are significant. In fact, if you are overweight, it is better to stay in that condition than it is to lose weight and then several months later regain it all. "Yo-yo" dieting takes a heavy toll on the body. The flow of bile, a digestive fluid, is greatly altered during periods of weight loss. During these periods the bile becomes thick, and there is an increased tendency in the gallbladder to form gallstones from this thickened fluid.

It has been shown in experimental animals that "yo-yo" dieting can also have adverse cardiovascular effects. Weight loss causes a mobilization of fat in the form of free fatty acids. This elevation, if brief, is not likely to be harmful, but many diet programs result in longer-term elevation of free fatty acids, and in some of the programs with a very low or absent carbohydrate intake an actual ten-dency toward acidosis and a condition called "ketosis" develops, with loss of water and salts from the body in the urine.

All of these changes in the body's chemis-try accelerate the development of atheroscle-rosis and the formation of blood clots. They also usually lead to hyperlipidemia, elevation of blood fats (triglyceride and cholesterol), especially when not enough carbohydrate is present in the weight-loss diet.

No one should attempt to lose weight with-out first having a reasonable plan for *long-term* weight maintenance once the weight is lost. More important than getting the weight off is *keeping it off*.

The *type* of diet you select may also have a lot to do with not being able to maintain weight-loss over the long term. The worst re-sults come from the so-called "starvation" or low-carbohydrate "ketogenic" diets. The ketogenic diets are those high protein/low carbohydrate diets which have been so popu-lar in recent years under a variety of names. The reason for their popularity is that they *do* result in rapid weight loss, some of which is just water loss from the body. The most sig-nificant problem with these diets—apart from the fact that they are too low in carbohydrate —is that the weight loss that results from them comes too much from lean body mass (muscle and water) rather than from fat.

These types of diets have a number of con-sequences you should be aware of. Weight, when it is almost inevitably regained, comes back as 65 to 70 percent fat in the typical individual. Since muscle is more active met-abolically than fat it takes more calories to maintain muscle than it does to maintain fat. The higher the fat-to-muscle ratio, therefore, the *fewer* calories it will take to maintain weight.

Theoretically, what this boils down to is that, yes, you can lose weight rapidly on crash, starvation, and ketogenic diets, but you will lose lean body mass as well as fat. And then when you regain weight, you get back the fat as fat and also some of the lean body mass as fat. That sets you back further than ever because all the new fat gives you a body with less lean body mass, which will then require even fewer calories to maintain your weight. So, unless caloric intake contin-ues to be stringently restricted, you will gain weight with greater ease than ever before.

The same number of calories that used to *sustain* you now *inflates* you! Your struggle is now more difficult than ever. If you had kept more of your lean body mass and lost more fat instead, you would, after having arrived at your target diet, been able to eat more and maintain that target weight more easily.

TABLE 20
Composition of Tissue Lost on Different Diets

	Lean Body Mass (Percent of Weight Loss)	Fat
Starvation or fasting	68	32
Ketogenic diets (less than 1000 Calories)	65	35
Mixed food diets (less than 1000 Calories)	40	60
Mixed food diets (more than 1000 Calories)	32	68
Mixed food diets plus mild exercise (more than 1000 Calories)	21	79

Table 20 shows you the composition of tissue lost on different short-term weight-loss programs. Note that on the starvation/ketogenic diets an enormous 65 to 68 percent of the loss was from lean body mass and only 32 to 35 percent was from fat. When there was a somewhat more balanced (mixed) diet but one that was still very restricted calorically (providing 800 to 1000 Calories), there was some improvement. There was even more improvement with a mixed diet providing more than 1000 Calories. The greatest amount of weight lost as fat was achieved when a mixed diet providing more than 1000 Calories was combined with a program of mild exercise.

We have found that the diet program which promotes maximum weight lost as fat is one that is made up of a variety of foods, is 800 to 1200 Calories for women and 1200 to 2000 Calories for men. Our diet programs are always accompanied by increased physical activity. This can take the form of walking for 30 minutes per day, swimming, jogging, bicycling, rowing, tennis, etc. The purpose of the increased exercise is twofold: (1) The loss of muscle tissue (lean body mass) is lessened during weight loss if the muscles are put to work and (2) exercise tends to inhibit the appetite and the desire for food.

Let's look at an example, based on theoretical computations from short-term metabolic studies, to see what type of diet might serve you best. Let's take a forty-five-year-old woman who is 5 feet 4 inches tall and now weighs 170 pounds. She wants to lose 45 pounds to attain her goal of 125 pounds. How can she do it?

A. She can choose a 500- to 800-Calorie, *very low carbohydrate* diet and lose 45 pounds in less than four months. At the end of that period, 51 percent of her body weight will be fat tissue and 49 percent will be lean body mass. Because of that relative distribution of fat versus lean tissue, she will have to restrict herself to a mere 1553 Calories to maintain her target weight. Any more than that and she will gain the weight right back and then some. And, in fact, we can tell you with virtual certainty that this woman *would* rapidly gain weight; try living permanently on 1553 Calories and you'll quickly agree.

B. She can choose a 1200-Calorie diet, along with a program of mild, regular exercise (expending 200 extra calories per day). She will lose 45 pounds in five months. At the end of that time, 35 percent of her body weight will be fat tissue and 65 percent will be lean body mass, a great improvement over the result of option A, above. This time, because of having more lean body mass, which has a higher metabolic activity, and because of the exercise, she will need 2035 Calories to maintain her target weight.

Which choice makes the most sense? Which is most likely to succeed over the long run? Which is the healthiest? Which is the most enjoyable and the easiest to deal with on a *permanent* basis?

If you've chosen option B, then you have chosen one of the weight loss/maintenance programs we've developed for the New American Diet.

Weight Loss/Weight Maintenance within the New American Diet

The New American Diet, especially when accompanied by mild exercise, can promote maximum loss of weight as fat. And, partly because it is so low in fat, it is ideal for weight maintenance. Another reason it is ideal for weight maintenance is that, given its composition, it may take more excess calories to produce weight gain than do higher-fat, lower-carbohydrate diets. It has been our experience that many people who have reached Phase Three of the New American Diet for the prevention of heart disease also experience some weight loss without consciously trying to lose weight.

Some of the comments contained in the first chapter of this part of the book (pages 55–66) are typical in this regard. Overweight individuals who had tried numerous other diets without long-term success report that they have steadily lost weight on our program, sometimes "without even trying." This

way of eating cuts back on fat yet leaves the individual feeling fuller because of the abundance of bulk that complex carbohydrates and fiber (grains, beans and vegetables) provide.

We firmly believe that the overwhelming majority of those who follow the New American Diet will maximize their potential for achieving and maintaining their desired weight. This is so because of its composition and because it is a way of eating over one's lifetime and not just for a few months. In short, it promotes a *permanent* change in dietary life-style. The same diet that for most people will result in desired weight loss is also used for weight maintenance, as well. Thus, unlike so many of the other programs, one doesn't revert to a high-fat diet after the weight is lost.

Note that starting the New American Diet before the age when creeping obesity may beset you has all of the hallmarks of a diet that would prevent obesity in the first place. These hallmarks are: It is low in fat and sugar; it contains a lot of fiber which makes meals bulky and filling, your plate is full (loaded), yet the foods it contains have fewer calories than if it were loaded with high-fat foods. Our motto for you is "better and easier to *prevent* obesity than to deal with it after it develops."

People who are slightly or mildly overweight will perhaps be content to work gradually toward the end-point goals of the New American Diet and let the pounds fall where —and when—they may, over a period of time, without making any conscious or specific effort to lose weight. We recognize, however, that there are some, especially among those who are more significantly overweight, who will want to shed some of their excess pounds *before* getting into our standard life-long program without caloric restrictions. Such individuals often need a lot of positive reinforcement—in the form of relatively fast weight loss—in the beginning, in order to muster sufficient motivation to take on a life-long weight-maintenance program.

For those individuals, we offer the New American Diet with reduced-calorie guidelines. These reduced-calorie weight-loss suggestions are simply the basic mixture of foods offered in our diet at reduced calories, a mixture or formula that is the product of our decades of research. These reduced-calorie guidelines are found in table 21—for both men and women.

TABLE 21
Reduced Calorie Guidelines for Men and Women

	For Women 1000–1200 Calories	For Men 1800–2000 Calories
Lean meat, fish, poultry (oz./day)	3	3
Low-fat dairy products (svgs./day)*	1–2	2–3
Bread or grain products (svgs./day)†	6–7	13–14
Fruit (pieces/day)	3	4
Vegetables (cups/day)	2	2
Fat, visible and hidden (svgs./day)‡	2	5

* One low-fat dairy product serving = 85 Calories. (1 cup skim milk or skim-milk yogurt, ½ cup 2% milk, low-fat plain yogurt, or low-fat cottage cheese, or 1½ to 2 ounces of these cheeses: Lite-line, Lite n' Lively, Weight Watchers, part-skim ricotta, Reduced Calories Laughing Cow)
† One bread serving = 68 Calories (1 small baked potato, ½ cup macaroni or other pasta, ⅓ cup rice, 1 slice bread, 1 corn tortilla, ½ flour tortilla, ½ bagel, ½ cup cooked cereal, 1 cup dry cereal, 1 4-inch pancake)
‡ One fat serving = 45 Calories (1 teaspoon or pat of margarine, oil, mayonnaise or Miracle Whip, 2 teaspoons imitation or light mayonnaise, salad dressing, peanut butter or diet margarine, 1 tablespoon low-calorie salad dressing)

The kind of results that can be expected are illustrated in the example cited earlier. In that example, the daily caloric intake—for a woman in that case—was 1200, combined with a mild exercise program. We often tailor programs for individuals, and you can do some experimenting on your own, if you like, but the commonest regimens we offer provide for 1000 to 1200 Calories for women and 1800 to 2000 Calories for men. Don't conclude that if cutting back moderately on calories is a good thing then cutting back drastically is even better. As we've explained, this is *not* the case. Do not, ordinarily, consume many fewer calories than those recommended in table 21.

Stick closely to the serving guidelines in table 21. Don't conclude that if you give up one of the bread/grain servings you can add an extra fat serving. You *can't*. Note that the *total* amount of *lean* meat, fish, shellfish or poultry for the day is 3 ounces. You need to avoid all higher-fat meats entirely.

Feel free to use the recipes in part 3. To help ensure that you stay within the caloric guidelines, consult the Nutrient Analysis Chart in the Appendix, which tells you the number of calories contained in each recipe. For women, table 22 provides a sample week of 1000-Calorie-per-day menus. For men, see table 17, pages 161–63, for a week of New American Diet menus providing 2000 Calories daily.

If you stick with these reduced-calorie menus you can be assured of the following: (1) You *will* lose weight; (2) you will be getting not only a nutritionally balanced diet but also one that confers the same disease-prevention benefits of the New American Diet at higher calories; (3) you will be eating the *kind* of diet that has been scientifically demonstrated to promote the most weight loss in

TABLE 22

New American Diet Phase Three Meal Plans—1000 Calories

	DAY 1	DAY 2	DAY 3	DAY 4	DAY 5	DAY 6	DAY 7
Breakfast	Orange Whole wheat English muffin, ½ Soft margarine, 1 tsp. Skim milk, ½ cup	Cantaloupe, ¼ Puffed Wheat, 1 cup Skim milk, ½ cup	Fresh raspberries, ½ cup Whole wheat raisin bread toast, 2 slices Soft margarine, 2 tsp.	Sliced banana, ½ in Plain low-fat yogurt, 4 oz. Cereal Bran Muffin Orange marmalade, ½ Tbsp.	Pink grapefruit, ½ Skinny hash browns: Shredded potatoes, 1 cup Vegetable oil, 1 tsp.	Honeydew melon, ¼ Oatmeal, ¾ cup Skim milk, ½ cup	German Oven Pancake, ⅓ with Blueberries, ½ cup and Peaches, ½ cup and Powdered sugar, 1 tsp.
Morning Snack		Cereal Bran Muffin					
Lunch	Greek Lentil Soup, 1 cup Melba Rounds, 3 Reduced Calories Laughing Cow, ¾ oz. Green grapes, ½ cup	Burrito: Flour tortilla (8") Refried Beans, ½ cup Lettuce, ½ cup Chowchow, ¼ cup	Chili Bean Salad, ½ cup served in Whole wheat pita bread, ½ Orange	Four Star Pasta Salad, ½ svg. Corn on the cob, 1 small piece Soft margarine, 1 tsp. Apple	Salad bar: Lettuce, 1 cup Cherry tomatoes, 4 Radishes, 4 sliced Cucumber slices, ¼ cup Kidney beans, ¼ cup Dressing: Vinegar, 4 tsp. Oil, 2 tsp. Wheatberry roll	Minestrone Soup, 1 cup Corn Bread, 1 piece (3" x 3") Fruit Cup: Banana, ¼ cup Grapes, ¼ cup	In Restaurant: Crab Louie: Crab, 3 oz. Lettuce, 1½ cups Carrots (grated), ¼ cup Cucumber, ¼ cup Tomato, ½ Black olive Thousand Island Salad Dressing, ¼ cup (brought from home) Whole wheat roll
Afternoon Snack			Soda crackers (unsalted tops), 6				

NOTE: Recipes that are in italics can be found in part 3.

TABLE 22—Continued

	DAY 1	DAY 2	DAY 3	DAY 4	DAY 5	DAY 6	DAY 7
Dinner	Cashew Chicken, 1 svg. Steamed rice, ¾ cup Lettuce salad, 1 cup Red French Salad Dressing, 2 Tbsp. Fresh sliced pineapple, 1¼ cups	Turkey-Vegetable Chowder, 1 cup Baked potato Soft margarine, 1½ tsp. Carrot-Raisin Salad, ½ cup	Lively Lemon Roll-Ups, ½ svg. Steamed carrots, ⅔ cup Sunshine Spinach Salad, 1 cup Whole wheat dinner roll Apricot Meringue Bar	Pizza Rice Casserole, ½ cup Baked squash, ½ Whole Wheat French Bread, 2 slices (2" diameter)	Parmesan Yogurt Chicken, 1 svg. Fettuccine, ¾ cup Steamed broccoli, ½ cup Whole wheat dinner roll	Baked Snapper with Spicy Tomato Sauce, ½ cup Baked potato Soft margarine, 1 tsp. Steamed zucchini, 1 cup Caraway dinner roll Pinto Fiesta Cake, ½ svg.	Spaghetti, ¾ cup with Marinara Sauce, ½ cup Lettuce salad, 1 cup Western Salad Dressing, 2 Tbsp. Steamed green beans, ½ cup Whole Wheat French Bread, 2 pieces (2" diameter)
Evening Snack	Popcorn (air-popped), 2 cups, with Soft margarine, 1 tsp.	Banana, ½		Graham crackers, 2 Skim milk, ½ cup	Apple		Popcorn (air-popped), 3 cups with Soft margarine, 1 tsp.

Nutrient Composition	DAY 1	DAY 2	DAY 3	DAY 4	DAY 5	DAY 6	DAY 7	Average	Phase Three Goal
Calories	1198	1072	982	1008	995	1037	965	1037	1000
Protein, % Calories	17	15	17	15	18	17	20	17	15
Fat, % Calories	18	19	21	20	24	17	23	20	20
Carbohydrate, % Calories	65	66	62	65	58	65	57	63	65
Saturated Fat, % Calories	4.0	4.7	4.4	4.8	4.8	3.3	4.4	4.3	5.0
Polyunsaturated Fat, % Calories	5.6	5.6	6.8	5.1	9.1	5.6	7.8	6.5	8.0
Cholesterol, mg*	38	29	58	38	65	56	89	53	<50†
CSI	7	8	8	7	9	7	9	8	8
Sodium, mg	1140	927	1015	774	747	806	1079	927	863
Potassium, mg	2690	2869	1457	2568	2026	2970	1452	2290	1950
Calcium, mg	434	543	377	627	300	475	329	441	400

* Mg = milligram.
† < = less than.

177

the form of fat while minimizing loss of lean body mass; (4) the design of the diet is such that, again from a scientific perspective, you will be able to eat more food without gaining weight once you've achieved your ideal body weight than if you had gone on a diet that resulted in greater loss of lean body mass; (5) you will have begun to learn a new life-style of eating while losing weight, one that can be continued for weight maintenance at higher caloric levels on a permanent basis.

You can expect to lose about 1 to 2 pounds per week on these weight-loss regimens, in most cases. We readily concede that you might lose weight twice as fast on very low-carbohydrate diets, starvation or ketogenic diets. You might lose 45 pounds in three or four months instead of five months. But, in view of everything you've learned, is losing that weight a few months faster worth it, given the health risks and the high probability that your rapid weight loss will be of short duration and will be followed by more weight gain?

Once you've achieved enough weight loss that *you* feel good about it, continue the basic New American Diet program, with no caloric restrictions, proceeding at your own rate. If you want to minimize your chances of regaining any significant amount of weight, *start* with the Phase Two guidelines, even Phase Three if you desire. It is definitely possible, even easy, to fill yourself up without gaining weight.

Remember, if you are obese, you are suffering from a physical disease. Our main aim is to *prevent* disease, but those who are already suffering from the disease of overconsumption can certainly benefit a great deal from following our program. They will want to progress to Phase Three more rapidly. Since motivation will be higher this may be fairly easy to achieve.

Help Yourself Even More with Exercise

A program of exercise can benefit just about everyone, especially those who struggle with their weight. The benefits of moderate, regular exercise—the sort that helps condition the heart and lungs—remain to be conclusively demonstrated from a scientific point of view. The well-controlled, long-term experiments that are needed to settle this issue simply haven't been done, although there is finally movement in that direction.

We are convinced, however, that regular, moderate exercise will help burn calories and that by itself will promote—and speed—weight loss. In addition, exercise seems to diminish appetite in many people, enhances a feeling of psychological well being and promotes good muscle tone. It also maximizes the amount of weight which is lost in the form of fat while minimizing the amount lost in the form of lean body mass. This is very important to the dieter because muscle burns a large percentage of the calories we use every day. As pointed out earlier, this means that *after* you've lost weight you'll be able to consume more calories and still keep your weight down, if you've retained a lot of muscle mass.

When people think of exercise they often conjure up a picture of a marathon runner or a professional football or basketball player. Few think in terms of the person who is able to weed the garden without getting a back injury or climb the stairs without getting very short of breath. The exercises we recommend are those which can be done without getting seriously out of breath and which can be increased in duration and intensity over a period of time.

We do not believe that you have to check your heart rate to make sure it is elevated to

TABLE 23
The Caloric Expenditure of Various Physical Activities

Activity	Calories/ 15 Minutes	Activity	Calories/ 15 Minutes
Horseshoe pitching	40	Cycling, 5.5 mph	68
Sailing	56	9.4 mph	105
Horseback riding, walk	45	Swimming	120
Brisk walking, 3 mph	60	Stair climbing	93
Gardening, weeding	75	Skating, ice, roller	104
Digging	129	Rope skipping 60–80 skips/min.	144
Table tennis	104	Skiing, cross-country	144
Dancing, waltz	86	Jogging, 11-min. miles	142
Volleyball	53	Tennis, singles	114
Golf	89	Squash	223

certain levels for certain periods of time in order to derive aerobic benefits. The kind of exercise we recommend *is* aerobic—exercising the heart and lungs—but measuring the heart rate accurately is difficult to do; there are, apart from human error, too many variables that affect this rate. Instead, we rely on scientific evidence in men that the amount of activity associated with reduced risk of having a heart attack is that which uses up 2000 Calories or more per week. Thus, we recommend that men *gradually* increase their physical activity with the end-point goal being to exert an extra 2000 Calories of physical effort each week or about 300 Calories per day.

Women, being smaller, should expend about 1500 Calories per week or just over 200 Calories per day. Admittedly, there is no scientific data relating the amount of exercise and heart disease in women, but the above calculations for women, derived from the figures for men, are based upon the smaller size of women and appear reasonable.

The best and safest way for people to burn calories is to engage in activities in which large muscle groups (arms and legs) are used, and which can be sustained continuously for

a relatively long period of time (15 to 60 minutes). Continuous, long-term activities such as walking, bicycling and swimming use body fat as an energy source and thus contribute to control and maintenance of "desirable" body weight. Table 23 lists average energy costs of various activities for each 15 minutes of activity, based on a body weight of 140 pounds. If you are heavier than that you'll expend somewhat more energy, but, for all practical purposes, these figures can be used by everyone.

Getting 2000 Calories' worth of exercise in a week is not that difficult! Table 24 shows one way to get there.

Build up your endurance *slowly* and *consistently*. In other words, don't start doing 20 or 30 minutes of exercise right from the beginning. It may take you several weeks or months to get to that point comfortably. Begin with 5 to 10 minutes of *continuous* exercise daily. Your capacity for exercise—and your ability to speed up the pace—will improve over a period of time. Gradually increase both the duration and the intensity of your exercise.

We believe that nearly everybody can benefit from this kind of exercise program. If you have any particular concerns about your

TABLE 24

Activity	Calories
Walking, 3 mph (brisk pace), 30 minutes *each* day, 7 days a week	840
Taking stairs instead of the elevator a total of 3 min. each day, 5 days a week	93
Gardening, 2½ hours on a weekend	750
Bicycle riding, leisurely pace, 30 minutes 3 times a week	408
TOTAL	2091

health or a history of heart disease yourself or in your family—consult your physician before starting any exercise program. Exercise is an optional part of this program, but it's an option we believe most people will want to go for. And if you are overweight, we believe the benefits of exercise can be very substantial—both physically and, in many cases, psychologically.

11

SPECIAL SITUATIONS:

EATING OUT/ENTERTAINING/HOLIDAYS/ CAMPING/PREGNANCY AND BREAST FEEDING/INFANTS/VEGETARIANISM

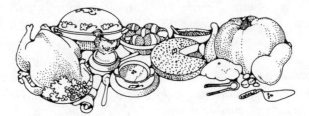

Handling Special Occasions/Situations

Guidelines of any kind are easiest to follow on "typical" days. But not all days are typical. We all know there are crosswinds of special situations and occasions out there ready to blow us off course. When it comes to guidelines related to eating, those special situations include meals in restaurants, vacations, business trips, Christmas, Thanksgiving, birthdays, weddings, anniversaries, dinner invitations, church potlucks, family reunions, club banquets, etc. Ultimately, just how many of these special occasions you're going to have is up to you, but in this chapter we'll provide you with tips and other information

which will help you steer a relatively safe course through choppy seas.

In the beginning, of course, nearly *every* day will be a special occasion, from the standpoint of the New American Diet goals. What we mean is that when you first start this program you will be eating food regularly which we regard as "special occasion" foods—such as extra meat, typical cheeses, ice cream, chocolate and salty foods. But, gradually, as you begin to make more and more changes, you'll find yourself eating less of these special occasion foods and on fewer occasions. Until this begins to happen, you will probably not feel like changing the way you eat in special situations. We find that it often takes people eight or nine months before they are ready to tackle special situations.

In this chapter we will pose a number of situations or scenarios you are likely to encounter—the kind that give many people a lot of trouble. We'll show you how to deal with these situations in practical, positive nonconfrontational ways.

Eating Out—In Restaurants

Scenario #1. Your job requires you to attend two or three business breakfasts and/or luncheons a week. You can't imagine how you can make all of this restaurant eating fit in with new American Diet goals. What do you do?

This is a very common problem and not nearly so hopeless as many initially surmise. You can eat out in restaurants with some regularity and still keep overall fat intake down. Here are two suggestions: The first is to make careful choices. This may seem obvious, but some people just assume there are no good choices in restaurants and so they dive into the bacon, eggs and cheeseburgers without even looking for better selections. In reality, almost *every* restaurant has something on the menu you can make work for you.

More and more restaurants are offering a wide variety of vegetable and fruit salads and salad bars. And even those restaurants that specialize in meat dishes usually also offer some with fish and chicken. If you eat out a lot in the course of business you will want to cultivate a few restaurants that offer foods similar to those recommended in the New American Diet program. Restaurants that feature ethnic foods are likely choices, but be careful even here because many of these establishments lean toward special occasion foods, too. So choose accordingly.

Most people initially need help in making low-fat menu selections. Often something as seemingly harmless as a salad somehow gets transformed, between the kitchen and your table, into a high-fat monster swimming in a salad dressing that is one-half to three-fourths fat. Enlist the help of your waiter or waitress. Do not hesitate to ask how certain foods are prepared. For example, is the fish deep-fried (which means lots of fat), poached, baked or broiled? Request that salad dressings be served on the side. You'll be surprised by how "a little dab'll do ya." Some people skip the salad dressings entirely and ask for lemon wedges instead, which make a nice substitute seasoning. Similarly, if you ask for a baked potato, request that the butter or sour cream be on the side so that *you* are in control of the amount of fat that is added.

For those business breakfasts, toast, or better yet, English muffins, can be ordered dry or with jelly or honey instead of soaked in butter. But again you'll have to speak up and specify that you want it served this way. And if your waffles or pancakes come with a huge glob of butter, don't hesitate to transfer said glob to the saucer under your coffee. Waiters, waitresses and even friends can be intimidating. When ordering, be friendly but firm and confident. By gently taking charge instead of being passive, you will probably get friendlier and better service than ever before.

Even by making the best possible choices in restaurants, of course, you're still going to have trouble fully conforming to New American Diet goals. Hence our second suggestion: Don't try to evaluate your food intake a meal at a time but instead consider what you eat in a day, a week or even several weeks at a time. In this way you can make things balance or average out over time. If, for example, you eat one particularly high-fat meal you can make your other two meals for that day even lower in fat than usual. Or if you have one particularly indulgent week you can make the next week especially "lean."

If you know you're going to have a business luncheon and that it's going to be tough holding down the fat, you can get a head start by having an especially low-fat breakfast (such as fruit, cereal with skim milk and toast with preserves or honey). And you can plan to have a very low-fat dinner that day, one of the meatless, cheeseless variety, such as spaghetti with Marinara Sauce, tossed salad with low-fat dressing, broccoli, unbuttered French Bread and fruit *or* baked fish or chicken, baked potato with dilled yogurt or Mock Sour Cream, romaine salad, whole wheat rolls and fruit.

Another way to deal with eating lunch in a restaurant is to plan ahead of time not to fill up. This is what many politicians and people on the lecture or banquet circuit do. Then supplement lunch with your own low-fat foods. These can be taken with you, if that fits into the situation, or you can eat a low-fat snack before or after lunch. Good choices are fresh fruit, soda crackers (unsalted tops), fresh vegetables, low-fat yogurt, etc.

Scenario #2 You are going on a two-week vacation. It will not be possible to make choices so that each day or even a week will average out to be low-fat. What are you going to do?

In this case, even if you normally try to make things balance a day or a week at a time, you'll have to try to make things average out over a period of say a month. Again, you can get a head start on this by being particularly careful the week *before* you go on vacation—eating as many meatless main

dishes as possible, avoiding desserts and so on. And then while you are on vacation you can still make an effort to select as many low-fat foods as possible. A good rule is to choose no more than one special occasion food per meal.

Thus, if you select a steak—and we suggest you choose a small one—complete the meal with lower-fat choices. In other words, do not choose a steak, plus sour cream and/or butter for your potato, plus Roquefort dressing for your salad, plus butter for your bread, plus cheesecake for dessert. Such a meal, apart from being the antithesis of New American Diet goals, puts you in distinct danger of having a "fat attack."

A "fat attack" is that dreaded event that occurs when you eat more fat than you are accustomed to eating; after you've been following the New American Diet guidelines for a while even meals that were once typical for you can bring on these attacks which are characterized by indigestion and gas and may, in some cases, last all night.

One final vacation tip: If you'll simply avoid *all* cheeses and desserts for the duration of your vacation you shouldn't have too much trouble holding down the fat.

Scenario #3. You are remodeling your kitchen and cannot use your stove for a week. The pressure is on to pick up quick meals at fast-food outlets. What should you do?

Fast-food restaurants are a temptation to nearly everyone. Our opinion is that they are here to stay, so it's up to each of us to "control" them and not to let them "control" us. The sort of food *averaging* we discussed above is one of the answers to the problem posed in this scenario. Don't fill up on fast foods; have something low-fat along in the car or when you get back home. Keep carrot and celery sticks with a good dip in your still functional refrigerator, along with fresh fruit and other low-fat snacks. Instead of having both a hamburger and a milk shake at the fast-food restaurant, have just the hamburger and stop by an ice-cream store afterward to have a dip of sherbet, sorbet or frozen low-fat yogurt. Later that evening, if you're still hungry, have popcorn or cereal with skim milk.

Some fast-food places are now offering lower-fat food choices. And, remember, not *all* foods contain the same amount of fat even in fast-food restaurants. Reasonably low-fat choices include bean burritos (but not deep-fried), tacos, tostadas and plain hamburgers (but not cheeseburgers). Choose salad with low-calorie dressings, if possible, to help dilute the fat.

TABLE 25

Pizza	CSI*	Calories
Spicy Cheese Pizza†	9	546
Green pepper, mushroom and onion	13	696
Vegetarian (green pepper, mushroom, onion, black olive)	13	695
Black olive	14	692
Canadian bacon	17	752
Pepperoni	21	806
Hamburger	22	843
Sausage	24	891
Cheese (contains twice as much cheese as other pizzas)	24	809
Combination (salami, pepperoni, hamburger, sausage, olives, mushrooms)	30	999

* Cholesterol-Saturated Fat Index; the lower the better.
† Recipe can be found in part 3.

As for pizza, that American fast-food favorite, yes, it *does* make a difference what type you select. Table 25 shows the number of calories and the CSI of a variety of types. Remember, the lower the CSI, the better the

choice. (The portions here are three average slices of a 14-inch pizza.) If you order pizzas with half the usual amount of cheese, the CSI will be quite a bit lower.

Entertaining

Scenario #4. It's time for you to make good on some of your social obligations and have friends over for dinner. Most of them, so far as you know, eat the typical American diet. What do you serve?

Trying lower-fat, lower-cholesterol, lower-salt, less-sweet foods on your family initially requires courage, stamina and high self-esteem. And as for trying these foods on company, many of you would no doubt rather meet Jack the Ripper in a dark, fog- shrouded alley—at least in the beginning.

Can it be done successfully? Yes, it can and has—countless times.

Let us emphasize, though, that you should try all *new* recipes on your family *first*. Only when you feel confident about how the recipe will turn out and only when you and your family really like the result should you venture into serving the dish to friends. Concentrate on those dishes that you *know* will bring you compliments. There is no confidence booster like praise. Then gradually become more daring in what you serve guests—as your confidence and your repertoire of hit recipes grow. Continue, of course, to be sensitive to the tastes of your guests. You want to please them, without compromising your own objectives, not to preach to them or try to convert them to a way of eating they may not be interested in or ready for.

Feel good about even the smallest things you try. You have to start somewhere. Offer

Mock Sour Cream with chopped green onions to accompany your favorite tried-and-true enchiladas. Or perhaps you could serve Apple Loaf Cake for dessert along with a meal you typically serve to guests. Other easy ways to *begin* serving modified foods are these: serve Dill Dip in a hollowed-out red cabbage with fresh vegetables or Popeye's Spinach Dip with ak-mak crackers to start the meal. Offer a lower-fat salad dressing, such as Red French Salad Dressing. Or end the meal by serving a loved fruit dessert such as Fruit Salad Alaska or Pears in Wine, instead of your "famous" cheesecake. Your guests will appreciate the savings in calories, and you may soon find yourself famous for some new, lower-fat desserts.

Offering *choices* to your guests is another easy way to begin serving lower-fat foods. Serve *both* sour cream and Mock Sour Cream to put on baked potatoes. To accompany warm Apple Crisp, offer both Yogurt Dessert Sauce and whipped cream. For salads, you might offer both store-bought Ranch Salad dressing and our Western Salad Dressing, a low-fat, low-salt version of ranch. As you become more skilled, you can offer more low-fat items and fewer choices. A good goal to aim for is to serve no more than one higher-fat item when you entertain. If you stop to think about it, you'll realize that very often just about *every* item you typically serve guests is a special occasion food (high-fat red meats, regular cheeses, high-fat dairy products, chocolate, etc.). Start cutting back on these until finally you are able to serve meals to guests, with confidence, that meet the Phase Three New American Diet goals. In fact, some of our patients tell us that in their social circles it is the "in" thing to serve low-fat, low-calorie meals, i.e., they have become a status symbol of a new life-style.

Being Entertained

Scenario #5. You've been invited to dinner at the home of some people you just recently met. They have no idea you are in the process of changing to a lower-fat way of eating. When you arrive at their home you find them beaming with pride at a table laden with all of their old family favorites, most of which, as it turns out, are swimming in fat—from the hors de'ouevres to the desserts. What do you do, short of feigning a heart attack?

Probably not much right then! The first thing to do is to consider your food intake for the whole day (or the next day) and not just for the high-fat feast at hand. As previously discussed, you can make even this meal average out. In all likelihood you will already have anticipated that the meal might not be like the ones you have at home—so you can prepare by being very Spartan about your fat, sugar, salt intakes *before* you go to dinner.

You can also take precautions by not arriving for dinner in a ravenous state. This will prevent you from going back for seconds and may enable you to eat a little less of even your first serving.

Passing up the appetizers is often a good idea, as these are usually very high in fat. Declining dessert or requesting a small portion is another good ploy. This is perfectly acceptable socially.

And with more people changing their dietary habits all the time, who knows, you may soon arrive at your friends' home to discover that they, too, are changing to a lower-fat way of eating.

Holidays

Scenario #6. You do pretty well in following New American Diet goals most of the year, but in the holiday season you seem to lose all control. How can you break this pattern?

It *can* be done. Holidays do pose a real problem, but there is hope. Figure 32 provides a number of tips you may find useful during the make-merry season.

In addition to those tips, here's another one we frequently whisper to the desperate during the holidays: *only the cook will know.* Here are some examples of what we mean:

In pumpkin pie, desserts or any recipe—
—Replace each whole egg with 1½–2 egg whites. You'll save 480 milligrams of cholesterol in an average pie and believe us only the cook will ever know!
—Use skim evaporated milk for cream or regular evaporated milk. This substitution for light cream will cut the fat by 9 teaspoons per cup. (405 Calories from fat!)

TIPS FOR HOLIDAY SURVIVAL

When you make holiday treats, modify the recipes to be lower in fat, sugar and salt.

Before eating, always ask: "Am I really hungry?" If not, do something else. If yes, eat and thoroughly enjoy, paying attention to how the food tastes.

Deal with food at work by:
—placing it in the context of the whole day's or week's intake; if you eat snacks at work, make trade-offs at other times . . .
—being brave enough to offer your co-workers a *delicious* low-fat treat . . .
—avoiding being where the food is unless you plan to eat it.

If you're overloaded with food gifts, consider giving some away to people less fortunate than you, or freezing it and doling out small quantities.

When you are in charge of food always be sure a low-fat alternative is available.

Give yourself a nonfood treat: get a massage, plan a special hike, read a novel, spend a quiet evening alone.

Turn candy- and cookie-making time into nonedible projects like making wreaths, dough art tree decorations or a gingerbread house.

Take a daily walk! It will calm your nerves and rejuvenate your body.

Remember, you are in charge of what you eat regardless of other people's comments about how much or how little you are eating. You don't have to eat to please others.

Instead of the holiday meal being the main focus create a new family tradition:
—play in the snow
—have a day of hiking or skiing
—help serve a holiday meal in the community

Make all at-home meals especially low-fat so that higher-fat foods at social events can be enjoyed without guilt.

Don't leave holiday munchies out. Put them away after serving.

At social events always have a glass of water (with ice and a twist of lemon or lime) in your hand. Take *very* small portions of food especially when there are lots of choices. Visualize beforehand what you want your plate to look like when it's full. And, look forward to the occasion as time to socialize with friends as well as time to eat.

Figure 32.

In dips, spreads and other recipes—

—Replace real mayonnaise with imitation or light mayonnaise or blended cottage cheese. If you use imitation mayonnaise, you'll cut the calories in half. If you use low-fat cottage cheese, you'll save 15 teaspoons of fat or 668 Calories from fat per cup!

—Use low-fat yogurt or Mock Sour Cream for sour cream. You'll save 8 teaspoons of fat (360 Calories from fat) with a one-cup substitution.

—Substituting margarine for butter saves 495 milligrams of cholesterol per cup. Will those cookies taste that much different? If so, try adding Butter Buds for a buttery flavor.

Holiday parties and open houses are the way many of us share the holiday spirit with neighbors, friends and co-workers. Here are some suggestions for New American Diet party fare from our recipes (in italics) in part 3:

Drinks
  Cranberry Wassail
  Mulled Cider
  Quick Hot Spiced Cider
  Fruited Punch

Gourmet
  Spicy Stuffed Mushrooms
  Cold *Salmon Mousse* with low-fat crackers
  A whole decorated cold poached salmon
  "Egg Salad" Sandwich Spread or shrimp salad–filled *Cream Puffs*
  Eggplant Delight with low-fat crackers
  Apricot Meringue Bars
  Strawberry or *Blueberry Ice*
  Baba Au Rhum

Ricotta Cheesecake (bake in square pan and cut into small squares) or *Creme de Menthe Cheesecake*

Quick to Make
  Grandma Kirschner's Date Nut Bread
  Pumpkin Harvest Loaf
  Cranberry Bread
  Vegetable tray with *Dill Dip*
  Fresh fruit platter
  Ricotta cheese spread for breads and fruit
  Popeye's Spinach Dip with low-fat crackers
  Miniature turkey sandwiches (small whole wheat or rye buns, or use cocktail rye bread, serve with thin sliced turkey breast, assorted mustards, lettuce and alfalfa sprouts)
  Bean Dip and guacamole with Baked *Corn Chips* or baked flour tortilla chips

A favorite holiday dinner you may wish to try:

  Antipasto
  Roast turkey with fresh cranberry relish
  Mashed Potatoes
  Turkey Gravy
  Chinese Salad Rich Style
  Steamed broccoli
  Whole Wheat Refrigerator Rolls
  Apple Loaf Cake and/or *Pumpkin Pie* with *Yogurt Dessert Sauce*

Camping

Scenario #7. You and your family like to take hikes and camp out frequently. A lot of trail food tends to be very high in fat. How do you get around this?

Since hiking and camping are increasingly popular, some advice is in order about eating on the trail. Trail food does not *have* to be high in cholesterol, fat, salt and sugar in order to taste good, be easy and fast to prepare and provide quick energy. For your day hikes, backpacking and car camping trips, forget the bacon, eggs, wieners, cheese and chocolate bars. Here are some of our suggestions for the trail:

Snacks: fresh fruit, low-fat, low-salt crackers, hardtack bread, popcorn, hot chocolate mix, your own mix of dried fruits and a few unsalted nuts, carrots sticks, celery with Reduced Calories Laughing Cow cheese or whipped part-skim ricotta, fruit leather.

Breakfast: pancakes (prepared from mix) with dried fruit added and hot cocoa; or fruit cobbler (steam-baked in a covered pot) made from *Baking Mix* (see recipe, part 3) and reconstituted dried fruit; or biscuits with jam and fruit; or hot cereal (oatmeal, mixed grains) with nonfat dry milk and fruit; or skinny hash browns (stored in Ziploc bags), fruit and bran muffins.

Lunches: pita bread stuffed with our premade *Chili Bean Salad* (packaged separately in plastic); or instant tabouli mix; or instant hummous; or peanut butter and jelly sandwiches (two per person); or bagels with Reduced Calories Laughing Cow Cheese.

Dinners: Instant macaroni and cheese (omit the margarine and use skim milk); or spaghetti noodles with prepared Italian sauce; or fettuccine or other pasta, with any packaged sauce.

An example of a simple but complete camp-out dinner would be canned chili with beans, wheatberry rolls, chopped lettuce with low-calorie dressing, gingersnaps and canned peaches.

Another example is our "Two Pot Camp Dish": prepare instant rice in one pot (about 2 cups uncooked rice for four people) and, in another pan, brown a little *very lean* ground beef (½ pound for four people) with onion. Mix with prepared rice a can of mushroom soup and heat through. Serve with carrot and celery sticks and fresh fruit. Later, eat popcorn as a snack around the campfire.

Or, if you want a gourmet—yet quick—camp repast, consider our "Ten-Minute Fish Dinner." You can prepare the sauce at home and reheat it over the camp stove or campfire. Add the fish and ten minutes later dinner is ready to eat. To complete the menu add raw vegetables, whole-grain bread and flavored coffee or cocoa made with skim milk for dessert. The recipe for this can be found in part 3 under *Cioppino.*

Pregnancy and Breast Feeding

Scenario #8. You are pregnant. You receive advice from several sources to eat more eggs, meat and milk in order to "get enough protein, iron, and calcium" during this critical period. Do you really need to do this?

The answer is no. The advice is well-meant, no doubt, and proceeds from a general understanding that pregnant women need extra calories (about 300 extra per day) and a protein intake sufficient to sustain the pregnancy (about 74 grams daily). What many people do not know, however, is that the typical woman in the United States is already eating at least this much protein and often far more. And, remember, the New American Diet is *not* lower in protein than that of the typical American Diet.

The Food and Nutrition Board of the National Academy of Sciences recommends that pregnant women, on average, consume 2300 Calories per day and that women who breast-feed their infants consume 2500 Calories per day. It recommends that the pregnant woman get a minimum of 74 grams of protein daily and that the lactating (breast-feeding) woman get at least 64 grams.

TABLE 26
The New American Diet in Pregnancy

New American Diet Menu	Food	Amount	Protein (gm)*	Iron (mg)†
	Breakfast			
Calories: 2345	Orange juice	1 cup	2	0.2
Fat: 57 gm* (22% of calories)	Oatmeal with	¾ cup	4	1.1
Cholesterol: 96 mg†	Raisins	2 Tbsp.	1	0.6
Protein Sources:	Toast, whole wheat	1 slice	3	0.8
Milk 29%	Margarine	1 tsp.	—	—
Meat/fish/poultry 20%	Skim milk	1 cup	8	0.1
Grains 20%				
Legumes 14%	**Lunch**			
Vegetables 16%	*Greek-Style*			
	Garbanzo Soup			
	(⅙ recipe, about 2 cups)		14	5.8
	Raw veggies		1	0.4
	Bran muffin	1 large	3	1.5
	Yogurt and	1 cup	12	0.2
	Blueberries, fresh	½ cup	1	0.8
	Snack			
	Skim milk	1 cup	9	0.1
	Dinner			
	Tangy Snapper	¼ recipe	20	1.4
	Super Stuffed Potato	1	10	1.4
	Whole Wheat Muffins	2	7	1.2
	Margarine	1 tsp.	—	—
	Lettuce salad	1 cup	1	0.3
	Italian dressing	1 Tbsp.	—	—
	Sherbet	½ cup	1	—
	Evening Snack			
	Popcorn (no margarine or oil)	3 cups	3	0.6
	Apple	1 large	—	0.6
		TOTAL	99	17.3

NOTE: Recipes that are set in italics can be found in part 3.
* Gm = gram.
† Mg = milligram.

190 THE NEW AMERICAN DIET

Table 26 shows a sample 2345-Calorie New American Diet daily menu for pregnant women. A typical American diet menu containing the same number of calories would provide about the same amount of protein—which, at 99 grams, far exceeds the requirement. But along with the protein, the standard American/Western world fare would also, typically, deliver more than 500 milligrams of cholesterol and 111 grams of fat (44 percent of total calories), while, as you can see from table 26, the diet's 2345-Calorie menu contains only 96 milligrams of cholesterol and 57 grams of fat (22 percent of total calories). And you can actually get more iron in this diet than in the typical U.S. diet. Calcium is also supplied in entirely adequate amounts.

What is not yet well-known, even in medical or nutrition circles, is that there are a number of advantages to following the New American Diet goals throughout pregnancy:

1. Every woman's blood cholesterol goes up temporarily during pregnancy (for example, many rise from 180 to 250 milligrams per 100 milliliters of blood). This elevation is not risky in most women but it could be in some. With the New American Diet, levels will not rise as high.
2. The amount of cholesterol that is in the bile will be decreased by following the New American Diet. This decreases the risk of developing gallstones, something very common in U.S. women who have had several children.
3. Constipation, a frequent problem during pregnancy, is reduced through the New American Diet's high reliance upon fiber-rich foods (whole grains, fruits, vegetables, legumes).

4. The New American Diet may help avoid excessive weight gain.
5. The diet provides more iron and folic acid, both important in pregnancy, than does the typical U.S. diet.
6. The New American Diet does not have to be changed or specially tailored to be suitable for use during pregnancy—except to the extent that 2300 Calories are required daily. Though the diet supplies more iron than the typical U.S. diet, pregnant women may need to take an iron supplement during pregnancy.

If you decide to breast-feed your child—a good idea in our view—the New American Diet serves very well, although you will want to increase your caloric intake from the 2300 Calories you took in during pregnancy to 2500 Calories during the breast-feeding period.

Infants

Scenario #9. The new baby is starting to eat and is about finished with breast feeding. Now what? What kinds of food—and milk—do you feed the baby?

With the ever-changing ideas about how, when and what to feed babies, it is no wonder that there is a lot of confusion on this issue. It's not really particularly complicated, however.

First, we feel strongly that babies should get breast milk or the equivalent until the natural time of weaning—usually 1½ to 2 years of age. Then switch to *skim milk.* (Remember, it has as much calcium and protein in it as whole milk.)

Second, we also feel very strongly that,

aside from breast milk, any other foods given them should be low-fat. It does not make sense to introduce high-fat foods with the idea of then changing to low-fat later on. (Note that most baby food is already low in salt. The mothers of America insisted upon this over a decade ago and the food manufacturers complied.)

As we've pointed out many times, what we *like* to eat is largely learned. Just follow the guidelines of the New American Diet and feed your infants as you feed yourself, right from the time they start to eat solid foods. You'll be giving your children a real head start.

Vegetarianism

Scenario #10. Your family, or some member of your family, decides to become vegetarian. How well does this square with the goals of the New American Diet?

It is clear that a considerable amount of food in the New American Diet comes from the vegetable kingdom. Still, it is not a vegetarian diet. Low-fat animal products, including lean meat, are used as condiments to provide flavors for the pastas, many cereal products, beans, vegetables and potatoes. New American Diet concepts can, nonetheless, certainly be used by people who adhere to vegetarianism—depending upon which school of vegetarianism they follow.

Some vegetarians eat fish but consume no poultry or red meat. This concept fits in nicely with the New American Diet's emphasis on fish consumption and deemphasis on red meats. Some others are ovolacto vegetarians. These people do not eat *any* meat, poultry or fish but do consume eggs, butter, cheese, milk and other dairy products. Depending upon the quantities of these products consumed, each individual might find it very difficult to meet the goals of the diet. If they switched to low-fat or nonfat dairy products and to egg whites and/or egg substitutes, the ovolacto vegetarians could meet the goals of the diet.

The strict vegetarian who does not consume *any* food product derived from *any* animal could also meet New American Diet goals. Such individuals, however, might be in danger of developing a specific nutritional deficiency. This is a deficiency in vitamin B_{12} (the antipernicious anemia vitamin), important both for forming blood cells and proper functioning of the nervous system. We have been extremely careful to be certain that the New American Diet fulfills all known nutritional requirements. But a pure vegetarian would need to take vitamin B_{12} supplements to meet all nutritional needs. Vitamin B_{12} is found only in foods of animal origin. It is found in ample amounts in skim milk, in fish and shellfish and in all low-fat animal products. The body's requirements for the vitamin are very small. Thus only small amounts of animal foods are needed to satisfy the requirement.

12

MEDICAL TESTS TO MONITOR YOUR PROGRESS

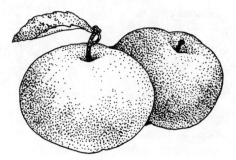

To Test or Not to Test? (That's *One* of the Questions)

"Do we need to get our blood tested to find out whether we're doing the right things?" That is a question that is on the minds of many people who participate in our program. The quiz that we provided in part 1 and reintroduced you to at the conclusion of each phase of the New American Diet can help you determine the extent to which you are achieving the program goals. But you may still wonder what effect all of your efforts are actually having on the concentrations of cholesterol, triglyceride and lipoproteins (LDL and HDL cholesterol) in your blood and on your blood pressure.

There are relatively simple blood tests to help you determine these things. It is not essential that you have these tests, although if you have any history of heart disease or hypertension in your family, regular medical monitoring, including these tests, is certainly advised. For others, the tests are optional, but an increasing number of physicians recommend some of them during any routine physical exam.

We have nothing against these tests and recommend them ourselves under certain circumstances. In general, however, they are just what we've labeled them—optional for most people. If you are conscientious in following the goals of the New American Diet, your intake of fat and sodium will be low, and you will have maximized your potential for lowering your blood fats and blood pressure by diet. This will be reflected in your blood values and your blood pressure in most cases. Many people know this but still want the reassurance blood tests provide. If you are one of those people, you'll have still other questions, some of which we answer below.

What Tests Should I Have?

The only lipid tests, under normal circumstances, that need concern you are those related to cholesterol and triglyceride. When blood is drawn there is often a standard panel of tests to which the blood is subjected. These tests usually include those for total cholesterol and triglyceride. Often, at additional cost, you may also find out the concentrations of HDL cholesterol and LDL cholesterol in your blood. You will recall from our previous discussions that HDL is the "good guy" that helps safely transport excess cholesterol to the liver and out of the body, while LDL, in excess, is the "bad guy" that carries cholesterol to the arteries where it can be deposited, contributing to atherosclerosis.

The amount of cholesterol that is ultimately deposited in the artery is determined by a number of factors. The higher the LDL cholesterol level the more that is deposited. Cigarette smoking, high blood pressure (hypertension) and high blood sugar (diabetes) all increase the amount of cholesterol that is deposited in the artery wall. In fact, these seem to drive more cholesterol into the artery much faster than would be the case in people who have the same blood cholesterol level but who do not smoke, have hypertension or diabetes. The last factor is that there is great variability in the amount of cholesterol that gets into the artery wall at any given blood cholesterol level. What controls this is un-

known although there is some evidence that suggests that the HDL cholesterol level is important. High levels of triglyceride are another risk factor but probably not as important as cholesterol, LDL and HDL.

In addition to total cholesterol, triglyceride and possibly HDL and LDL cholesterol, you should also be interested in monitoring your blood pressure, especially as you reach middle age and later.

How Can I Judge the Results?

This is a very good question. There is a lot of confusion over the interpretation of lab results. When you get the total cholesterol concentration in your blood measured, for example, your doctor and/or the lab report may very well indicate that "normal" is anywhere between 150 and 300 milligrams per 100 milliliters of blood. In fact, however, all this tells you is the range or distribution of cholesterol levels in the U.S. population, a population which has excessive coronary heart disease, stroke, etc. This range is *not* reflective of what a truly healthy population relatively free of these diseases should exhibit. That range would be from 110 to 200 milligrams per 100 milliliters.

To be blunt, "normal" may not be normal but only average for a coronary-diseased population. Why is there this discrepancy? The fact is that the latest research findings take time to filter down completely to the grassroots level even in medical practice. Doctors are gradually changing their views as new findings are reported and confirmed and as they become convinced that they should be concerned about cholesterol. The recent

Consensus Conference on Cholesterol at the National Institutes of Health showed how unanimous is the weight of scientific opinion that blood cholesterol levels above 200 milligrams per 100 milliliters for most adults and above 170 milligrams per 100 milliliters for children need attention. And the report of this conference suggested that diet was the best way to go.

Remember always to fast (meaning not eating or drinking except for water) for twelve hours before having your blood drawn for any of these tests. Otherwise, what you eat or drink before testing will affect the outcome and give you results that can't be compared to anything. Also, it's a good idea, as you track your results over a period of years, to try to have your tests done at the same laboratory as there are variations in techniques and thus sometimes in results at different labs. Do not rely on a single value. There is day-to-day variation and any laboratory will occasionally make an error. So if there is any question about your results, have another sample taken later.

When you get your results, the following will help you judge where you are at:

For children and young adults under the age of 25, a total blood cholesterol level of below 180 milligrams per 100 milliliters of blood is what we like to see. For adults age 25 to 44, we look for a level below 200. For those 45 or older, we aim for levels below 220. Ideally, however, everybody should be below 180 regardless of age.

As for triglycerides, we set the upper limit at 140 milligrams per 100 milliliters of blood —for everybody. The triglycerides are blood fats which, under normal circumstances, transport energy to the cells of the body. When the concentrations of these fats become elevated, however, they become risk factors (though not as potent as elevated cholesterol) in heart disease, obesity and diabetes. We find that the protective "good" particle, HDL, is frequently depressed when triglyceride concentrations are high.

If you opt for the HDL and LDL cholesterol tests, these are the results we hope for: HDL should be *above* 40 milligrams per 100 milliliters of blood in men and above 50 in women; LDL should be *below* 126. (If your HDL is below 30 you should probably consult a physician who specializes in treating people with high concentrations of blood fat.) Sometimes the lipoproteins are expressed in a ratio (LDL cholesterol/HDL cholesterol). What we want, in this case, is a ratio of LDL to HDL between 2.0 and 3.2.

Some of you, probably less than 5 percent, may have very high values of cholesterol and triglyceride. The cholesterol level may be above 280 milligrams per 100 milliliters of blood and the triglyceride above 300 milligrams per 100 milliliters of blood. The New American Diet will help you lower these high values, but you may have a more serious genetic form of hyperlipidemia (high blood fat) and may require the help of a specialist in this area (someone in "lipid metabolism"). The New American Diet provides, however, the initial treatment for all forms of genetic hyperlipidemia.

As for blood pressure, this test is accomplished quickly and easily. Medical authorities universally agree that an adult blood pressure of 140/90 (expressed as "140 over 90") or higher warrants concern and intervention, which, initially, will probably be dietary in nature, beginning with a reduction in consumption of salt.

Is It Ever Too Early or Too Late to Have These Tests?

The real question at issue here is this: Is it ever too early or too late to try to prevent disease or improve health? Our emphatic answer to this is *no*. When it comes to holding down cholesterol and triglyceride levels, the younger you start the better. As we age, cholesterol concentrations tend to increase due largely to decades of consuming the high-cholesterol, high-fat Western world diet. A cholesterol level of 170 in childhood may well become 250 or even more at age 55. Figures 33 and 34 show the age-related changes in the blood cholesterol, LDL cholesterol, HDL cholesterol and triglyceride values from our family study. Locate your place on these fig-

ures. Note the higher HDL levels in women, one reason, incidentally that premenopausal women have less coronary heart disease than men of comparable age. By following an imaginary line parallel to the line on the graph, you can then get an idea of what your levels were when you were younger and project what they will be in the future—that is *unless* you change your eating habits. The New American Diet helps prevent this otherwise inevitable increase with age.

On the other hand, it's almost never too late to get started on the New American Diet, either. You may need even more encouragement, of course, if you start late and know that your cholesterol levels are already considerably elevated. You should be aware, however, that you might not get the same results, starting later in life, that you might

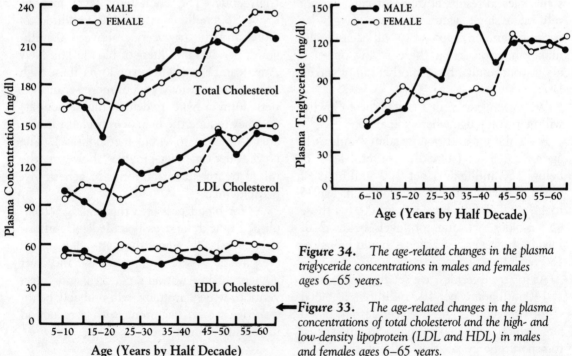

Figure 34. *The age-related changes in the plasma triglyceride concentrations in males and females ages 6–65 years.*

Figure 33. *The age-related changes in the plasma concentrations of total cholesterol and the high- and low-density lipoprotein (LDL and HDL) in males and females ages 6–65 years.*

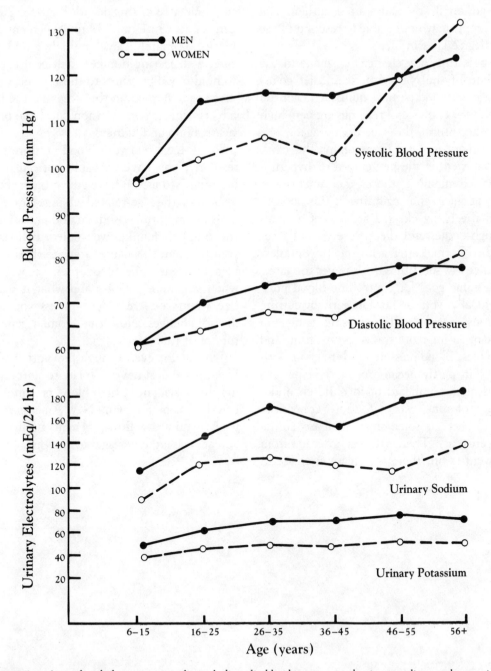

Figure 35. *Age-related changes in systolic and diastolic blood pressure and urinary sodium and potassium excretion in male and female subjects to 65 years old.*

have gotten if you had started earlier. The body simply may not be able to respond to the same degree later in life.

Despite this, any change you make in the direction of the New American Diet goals, *will* help you, and perhaps quite significantly. Even if your cholesterol readings are very high in the beginning, don't be discouraged. The New American Diet is useful for the *treatment,* as well as the prevention of hyperlipidemia. Remember those experiments we talked about in the beginning of this book in which the badly clogged arteries of animals fed high-cholesterol diets were partially restored to normal after a low-fat, low-cholesterol diet was substituted? It's never too late!

The same goes for controlling blood pressure. Ideally, you should start early by cutting salt consumption and increasing potassium intake by eating more grains, beans, fruits and vegetables. Blood pressure tends to go up with age, again partly because of diet. Hypertension is almost unheard of in children under the age of nine except for rare congential causes. There is some small increase during the teen years. Then with each decade from the twenties on, there is a steady increase in the incidence of this disorder. About 20 percent of all whites and 30 to 40 percent of all blacks ultimately develop high blood pressure, a staggering number. Our goal is to try to hold blood pressures to those levels we enjoyed as children and thus to avoid the many adverse effects hypertension can have on the heart, brain and kidneys.

If you have had your blood pressure taken regularly, you have probably noticed that it has increased as you have grown older. Figure 35 shows the age-related changes in blood pressure and urinary sodium and potassium in the sample of families we studied. By locating your place on this figure, you can then get an idea of what your blood pressure was like when you were younger and what it will be like when you are older—unless you make dietary changes. Note that women generally run lower than men.

But, again, even though prevention is the ideal, it's almost never too late to start checking the onslaught of high blood pressure. You can do this by following New American Diet goals. And you will reap benefits no matter if you are age fifteen or age seventy-five.

PART

3

The Cookbook
Recipes for
the New American Diet

Developed under the direction of

Sonja L. Connor, M.S., R.D.
and
William E. Connor, M.D.

Produced by the Family Heart
Study Nutrition Staff

Nancy Becker, M.S., R.D.
Joyce R. Gustafson, B.S., R.D.

Sabine M. Artaud-Wild, B.S., R.D.
Sandra R. Bacon, R.N.
Carolyn J. Classick-Kohn, M.S., R.D.
Donna P. Flavell, B.A., R.D.
Lauren F. Hatcher, M.S., R.D.
Holly J. Henry, M.S., R.D.
Martha P. McMurry, M.S., R.D.
Chere B. Pereira, B.S.
Susan R. Vaughan, B.S., R.D.

We appreciate the following publications which have provided inspiration for several recipes: *Laurel's Kitchen, Joy of Cooking, Sunset* magazine and cookbooks, *Betty Crocker's Cookbook, Diet for a Small Planet,* and *Oregon Trawl Fish and Shrimp Story.*

Special Thanks

This cookbook would not have been possible without the help of many people.

We are especially grateful to:
The Family Heart Study Participants who have shared newly found recipes and ideas in the spirit of adventure and openness to change. The 233 families who made up our study cheerfully embarked upon a five-year plan to alter their eating styles. These recipes reflect years of experimentation in both adapting family favorites and trying new foods.

We also wish to thank:
Typists—Marcia Hindman, Mary Wallis, Joanne Skirving, Heather Henderson and Paula Bisaccio
Cooks who prepared recipes for testing:
  Clinical Research Center Metabolic Kitchen Staff
    Vicki Norton, B.A.
    Peggy Smith, B.S.
  Family Heart Study
    Susan Watts
    Beth Scherman
Dietetic Interns at The Oregon Health Sciences University who helped develop new recipes.
Family, friends and colleagues who were willing to experiment and who ate many a strange-looking meal on the way to ultimately developing some great recipes.

INTRODUCTION

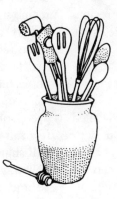

The Family Heart Study staff and families are proud to offer a rich collection of low-fat recipes. Together for the last seven years we've been testing, tasting, calculating and changing hundreds of new dishes. Our sources have been many and reflect the varied tastes and food experiences of our families, patients and staff members.

In creating this cookbook we've kept in mind several factors. The first was nutritional composition. Our recipes are low in fat and cholesterol. Minimal use of oils and margarine has kept most of the recipes under 5 grams (or 1 teaspoon) of fat per serving. Main dishes contain generally less than 10 grams of fat. The cholesterol content of our recipes is less than 100 milligrams per serving, many of them being cholesterol-free!

In addition, we've made every effort to keep the sodium content of recipes to a minimum. We suggest you use Lite Salt, a mixture of potassium and sodium chloride or one of the many salt substitutes rather than regular table salt. In our efforts to make these recipes as low in sodium as possible, we may have gone a bit below your salt threshold. If this is the case do add a little Lite Salt rather than give up the recipe. The recipes containing broth, bouillon, canned beans, seasonings from rice mixes or other convenience foods are higher in sodium than other recipes. By including these recipes along with others lower in sodium, we have found that the overall sodium content of a week's menus can meet the goals of the New American Diet. Besides, in the near future there will be more products on the market, low in sodium and tasting good.

You'll find generous amounts of grains, beans, potatoes, bread and pasta suggested, as well. This is in keeping with the New American Diet goal of increasing the use of plant products to boost complex carbohydrate and fiber intakes.

Another consideration has been ease of preparation. We've tried to simplify recipes that have many steps and minimize the use of unusual ingredients. We believe this collection of recipes will provide ideas for basic family fare as well as for those special occasions that warrant more time and effort.

You'll find several recipes that are labeled "Quick" and "Easy"; this is to help you identify those recipes that take 30 minutes or less to prepare (Quick) and those that can be tossed together in a few minutes but take an hour or so to cook (Easy).

The process of compiling this cookbook has been very exciting for everyone involved. We've tasted, discussed and analyzed every one of these recipes. You can imagine the prejudices and personal tastes that had to be confronted before we were able to reach a consensus. As it is, you may feel that some recipes taste better (or work better) than others. We welcome feedback and additional recipe suggestions.

Part of the excitement of working with these recipes was the realization that we all had favorites that were too high in fat and cholesterol, yet many could be salvaged with some imaginative modifications. It's been an eyeopener for all of us to learn to pare fat, use less salt and be creative. We hope that you will share our enthusiasm for cooking in this new way.

Enjoy!

BUT WHERE DO I START?

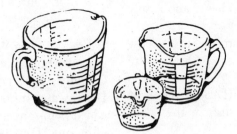

It is one thing to take a new cookbook and pick out recipes to try. It is entirely another thing to pick out recipes to try from a cookbook of a new cuisine. And low-fat cooking is just that. The most commonly asked question is "But where do I start?" To help you tackle this new world of recipes we have compiled suggestions from twelve people who have been cooking "low-fat" for two to seventeen years.

From Lauren: Works full time; runs every day after work; cooks very well for herself and husband, Paul.
—Skinny "French Fries" (A family favorite.)
—Beef and Bean Ragout (An everyday dish; I make a double batch and freeze.)
—Baked Corn Chips (Everyday snack.)
—Bean Dip (Great for burritos as well as for a party dip.)

—Bean Hot Dish (Good potluck recipe— omit beef for lunches.)
—Lemony Chicken Kabobs (BBQ for company)

From Sandy: Spends lots of time chasing Brian and cuddling Jonathan; cooks great food for herself, Kelly, her husband, and Brian.
—Chili Bean Salad (Wonderful for picnics.)
—Broccoli with Rice (Family favorites for meatless meal.)
—Marinara Sauce (An absolute "must" to have on hand for spaghetti, lasagna, manicotti, etc.)
—Spicy Chicken with Spinach (We love it!)
—Parmesan Yogurt Chicken (Kelly raves about this recipe.)
—Beef Tomato Chow Yuk (This has become a quick company standby and is delicious.)

—Easy Oven Lasagna (For the "I love lasagna but am too lazy to make it crowd.")
—Sesame Halibut (This recipe is great for the skeptical fish eater.)

From Joyce: Our expert on feeding teenagers. Ken and Tom flew the coop recently. Joyce now cooks wonderful dishes for herself, her husband, Dick, and lots of company.
—Super Stuffed Potatoes (Guests and family alike really like these.)
—Marinara Sauce (I was surprised it is so easy to make and tastes so good. Our favorite on fresh pasta.)
—Lively Lemon Roll-Ups (Dick wants us to put two stars by this dish in the cookbook.)
—Cioppino (Now a regular first-night item on camping trips. I make and freeze the soup base at home, pick up fresh fish as we leave town and put it on ice. Dinner only takes a few minutes to serve when we arrive hungry.)
—Acapulco Enchiladas (Our ski group now has asked this to be on the permanent menu for our annual New Year's trip.)
—Four Star Pasta Salad (So unusual and makes a lot so is great when you have a big crowd.)

From Nancy: A great cook who has been the inspiration behind the cookbook. Work, political activities and cooking for her weekly dinner collective all keep Nancy hopping.
—Whole Wheat French Bread (I don't often make bread, but this one is so spectacular that I make sure to include it in a company dinner. It's also foolproof!)
—Greek Lentil Soup (I make this one often.)
—Mushroom Barley Pilaf (There aren't too many barley recipes that come out as

well as this one does. It works well as a side dish or as a main dish.)
—Country Captain (I have been making this dish for company for years.)
—Stuffed Sole (This fish roll-up recipe is easy to make, is very, very good and the ingredients are cupboard staples—bread crumbs, carrots, parsley.)
—Vanilla Pudding (There's nothing better than vanilla pudding and fresh berries!)

From Sherry: Without a doubt the greatest user of whole grains and beans on our staff. Currently she's cooking tasty dishes for son Damon and husband Jim, and has recently added twin sons to her family.
—Skinny "French Fries" (This recipe is quick and easy.)
—No-Meat Enchiladas
—Cashew Chicken
—Chicken and Tomatoes in Black Bean Sauce (I substitute ½ tablespoon black bean and chili sauce for the fermented beans.)
—Broccoli Lasagna Rolls

From Donna: She has the ability to make really good dishes without a lot of ingredients and a lot of fuss. Her kids, Anne and Steve, and hubby, Tom, get good eats at her table.
—Cashew Chicken (This is probably everybody's favorite! With this recipe, I learned something of the art of stir frying and now can come up with many different combinations, depending on what's on hand.)
—Cheese Stuffed Manicotti (This is our family favorite right now. There's usually a little left over which is great for the next day's lunch.)
—Skinny "French Fries" (Easy to prepare. Be

sure to make a bit more than you think you'll need.)

—German Oven Pancake (This is always considered a treat at our house. Very impressive for company.)

—Acapulco Bean Casserole (A good standby and a favorite with kids.)

—Lively Lemon Roll-Ups (This is a great recipe—very attractive as well as tasty.)

From Barb: With eight children, she is the person on our staff who has cooked the most. Barb goes for convenience, but never cuts corners on taste and quality.

—Broccoli with Rice (This is good as a luncheon dish, a potluck favorite and a main dish with a little cubed chicken.)

—A Barrel of Muffins (Dough is always ready to pop in oven and 20 minutes later, fresh baked muffins for friends.)

From Chere: Her cooking life changed a bit with the birth of Birch. Chere is imaginative in her cooking for hubby, Cliff, and new son. Like the rest of the staff, they like good food.

—Bean Stroganoff (I was introduced to this when a friend made it on a camping trip and everyone really liked it.)

—Spinach Lasagna (People always remark that they've never had spinach in lasagna before and they really like it.)

—Poppy Seed Cake (This is nice baked in a tube pan, sliced horizontally and filled with lemon yogurt.)

—Frozen Fruit Yogurt (Everyone is always delighted when served frozen yogurt at our house.)

From Carolyn: Our new cook on the block. She cooks for Craig, who gave her a chuckle when he suggested that people should make changes in phases.

—Spicy Chicken with Spinach (Those of us who do not speak fluent "wok" find it easy to communicate with this dish.)

—Bean Hot Dish (This recipe is a great standby for last-minute picnics and potlucks.)

—Popeye's Spinach Dip (Finally, a dip that doesn't go directly to the hips!)

—Pinto Fiesta Cake (The last place one would look for beans is in a cake, yet here they are, unexpected and discreetly coupled with apple and cinnamon.)

—German Oven Pancake (I love this breakfast-brunch entrée because it is so much lighter than typical pancakes.)

—Parmesan Yogurt Chicken (This recipe is a good example of how versatile low-fat yogurt is.)

From Sabine: A great cook who can make any recipe "French." She has us all beat in knowing how to make delicious fish dishes and fruit desserts. After cooking for Anne, Phillip and Paul—now grown—she now enjoys cooking for friends.

—Eggplant Parmesan (Slice eggplant lengthwise and use only ¼ cup Parmesan to make it lighter.)

—Bean and Basil Soup (Grew up on it. Makes a whole meal when served with good bread and fruit.)

—Tomatoes "Provençale" (Goes well with chicken or fish; a favorite of my children.)

—Fish (The fish section of my cookbook is the one with the most food stains.)

—Fish à la Mistral (My "convenience" recipe. I always have cod in the freezer. Twenty minutes after I come home we sit down and eat this flavorful dish.)

—Salmon Mousse (The recipe I have used the most has been the Salmon Mousse. I serve it as an entrée, as a dip and take it to potlucks.)

From Tim: He doesn't cook much, but Jill, his wife, certainly does and well, too. They, along with Elizabeth and James, like the following recipes.
—Cheese Stuffed Manicotti
—Spinach Lasagna
—Broccoli with Rice
—Basic Stir-Fried Vegetables
—Tostadas

From Sonja: I am lucky Bill, Chris and Peter place high value for time spent on food preparation—so it's very rewarding for me to spend hours in the kitchen.

—Marinara Sauce (My most used recipe from the cookbook, a great recipe, 1000 uses, can be canned!)
—Whole Wheat French Bread (I make it three to four times a month—usually on Saturday—undercook it, freeze it, and it's just like fresh when heated.)
—Eggplant Parmesan (Bill has a fetish for eggplant and this is one of his favorites.)
—Broccoli with Rice (I have yet to find anyone who does not like this dish—very nice to serve with fish.)
—Fish Almondine with Dilly Sauce (Bill can eat this entire recipe.)
—Waffles (I make this recipe almost every weekend.)
—Spicy Chicken with Spinach (This is the current family favorite.)

TIPS FOR THE COOK

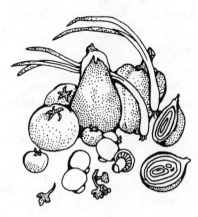

We view the principles of the New American Diet as guidelines for the gradual adoption of a new eating life-style. This may mean months or years. A new way of eating does not occur by decision only but by practice as well. To this extent we have provided the tools with which to practice—*recipes.*

Obviously, introducing new recipes and new foods into one's life-style can be met with all sorts of resistance. But many of us are convinced of the advantages of changing our diet in order to prevent heart disease and other diseases of overconsumption. Still, we know that some meals definitely go better than others. Are there tricks to the trade? Perhaps. Here are a few that work for us:

Go about changes slowly—You have heard this time and time again, but in our experience it cannot be emphasized enough. Hard-core milk drinkers, for example, take their beverages seriously so it is best to go from whole to skim milk cautiously. Many families have tried putting skim milk in the 2% carton with mixed results. Better to go a step at a time, 2%, 1%, etc.

Have good choices handy—For any changes to happen, the desirable foods must be near at hand. If potato chips are on the shelf, the family will reach for them and it will be back to the old habits. Our kitchens now contain popcorn, lower-fat cheeses, unshelled peanuts, dates, sunflower seeds and granola, with frozen yogurt, fresh fruit and ice water in the refrigerator. The trips to the junk counters have not been eliminated, but the better choices are closer to the TV.

Serve new dishes as a side dish first—We always try to have a surefire favorite with something really new or unusual. An eggplant dish with that suspicious name "ratatouille" seems much safer with a favorite chicken, mashed potatoes, fresh pineapple and the old standby, cookies.

Avoid repeating new foods too soon—It is easy to be excited about success, but give the memory of it time to grow. We have been very excited about bean cookery. As you know, there are numerous kinds of beans and ways to serve them. Now we hear the children ask if they will find beans in the fruit salad or popcorn. Bean soup, kidney beans in a salad and hummous (made from garbanzos) are all tasty, but it is probably best not to serve *all* of them in a week's time. And remember you need to get "acclimatized" to beans *gradually*.

Serve enough for everyone to get his/her fill—Remember, by serving lower-fat foods, you also *reduce* calories. Thus, by serving such things as lower-fat milk, mozzarella cheese, yogurt salad dressings, leaner meats, no chicken skin, fewer egg yolks and more sherbet, you are removing a lot of fat from the family's diet. These are all good steps for most of us who want to keep our weight down. However, for the growing teenager or the very active among us, additional foods must be eaten to replace the lost calories or someone will be saying: "I'm hungry; where are the candy bars?" Or worse yet: "Let's have some *good* foods tomorrow." If a teenager drinks three glasses of skim milk each day instead of the usual 3.8 percent, this is a reduction of 270 Calories in fat content alone! These can be made up by simply having another sandwich sometime along the way.

Enjoy your success and forget old habits—Stir-fried meals are very enjoyable for us, probably because they are easy to fix. The ultimate vote of confidence: "Folks, I'd like to invite some dinner guests who have unusual tastes; I'm sure *you'll* know some good things to fix for them!"

BASICS TO HAVE ON HAND

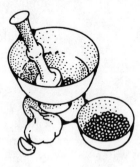

ON THE SHELF

Beans and peas, dry
  Kidney
  Garbanzo
  Black
  Soy
  Pinto
  Lentils
  Split Peas
Raisins, dates, dried fruits
Rice, white and brown
Bulgur
Pasta—spaghetti, eggless noodles, macaroni
  (whole wheat and white), several varieties
Barley
Unsalted nuts
  Walnuts
  Cashews
  Almonds
  Pecans
  Filberts
Unshelled, unsalted peanuts
Popcorn
Jams, jellies, maple syrups, honey, sugar
  (white/brown)
Unflavored gelatin
Falafel mix
Tabouli mix
Pancake mix (no egg yolk in mix)
Macaroni and cheese mixes
Peanut butter
Tahini (sesame seed butter or paste)
Whole wheat flour and unbleached flour
Angel food cake mix
Bouillon, cubes, granules or canned
Chicken broth, cubes, granules or canned
Powdered nonfat milk
Cornmeal
Cornstarch

Breakfast cereals,* uncooked (oatmeal,
  Ralston, Wheatena, etc.) and ready to eat
Baking soda and baking powder
Vegetarian burger mix
Pizza mixes
Beans, Canned †
  Pinto
  Kidney
  Garbanzo (chick-peas)
  Refried (vegetarian)
Tomatoes, canned (no salt added)
Tomato paste (no salt added)
Tomato sauce, regular, spaghetti, pizza, etc.
  (no salt added)
Green chiles, jalapeño
Salsa
Tuna fish, water-packed
Pineapple and other fruits, juice or water-
  packed
Vegetable oil
Molasses
Water chestnuts
Olives
Mushrooms
Bean sprouts

IN THE BREADBOX
Whole wheat bread, French bread
English muffins
Pocket bread
Lower-fat crackers* (graham, Bremner, Finn
Crisp, ak-mak, soda with unsalted tops, Wasa
Bread, Zwieback, rice cakes, Cracottes,
RyKrisp)
Tortillas (flour and corn)
Pretzels (unsalted)

IN THE REFRIGERATOR/FREEZER
Soft margarine
Egg substitute and/or eggs (use whites)
Lower-fat cheeses,* some of which are Light
  n' Lively, Green River, Olympia's Low Fat,

Lite-line, Kiel-Kase, Heidi Ann, mozzarella
  (imitation or part-skim), Scandic Mini
  Chol (Swedish low cholesterol), Hickory
  Farms Smokey Lyte, low-fat cottage cheese,
  Reduced Calories Laughing Cow
Low-fat yogurt
Skim milk (fresh and/or canned)
Buttermilk
Imitation or light mayonnaise or Miracle
  Whip Light
Low-calorie salad dressing/mix
Fresh lemons
Sherbet, sorbet and/or frozen yogurt
Assorted fruits and vegetables (fresh, frozen)
Parsley
Chicken or turkey breasts, skinned
Fish (red snapper, cod, fillet of sole, etc.)
Ground lean beef (10 percent fat)
Beef round steak or flank steak
Turkey sausage
Ground turkey

CONDIMENTS AND SPICES
Lower-sodium soy sauce (Kikkoman Lite Soy
  Sauce) *
Lite Salt *
Low-sodium ketchup
Tabasco sauce
Rosemary leaves
Oregano leaves
Garlic
Dill weed
Thyme leaves
Basil leaves

This is only a starter list

* Certain products are listed to provide examples of
food items on the market which are acceptable choices
for a person wishing to comply with the New American
Diet goals. Often there are other products of similar
composition with different trade names which are also
acceptable for use.
† Use low-sodium beans if available.

A GUIDE TO USING FOODS BOUGHT IN BULK

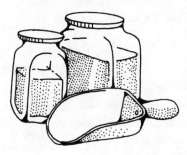

When buying food in bulk from bins rather than in tidy packages, you will notice that there are no directions for cooking! We hope this will acquaint you with a few of the many foods available in bulk as well as help you if and when you decide to take on the challenge of purchasing foods in large quantities.

BEANS

Regular Method. Soak beans overnight in 3–4 times their volume of water; *or* bring the beans and water to a boil, cover tightly and let sit for 2 hours. After the soaking process, simmer the beans (partially covered) until soft. Refer to table 27 for specific cooking times. Keep in mind that cooking time will vary depending on *how soft* you desire the beans.

TABLE 27
Cooking Times and Proportions

Beans	Water	Cooking Time
1 cup dry measure (yield approximately 2 cups)	3–4 cups	
Black beans		1½ hours
Black-eyed peas		1 hour
Garbanzos (chickpeas)		3 hours
Great Northern beans		2 hours
Kidney beans		2 hours
Lentils		¾–1 hour
Limas		1½ hours
Pinto beans		2 hours
Small white beans (navy, etc.)		1½ hours
Soybeans		3 hours or more
Split peas		¾–1 hour

Pressure Cooker. With this method, pre-soaking is unnecessary. Bring the washed beans to boil in 3–4 times their volume of water. (Fill cooker no more than half full.) Cover and bring to 15 pounds pressure. Cook beans for 15–30 minutes; cool immediately. *Caution: Don't* pressure-cook split peas, lentils or soybeans; they tend to foam and may clog pressure valve. Use table 27 to establish cooking times; smaller beans take less time, larger beans will need to cook for the longer period.

FALAFEL

Falafel is a "convenience food" from the Middle East. It's a spicy (curry) garbanzo bean powder that mixes with water to form patties or balls. Delicious served as a sandwich with pita bread, yogurt, tomatoes, and sprouts. Great for backpacking.

1. Mix 1 cup falafel with ¾ cup water (4 servings). You can add 1 egg white at this point to help keep things together (optional).

2. Let stand for 5–10 minutes. (When ready to use, it should be about the consistency of oatmeal cookie dough. Adjust proportions accordingly.)

3. Make into patties or tablespoon-sized balls.

4. Brush your cast-iron skillet with oil or preheat small quantities of vegetable oil in skillet. Cook patties until golden brown on both sides. Falafel patties may also be baked (on nonstick baking sheet) in oven at 350° for 10 minutes.

GRAINS

Keep in mind that there is great variability among the grains—and this will apply to their cooking times (see table 28) and amounts of liquid required, as well. The following is an oversimplification but it will help to some extent. Ultimately, when it comes to grains, your experience will be your best guide.

TABLE 28
Timetable for Cooking Grains

Grains	Regular Cooking
White rice, bulgur, cracked wheat and soft or partially cooked grains	15–20 minutes
Brown rice, barley and other medium grains (For millet use 4 grain: 1 water)	40–45 minutes
Whole wheat berries, whole rye, whole oats and other "hard" grains	1 hour or more*

*May be soaked overnight or simmered, then soaked for 2 hours to shorten cooking time.

Regular Cooking Method for Rice and Other Grains.

1. Rinse grain under cold water and drain.

2. Bring to boil twice as much water as grain you are cooking—for example, 4 cups water for 2 cups rice.

3. Stir in grain and bring mixture to a second boil.

4. Lower heat to simmer, cover tightly and cook until all the liquid is absorbed and grain is tender. (Don't uncover or stir until time is up.)

5. If rice or other grain is not tender when all of the liquid is absorbed, add hot water and simmer again.

Sauté Method. Common for bulgur or buckwheat groats but delicious with rice also.

1. Heat *small* quantity of oil in skillet or pot (just enough to toast the grain without burning it).

2. Sauté grain for about 5 minutes (or more), stirring often. (You may also sauté onions, garlic, celery, etc. with grain.)

3. Add hot water (2 times the volume of grain), bring to a second boil, lower heat, cover and simmer as above under regular cooking.

NUTS AND SEEDS

To roast from raw state: Place in a dry pan and roast over medium flame until desired brownness, or spread them on a baking sheet and toast them in a 200° oven.

TOFU

Tofu is bean curd—a bland, white soybean product. It resembles cheese curd in its texture. It is sold in slices (4 inches square by 1 inch thick) or slabs, comes firm or soft, and is kept refrigerated in a water bath. (Change water *daily*.) Tofu is found diced in Oriental cooking (soups, stir-fried vegetables, etc.); also good in spicy dishes like lasagna or served alone (breaded and skinny fried).

TVP

TVP is "Textured Vegetable Protein" (beef-, chicken- or ham-flavored soy product). Useful as a meat substitute or extender. We suggest either using in combination with meat or, if used alone, use in spicy dishes. Reconstitute with appropriate bouillon for better flavor. To reconstitute:

Add 1⅔ cups TVP to 1⅔ cups hot water. Let soak 3 to 5 minutes, stirring occasionally. (Makes approximately 1 pound product.)

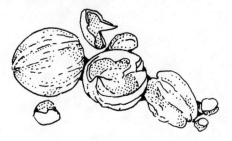

REDUCING FAT, CHOLESTEROL AND SALT

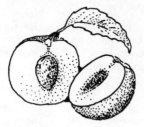

Choices are never easy. Here are some suggestions which show a progression toward the New American Diet goals.

PRESENT AMERICAN DIET	TOWARD THE NEW AMERICAN DIET	
Egg yolks	Make omelets and scrambled eggs with fewer egg yolks and more egg whites (e.g., 4 whites with only 1 yolk)	Bake or cook with 1–2 whites in place of each yolk Use egg whites, commercial egg substitute or *Homemade Egg Substitute*
Margarine on Bread Biscuits Pancakes Waffles	Use less spread—learn "art of scraping"	Breads from whole grains/fresh French bread with no spread Use honey or jam as spread on bread Syrup or fruit as spread on pancakes, waffles
Margarine on baked potatoes	Use less fat Use diet margarine	Use 　*Mock Sour Cream* 　*Western Salad Dressing* 　Plain yogurt—add dill, chives or green onions 　Low-calorie Italian dressing 　Low-fat cottage cheese 　Salsa

NOTE: Recipes in italics can be found in this section.

PRESENT AMERICAN DIET →	TOWARD THE NEW AMERICAN DIET →	
Margarine or oil to sauté or fry	Use minimal amount of oil—1 Tbsp. for stir-frying vegetables, hash browns or *Skinny Sole*	Use nonstick pan or spray Sauté without fat over medium heat Steam vegetables in small amount of boiling water—excellent for casseroles Microwave, covered Grill over charcoal Broil or bake meats with no frying Poach fish
Margarine, oil, shortening in baking	Use ½ to ¾ the amount the recipe calls for (not more than ½ cup fat per recipe)	Use recipes with only ¼ cup of fat or less (for 12 servings)
Mayonnaise or Miracle Whip (for use in tuna or potato salad, sandwiches, etc.)	Use ½ the amount Use imitation or light mayonnaise or Miracle Whip Light Mix imitation mayonnaise or Miracle Whip Light with plain low-fat yogurt	Use small amount of imitation mayonnaise Use *Tangy Salad Dressing* Mix low-fat cottage cheese with water-packed tuna fish for sandwiches
Salad dressings Thousand Island, blue cheese, Avocado, Sour Cream or mayonnaise type	Use less by mixing greens and dressing (add tomatoes, cucumber, etc. after dressing the salad) Make ranch dressing with imitation or light mayonnaise or Miracle Whip Light *Red French Salad Dressing* *Vinaigrette Salad Dressing*	Commercial low-calorie salad dressings Lemon juice or vinegar *Western Salad Dressing* Use low-fat yogurt to replace most of the mayonnaise or sour cream in recipes
Creamer for coffee (Coffee Rich, half-&-half or store-brand creamers)	Use less and use powdered creamer, 2% milk, Mocha Mix or Poly Rich	Powdered nonfat milk Evaporated skim milk Skim milk
Sour cream	Sour half & half Combine sour half & half with low-fat yogurt	Low-fat yogurt *Mock Sour Cream* in dishes which are not heated
Real whipped cream or whipped topping (Redi-Whip, Cool Whip, and others)	On special occasions— Use ½ the amount of topping Dream Whip made with skim milk	Vanilla low-fat yogurt *Yogurt Dessert Sauce*
Whole milk	2% milk for drinking and for cooking	1% or skim milk for all uses
Ice cream	Ice milk Soft-serve ice cream	Frozen Fudgsicle Frozen yogurt, sherbet Frozen ices or sorbets Light ice milk

PRESENT AMERICAN DIET →	TOWARD THE NEW AMERICAN DIET →	
Cheese in cooking: Cheddar Swiss Jack, etc.	Use smaller amounts of: Green River, Olympia's Low-Fat, part-skim mozzarella or ricotta Mix high-fat cheese with lower-fat cheeses	Use Lite n' Lively or Lite-line Use smaller amounts of imitation mozzarella, Cheezola, Scandic Mini Chol or low-fat cottage cheese in casseroles
Parmesan Romano	Use in small amounts—2 Tbsp. per serving	Use in smaller amounts—1 Tbsp. per serving
Cheese for appetizers and snacking: Havarti Brie Port Salut Cheddar Roquefort Feta etc.	Use Green River, Olympia's Low Fat or light cream cheeses sparingly Save cheese for special occasions—not to eat regularly as a snack	Use Reduced Calories Laughing Cow cheese or small amounts of herb-flavored, part-skim ricotta on low-fat crackers
Cheese in sandwiches or burgers: Cheddar Swiss Jack American slices	Use part-skim mozzarella or ricotta in small amounts	*Fruit and Nut Sandwich Spread* or Reduced Calories Laughing Cow Cheese Lite-line Lite n' Lively Use *Hummous* or *Salmon Mousse* in sandwiches
Cream cheese and Cream cheese spreads	Use Neufchâtel in small amounts	Save for very special occasions Whip part-skim ricotta for a spread Use light cream cheese in frostings
French fries Hash browns Tater Tots	*Skinny "French Fries"* Hash browns cooked in very little oil (1 tsp./svg.) *Homemade Tatertots*	Baked potato with *Mock Sour Cream* or low-fat yogurt or low-fat cottage cheese
Doughnuts Danish pastries Croissants	Eat less often Eat Muffins *Baked Doughnut Holes*	Bagels with Reduced Calories Laughing Cow cheese or part-skim ricotta or *Salmon Mousse* Toast English muffins *Soft Pretzels*
Snack crackers (most) *Ritz* *Triscuits* *Wheat Thins* etc.	As a special treat only	Bremner wafers, soda crackers with unsalted tops, unseasoned RyKrisp, ak-mak, popcorn, unsalted pretzels, melba toast, flatbread, Wasa, Cracottes or rice cakes
Chips *Potato* *Corn* *Doritos* *Fritos, etc.*	As a special treat only	*Pita Chips* *Baked Corn Chips* Popcorn

PRESENT AMERICAN DIET	TOWARD THE NEW AMERICAN DIET	
Potato chips on casseroles	Use ½ the amount Mix ½ chips and ½ cracker crumbs	Bread or cereal crumbs Cracker crumbs Plain bran flakes
Cookies Cakes Brownies (even those without egg yolk!)	Eat less often Reduce amount of nuts Serve without frosting Avoid coconut	Vanilla wafers, gingersnaps, graham crackers, fig bars, Animal Crackers, fortune cookies Fruit for dessert Angel food cake
Two-crust pie	Single crust made with soft margarine or Crisco or oil	*Graham Cracker Crust* *Apple Crisp* Cobblers with biscuit topping
Granola and Granola bars	Choose commercial granola without coconut or nuts Mix granola with Grape-Nuts Make *Our Granola*	Bran cereals, Puffed Rice, Shredded Wheat, Grape-Nuts, Wheat Chex, Rice Krispies or a combination of dry cereals with dried fruit Hot cereal
All chocolate and chocolate chips candy creams toffee	Save for special occasions Use less than recipe calls for. In baking replace 1 oz. chocolate with 3 Tbsp. dry cocoa and 1 Tbsp. oil	For treats eat Life Savers, jelly beans, hard candy
Pizza Sausage/Bacon	Canadian bacon, shrimp or vegetarian pizza	Make your own: *Spicy Cheese Pizza*, *Pita Pizza*
Peanut butter	Use as part of a *meal*, not a snack Omit margarine on bread when making peanut butter sandwiches	Spread thinly and use jelly or honey with the spread
Nuts and seeds (all kinds)	Use as *condiment* to add texture to casseroles and mixed dishes and not as a snack Use less in recipes	Use popcorn or unsalted pretzels as snacks Use ½ cup nuts or less per recipe in baked items (banana bread, etc.)
Lunch meat sandwiches (bologna/salami)	Chicken or turkey breasts Turkey wieners (less often) Turkey pastrami Turkey ham	Small amount of thinly sliced pressed turkey or chicken lunch meat with lots of vegetables
Ground beef 25%–30% fat (in casseroles)	Use less meat than recipe calls for (increase rice or pasta) Use 10%–20% fat beef	Use ground turkey or chicken Use 10% fat ground beef in small amounts or in combination with textured vegetable protein (TVP)
Gravy	Refrigerate meat juice; skim off the fat before thickening Use less often	Save for special occasions Make *Turkey Gravy*

APPETIZERS AND HORS D'OEUVRES

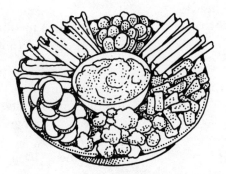

A meal with friends often calls for an opening act such as dips, canapes or "finger foods." Traditionally, these have been high in fat, cholesterol and sodium. Here we have gathered a selection of appetizers that come from the vegetable realm and contain no meat, fish or high-fat cheese.

Consider using an array of dips (such as Hummous or Bean Dip) with Baked Corn Chips or vegetable dippers rather than potato chips. Mock Sour Cream can be used with various herbs to create unusual creamy-based dips. For a snazzy effect, serve Dill Dip in a hollowed-out red cabbage. Bean Dip is also an excellent sandwich spread; with sprouts or lettuce, it can be an interesting (and filling) lunch. Any spread, such as Herbed Tofu Dip, works well with a salad or soup for a light supper.

Antipasto
Baked Corn Chips
Bean Dip
Broccoli Canapés
Chowchow
Cream Puff Shells
Dill Dip
Eggplant Delight
Great Little Snackers
Herbed Tofu Dip
Hummous
Marinated Mushrooms
Mock Sour Cream
Mushroom Nut Pâté
Onion Squares (see "Side Dishes" section)
Pita Chips
Popeye's Spinach Dip
St. Helens Appetizer
Salmon Mousse (see "Fish and Shellfish" section)
Spicy Stuffed Mushrooms
Steamed Buns

ANTIPASTO

This beautiful dish is a great appetizer and also a lovely salad. Can be made several days ahead and kept chilled.

VEGETABLES (Group 1)
  2 cups carrots
  1½ cups zucchini (1 small)
  6 cups cauliflower (small head)
  4 cups broccoli (small bunch)
  1 medium green pepper

DRESSING
  ½ cup chili sauce (tomato-based)
  1 tablespoon oil
  ¼ cup freshly squeezed lemon juice
  ¼ cup wine vinegar
  2–3 cloves garlic, minced
  ½ teaspoon dry mustard
  1 teaspoon oregano leaves
  1 teaspoon basil leaves

VEGETABLES (Group 2)
  1 can (6 ounces) black olives, pitted and drained
  1 can (6 ounces) artichoke hearts, drained and quartered
  ½ pound fresh mushrooms, sliced lengthwise, not thinly
  ½ of 13 ounce jar medium-hot chili peppers, drained
  1 pint cherry tomatoes

Chop or slice first 5 ingredients into attractive bite-sized pieces. Boil vegetables briefly until crisp-tender (5 minutes for carrots, 2 minutes for the others). Drain. In a saucepan, combine dressing ingredients and bring to boiling point. While hot, pour over boiled and drained vegetables in a large bowl. Toss gently, cool to room temperature, drain well and add Group 2 vegetables. (Drained dressing can be used elsewhere for a salad dressing.) Toss thoroughly and gently. Chill.

Makes 32 servings (½ cup each). This recipe makes a large amount, but the recipe divides in half easily.

✗ BAKED CORN CHIPS

  20 corn tortillas *
  Margarine (not more than 2 teaspoons)

Scrape each tortilla with a small amount of soft margarine. Cut tortillas, several at a time, into 8 pie-shaped wedges using kitchen shears. Arrange in a single layer on cookie sheet. Bake at 350° until crisp and slightly browned (10 minutes). Store in an airtight container.

Makes approximately 8 cups.

* Use thin tortillas (e.g., Diane's Corn Tortillas.)

BEAN DIP

This dip makes a marvelous burrito filling. To prepare, simply spoon bean dip inside a warm flour tortilla and roll up. (For an easier bean dip, combine several tablespoons of salsa with refried beans.)

  ¼ cup diced green chiles
  ¼ cup unsalted tomato sauce
  4 green onions, chopped
  ¼–½ teaspoon ground cumin
  ½ teaspoon garlic powder
  1 can (30 ounces) refried beans *

Combine chiles, tomato sauce, onions and seasonings in a saucepan and cook until onions are tender. Add beans and simmer until warmed through. Serve either hot or cold; may be topped with grated low-fat cheese.

Makes about 4 cups.

* Use low-sodium beans if available.

BROCCOLI CANAPÉS

Can also be made with raw cauliflower.

1 bunch fresh broccoli
2 teaspoons olive oil
⅛ teaspoon Lite Salt or less
12 stuffed olives, cut in half
Juice of 1 lemon

Wash broccoli and cut off flowerets into bite-size pieces. Sprinkle with olive oil, garlic powder and Lite Salt. Add stuffed olives and the juice of one lemon. Toss lightly with fork and cover. Marinate for several hours before serving. Serve with wooden picks for spearing.

Makes 16 servings (¼ cup each).

CHOWCHOW

From Phoenix, Arizona, where the sun does shine and shine and shine . . . Make this when tomatoes are nice and ripe.

2 tomatoes, finely chopped
3–4 green onions, finely chopped
1 can (4 ounces) diced green chiles (or less if a milder product is preferred)
1 can (2.2 ounces) black olives, sliced
1 tablespoon olive oil
1 tablespoon vinegar
½ teaspoon garlic powder

Combine ingredients and serve with the Baked Corn Chips, page 220.

Makes 8 servings (2 cups).

CREAM PUFF SHELLS

These are great when filled with "Egg" Salad Sandwich Spread.

1 cup skim milk
⅓ cup margarine
1 cup flour
⅛ teaspoon Lite Salt or less
8 egg whites, at room temperature or
** 1 cup egg substitute (commercial or Homemade Egg Substitute, page 241)**

Place milk and margarine in heavy saucepan. Bring to a boil and add flour and Lite Salt. Stir quickly with a wooden spoon. The batter looks rough at first, but suddenly becomes smooth, at which point you stir FASTER! In a few minutes the paste becomes dry and doesn't cling to spoon or pan. When a spoon pressed on dough leaves a smooth imprint, stop stirring and REMOVE FROM HEAT.

Let sit for about 2 minutes, then beat in egg substitute or egg whites one at a time. The proper consistency has been reached when a small quantity of dough will stand up on the end of a spoon. Spoon onto a lightly oiled cookie sheet in small ¾-inch balls. When pan is filled, moisten tip of your finger and smooth down any points (otherwise they will burn). Sprinkle all of pan lightly with water (a spray bottle works well).

Bake in 400° oven for 10 minutes. Reduce the heat to 350° and bake about 25 minutes more. Do not remove from oven until firm to the touch. Cool before filling. (May be frozen at this point for future use). Cut horizontally almost all the way through, and place a teaspoon of filling in each. Fill shortly before serving so puffs will not become soggy.

Makes 2 dozen 3-inch shells.

DILL DIP

Very attractive when served in a hollowed-out red cabbage.

2 cups low-fat cottage cheese
4 tablespoons buttermilk
1½ teaspoons freshly squeezed lemon juice

Mix above ingredients in blender until very smooth. Remove from blender and add:

½ cup imitation mayonnaise or ¼ cup mayonnaise
1 tablespoon finely chopped parsley
1 tablespoon finely chopped onion
¾ teaspoon Beau Monde seasoning
1½ teaspoons dill weed

Chill until very cold. To serve in hollowed-out cabbage, flatten bottom of the cabbage head by slicing off a piece so it will sit straight. Surround with fresh vegetables on a large platter.
Makes 3 cups.

EGGPLANT DELIGHT

An unusual spread for crackers—"easy caviar"

2 eggplants
¼ cup very finely minced onion
¼ cup very finely minced scallions
1 teaspoon finely minced garlic
¼ cup very finely chopped green pepper
1 cup very finely diced, peeled tomatoes
¼ cup olive oil
1 teaspoon sugar
1 tablespoon freshly squeezed lemon juice, or more to taste
Ground black pepper to taste

Preheat oven to 400°. Place the whole eggplants on a sheet of heavy-duty aluminum foil and bake for 1½ hours or until the eggplant "collapses." Let cool. Remove the pulp and mash it. (There should be about 3 cups.) Add the onion, scallions, garlic, green pepper, tomatoes, olive oil, sugar, lemon juice and pepper to the mashed eggplant and stir well to combine. Serve as a spread on low-fat crackers.
Makes 5 cups.

GREAT LITTLE SNACKERS

Tahini, a "butter" made from sesame seeds, adds a wonderful flavor to this spread.

1 teaspoon olive oil
1 large onion, chopped
1 can (16 ounces) garbanzo beans, drained *
¼ cup tahini †
¼ cup imitation mayonnaise
1 teaspoon lower-sodium soy sauce
1 teaspoon chili powder
1–2 tablespoons water, if needed

Alfalfa sprouts
Low-fat crackers (Bremner Wafers work well)

Heat oil in fry pan. Sauté onions until light brown. Put into blender and add drained garbanzo beans, tahini, imitation mayonnaise, soy sauce and chili powder. Mix until a smooth texture is obtained. Add water as needed to blend. Spread ½ tablespoon of this

---

* Use low-sodium beans if available.

† Tahini is sometimes labeled "sesame seed butter" and is usually available in supermarkets in the specialty food section.

mix on low-fat crackers and top with alfalfa sprouts. (Small rounds of whole-grain bread may be used instead of crackers.)

Makes about 2¼ cups spread (enough for 72 crackers). Leftover spread freezes well for a month when stored in tightly covered container.

HERBED TOFU DIP

½ of 22-ounce carton (11 ounces) firm
  tofu, drained
¾ teaspoon celery seed
1 tablespoon chopped fresh parsley
½ cup sliced green onions
2 teaspoons Dijon mustard
1 teaspoon prepared horseradish
½ teaspoon dill weed
¼ teaspoon onion powder
2 cloves garlic, minced
½ teaspoon Lite Salt

Pat tofu dry. Whirl in a blender until very smooth; start and stop motor often enough to push tofu into blades. Turn into a bowl and mix with seasonings. Serve with fresh vegetables.

Makes 1½ cups.

HUMMOUS

2 cups cooked and drained garbanzo
  beans (canned beans * can be used)
¼ cup tahini †
2–5 tablespoons freshly squeezed lemon
  juice
1 garlic clove, chopped fine
¼–½ cup water
1 tablespoon chopped parsley

Combine above ingredients (except parsley) in the blender and blend until smooth, adding water as necessary. Remove from blender and add chopped parsley.

SERVE AS DIP WITH:
  Low-fat crackers
  Pieces of Middle Eastern bread

OR AS A SANDWICH WITH:
  Middle Eastern bread (also called pocket
    or pita bread)
  Alfalfa sprouts

Makes 2½ cups.

* Use low-sodium beans if available.

† Tahini is sometimes labeled "sesame seed butter" and is usually available in super markets in the specialty food section.

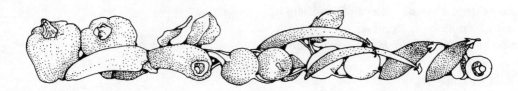

MARINATED MUSHROOMS

Spicy and juicy, these appeal to everyone.

**2 pints fresh mushrooms *or* 2 cans (6
ounces each) mushroom crowns,
drained
²⁄₃ cup tarragon vinegar
1 onion, sliced and separated into rings
1 clove garlic, minced
1 tablespoon sugar
½ teaspoon Lite Salt or less
2 tablespoons water
2 tablespoons oil
Pepper and dash cayenne**

Remove stems of mushrooms if using fresh
ones. Wash and pour boiling water over
mushroom crowns. Stir for 2–3 minutes.
Drain and marinate in remaining ingredients
overnight. When ready to serve, drain most
of marinade off and place mushrooms and onions in shallow serving dish. Serve with
wooden picks for spearing.
　Makes 10 servings.

MOCK SOUR CREAM

May be used for sour cream in any recipe that
doesn't require heating.

**1 cup low-fat cottage cheese
2 tablespoons buttermilk
½–1 teaspoon freshly squeezed lemon
juice**

Blend cottage cheese, buttermilk and lemon
juice in blender or with mixer until smooth.
Scrape sides of container often with rubber
spatula while blending.
　Makes 1 cup.

USES
As a dip for crackers, pretzels, breadsticks,
fresh vegetables or berries; as a dressing for
fruit or vegetable salads; as a topping for potatoes, cooked vegetables, tortillas, etc.; as a
spread for bagels.

NOTE: If a recipe requires the sour cream to
be heated, use *plain low-fat yogurt* directly
from the carton.

MUSHROOM NUT PÂTÉ

**1 pound fresh mushrooms, sliced
1 small onion, sliced
1 clove garlic, minced
⅓ cup slivered almonds, toasted
1 tablespoon oil
¼ teaspoon thyme leaves
Dash of tabasco sauce
1 tablespoon chopped parsley**

Steam mushrooms, onions and garlic in 3
tablespoons water. Remove from heat, drain
and reserve the liquid.
　Toast almonds by stir-frying in nonstick fry
pan for a few minutes. Coarsely chop almonds
in blender or processor; remove 1 tablespoon
and set aside. Continue chopping remaining
nuts, slowly adding oil until mixture is well
blended. Add reserved mushroom liquid if
mixture looks too dry. Add thyme, tabasco
and mushroom mixture and blend thoroughly. Remove from blender. Stir in the reserved nuts. Mold into loaf and sprinkle with
chopped parsley or spoon into attractive small
serving dish. Serve with low-fat crackers.
　Makes 2 cups.

PITA CHIPS

These are good with bean dip, with soups and in lunches.

Preheat oven to 325°. Split each of 6 pita breads into 2 round pieces (whole wheat pita bread has more fiber). Cut each half into 6 triangles with kitchen scissors. Arrange in single layers on cookie sheets. Sprinkle lightly with garlic powder, if desired. Bake for 8 minutes until chips are lightly browned and very crisp. Store in tight container.

Makes 8 cups.

POPEYE'S SPINACH DIP

Serve in a round loaf of bread which has been hollowed out!

    1 package (10 ounces) frozen, chopped
      spinach, thawed and squeezed dry
    ¼ package dry vegetable soup mix
    1¾ cups plain low-fat yogurt
    ¼ cup imitation mayonnaise
    1 can (8 ounces) water chestnuts,
      drained and chopped
    2 tablespoons chopped chives or green
      onions

Thaw spinach, drain and squeeze until fairly dry. Stir dry soup mix before measuring, to ensure that it is evenly mixed. Mix all ingredients together when spinach is ready. Chill and serve with raw vegetables.

For an unusual serving dish, slice top off a round loaf of unsliced sourdough bread and hollow out inside. Fill with cold dip. Save insides to use for bread crumbs, or cube and use for dipping.

Makes 4 cups.

ST. HELENS APPETIZER

Low-fat nachos!

    1 recipe Baked Corn Chips, page 220

    2 cups Refried Beans, page 281
    1½ cups plain low-fat yogurt *or* Mock
      Sour Cream, page 224
    1 cup shredded lettuce
    1 cup chopped tomatoes
    ¼ avocado, chopped
    Salsa (taco or hot sauce) as desired

Prepare Baked Corn Chips. Heat Refried Beans in a saucepan. Spread corn chips on an attractive serving dish. Spoon Refried Beans carefully over corn chips. (It will be uneven.) Layer yogurt *or* Mock Sour Cream, lettuce, tomatoes and avocado over beans ending with salsa.

Makes 12 servings.

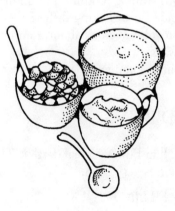

SPICY STUFFED MUSHROOMS

Use medium-size, very fresh mushrooms.

1 pound medium mushrooms (about 3 dozen)
1 tablespoon margarine
¼ cup finely chopped green pepper
¼ cup finely chopped onion
1½ cups finely chopped bread
¼ teaspoon Lite Salt or less
½ teaspoon thyme leaves
¼ teaspoon turmeric
¼ teaspoon pepper

Heat oven to 350°. Wash, trim and dry mushrooms thoroughly. Remove stems; finely chop enough stems to measure ⅓ cup. Melt margarine in skillet. Cook and stir chopped mushroom stems, green peppers and onions until crisp tender. Remove from heat; stir in remaining ingredients except mushroom caps. Lightly oil shallow baking dish. Fill mushroom caps with stuffing mixture; place mushrooms filled side up in baking dish. Bake 20 minutes in a regular oven or about 3 minutes in the microwave.

Makes about 3 dozen appetizers.

STEAMED BUNS

"Homemade Hom Bow"—a real dazzler. This meatless version is very good.

SAUCE FOR FILLING
2 teaspoons cornstarch
2 tablespoons water
½ teaspoon vinegar
½ teaspoon sesame oil
2 teaspoons lower-sodium soy sauce
¼ teaspoon sugar

FILLING FOR BUNS
1 clove garlic, minced
1 teaspoon peeled and minced fresh ginger root
½ teaspoon black bean sauce with chili *
1 teaspoon oil
3 green onions, minced
½ cup finely chopped, drained water chestnuts
2½ cups chopped Chinese cabbage

3 cans (7.5 ounces each) refrigerated buttermilk biscuits (makes 30 biscuits)

To prepare sauce for filling: Dissolve cornstarch in water in small bowl and add remaining sauce ingredients. Set aside.

To prepare filling: Mix garlic, ginger and black bean sauce with chili. Heat 1 teaspoon oil in skillet or wok. Add garlic mixture and stir until very hot. Add green onions, water chestnuts and Chinese cabbage. Stir-fry until cabbage is limp. Add cornstarch sauce and stir until thickened. This filling can be made ahead and refrigerated.

Roll out one of the canned biscuits on a floured board with a small glass or cup, until it is about 3 inches in diameter. Roll the edges out so that the center is slightly thicker. Place 2 teaspoons of the filling in the center. Bring up the edges of the biscuit so that they meet in the center and pleat them together, then press down on top so that the biscuit is an enclosed shell around the filling, with fluting around the top. Repeat this process with each of the 30 biscuits, then place them on waxed paper squares in a steamer. Steam as many as will fit in the steamer for 6 minutes.

Makes 30 steamed buns.

* Available in Oriental specialty stores.

BREADS AND MUFFINS

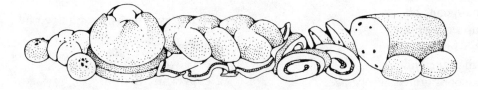

Because breads are important to include in every meal, you will find these recipes referred to many times throughout the book. They also make great snacks. This is only a small sample of the recipes that are generally available, but the recipes we have chosen to be in this section are low in fat and often high in fiber. If you serve them fresh and warm you will need no spread.

YEAST BREADS

Caraway Dinner Rolls
Honey Wheat Bread
Pita Bread
Soft Pretzels
Whole Wheat French Bread
Whole Wheat Refrigerator Roll Dough

MUFFINS

A Barrel of Muffins
Blueberry Bran Muffins
Carrot and Bran Muffins
Cereal Bran Muffins
Fruit and Nut Muffins
Natural Bran Muffins
Whole Wheat Muffins

SPECIALTY ITEMS

Baking Mix
Old-Style Wheat Biscuits
Pizza Crusts
Whole Wheat Tortillas

QUICK BREADS

Apricot Nut Bread
Corn Bread
Cranberry Bread
Grandma Kirschner's Date Nut Bread
Hearty Corn Bread
Lemon Nut Bread
Pumpkin Harvest Loaf
Quick Wheat Bread

Quick Breads

APRICOT NUT BREAD

Apricots and pecans make a lovely tea bread.

2½ cups flour
1 cup sugar
1½ tablespoons baking powder
½ teaspoon Lite Salt or less
3 tablespoons oil
½ cup skim milk
2 egg whites
¼ cup orange juice
4 teaspoons grated orange peel
¼ cup chopped pecans
10 large halves dried apricots, chopped

Preheat oven to 350°. Lightly oil and flour 9-by-5-inch loaf pan. Measure all ingredients into large mixer bowl; beat on medium speed ½ minute, scraping sides and bottom of bowl constantly. Pour into pan. Bake 35 to 45 minutes or until wooden pick inserted in center comes out clean. Remove from pan after 5 minutes; cool thoroughly before slicing.
Makes 1 loaf (16 slices).

CORN BREAD

Our motto is "If it has fat in it, don't put any on it!"

1 cup cornmeal
1 cup flour
1 tablespoon sugar
1 tablespoon baking powder
3 tablespoons oil
2 egg whites
1 cup skim milk

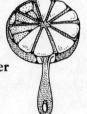

Heat oven to 400°. Combine dry ingredients in bowl and mix well. Beat oil, egg whites and milk together. Mix with dry ingredients until just blended. Pour into lightly oiled 8-by-8-inch pan. Bake 15 minutes or until done.
Makes 8 servings.

CRANBERRY BREAD

A holiday favorite—tart and flavorful.

2 oranges
2 cups whole wheat flour
2 cups white flour
1 teaspoon baking powder
1 teaspoon baking soda
2 cups sugar or less
3 egg whites
¼ cup oil
½ cup chopped nuts
2 cups ground or sliced cranberries

Preheat oven to 325°. Grate the rind off the oranges and reserve. Cut oranges in half and squeeze out the juice. Add enough boiling water to juice to make 1½ cups liquid. Combine juice and rind with all other ingredients. Place in two lightly oiled 9-by-5-inch loaf pans. Bake for 1 hour or until wooden pick inserted in center comes out clean.
Makes 2 loaves (32 slices).

GRANDMA KIRSCHNER'S DATE NUT BREAD

This bread is so good it does not need a spread and can be served as dessert!

1 package (8 ounces) dates
¾ cup coarsely chopped walnuts
1 cup raisins

1 teaspoon baking soda
1 cup boiling water
2 cups flour
1 cup sugar
1 teaspoon baking powder
2 egg whites

Preheat oven to 350°. Chop dates. Combine dates, nuts and raisins in bowl. Sprinkle baking soda over date, nut and raisin combination. Pour 1 cup boiling water over all of this. Cover the bowl and set aside while mixing rest of ingredients.

In another bowl mix flour, sugar, baking powder and egg whites. Mix together with pastry blender or two knives held together. Combine ingredients of both bowls; mix well. Bake in lightly oiled 9-by-5-inch loaf pan 1 hour.

Makes 1 loaf (16 slices).

HEARTY CORN BREAD

A lower-fat version of an old favorite.

2 cups cornmeal
½ cup whole wheat or white flour
¼ teaspoon Lite Salt or less
½ teaspoon baking soda
1 teaspoon baking powder
1 tablespoon brown sugar
1 egg white
1 tablespoon oil
2 cups buttermilk *or* 2 cups low-fat yogurt

Preheat oven to 425°. In a large bowl, stir together dry ingredients. In another bowl mix the wet ingredients. Combine the two and stir only until they are mixed.

Turn into an 8-by-8-inch lightly oiled pan. Bake for 20–25 minutes.

Makes 8 servings.

OPTIONS
Add more buttermilk for a moister product. Grated carrots, whole kernel corn or snipped herbs may also be added.

LEMON NUT BREAD

⅓ cup margarine
⅔ cup sugar
3 egg whites
2 teaspoons baking powder
¾ cup whole wheat flour
1½ cups white flour
1 cup skim milk
1½ teaspoons dried lemon rind
3 tablespoons chopped nuts

GLAZE
⅓ cup powdered sugar
3 tablespoons freshly squeezed lemon juice

Preheat oven to 350°. Cream together margarine and sugar. Add egg whites and mix thoroughly. Combine dry ingredients and add the above alternately with milk. Stir in lemon rind and nuts. Bake in a lightly oiled 9-by-5-inch loaf pan for 60 minutes or until wooden pick inserted in center comes out clean. Remove bread from oven. Mix powdered sugar with lemon juice until smooth and pour over warm bread. Allow to sit for 20 minutes, then remove bread from pan.

Makes 1 loaf (16 slices).

PUMPKIN HARVEST LOAF

Take the time to add the Lemon Glaze on top as it makes the bread very special! Freezes well.

1¾ cups pumpkin
½ cup egg substitute (commercial or Homemade Egg Substitute, page 241)
2 egg whites
¼ cup oil

1 cup sugar
2 cups flour
2 teaspoons baking powder
1 teaspoon baking soda
1¼ teaspoons cinnamon

Preheat oven to 350°. Beat together pumpkin, egg substitute, egg whites and oil. Add sugar, flour, baking powder, baking soda and cinnamon. Combine all ingredients and pour into 9-by-5-inch loaf pan that has been sprayed with nonstick spray, then floured. Bake 60 minutes or until wooden pick inserted in center comes out clean.

LEMON GLAZE
½ cup powdered sugar
3 tablespoons freshly squeezed lemon juice
½ teaspoon lemon rind

If a glaze is desired mix the ingredients and pour over warm bread while in pan. Let cool slightly and remove from pan. Dust with powdered sugar.

Makes 1 loaf (16 slices).

QUICK WHEAT BREAD

Baked in a round casserole dish and garnished on the top with sunflower seeds, this bread is a winner!

1½ cups whole wheat flour
1 cup white flour
½ cup quick-cooking oatmeal
¼ cup brown sugar
1 tablespoon finely shredded orange peel
2 teaspoons baking powder
½ tsp. baking soda
½ teaspoon Lite Salt or less
1¾ cups buttermilk *or* sour skim milk *
1 egg white
⅛ cup shelled sunflower seeds *or* ¼ cup chopped walnuts
1 tablespoon wheat germ
1 teaspoon honey
1 tablespoon sunflower seeds (optional) for garnish

Preheat oven to 350°. In a large bowl combine flours, oatmeal, brown sugar, orange peel, baking powder, baking soda and Lite Salt until well blended. Add milk and egg white; stir only until ingredients are moistened. Fold in the sunflower seeds or walnuts.

Lightly oil a 1½-quart casserole dish; sprinkle lightly with wheat germ. Pour batter into prepared dish. Bake for 50 to 60 minutes or until wooden pick inserted in center of bread comes out clean. If necessary, cover loaf with foil during the last 15 minutes of baking to prevent overbrowning.

Cool in casserole for 10 minutes; turn bread out onto wire rack. Brush top of loaf with 1 teaspoon honey and sprinkle with additional 1 tablespoon of sunflower seeds, if desired. Serve warm or cool.

Makes 1 loaf.

* To make sour milk, place 2 tablespoons lemon juice or vinegar in a 2-cup measure. Then add milk to make 1¾ cups.

Yeast Breads

CARAWAY DINNER ROLLS

These lovely dinner rolls can also have dill flavoring. They can be made early in the day and reheated at mealtime.

   2 tablespoons active dry yeast
   ½ cup warm water
   2 tablespoons caraway seeds *or* dill weed
   2 cups low-fat cottage cheese
   ¼ cup sugar
   ½ teaspoon Lite Salt
   ½ teaspoon baking soda
   3 egg whites
   2⅔ cups white flour
   2 cups whole wheat flour

Dissolve yeast in warm water. Add caraway seeds *or* dill weed. Heat cottage cheese just until lukewarm. Mix cottage cheese, sugar, Lite Salt, baking soda and egg whites into yeast mixture. Slowly add flours, mixing until dough cleans bowl.

Cover and let rise in warm place until double, about 1 hour. Stir down dough. Place in 24 lightly oiled muffin tins. Cover and let rise again until double, about 45 minutes.

Preheat oven to 350°. Bake about 25 minutes. Remove from muffin tins while warm. Makes 24 rolls.

HONEY WHEAT BREAD

We feel it is important to include our own version of a basic whole-grain bread although almost any yeast bread can easily be modified to be a low-fat, cholesterol-free, pleasant-tasting product. Don't be afraid to alter the types and amounts of sweetener and flours in this recipe according to your individual preference. (For additional variety, try kneading into the dough 1 cup of raisins, 1 cup of sunflower seeds, or ½ cup of cracked wheat or bulgur.)

   1 cup skim milk
   ¼ cup oil
   ¼ cup honey
   ½ teaspoon Lite Salt
   2 tablespoons active dry yeast
   1½ cups warm water
   2 cups white flour
   5½ cups whole wheat flour

Heat milk until bubbles form around the edge. Add oil and stir. Add honey and Lite Salt and stir until well blended.

In a large bowl, dissolve yeast in warm water for 30 minutes. Add milk mixture. Add all of white flour and half of wheat flour, about 3 cups. Stir until well mixed. Gradually add the rest of the wheat flour. Stir at first, then mix with hands until dough pulls away from sides of bowl. Let rest for 10 minutes.

Turn dough out onto a lightly floured board. Knead, push and fold until dough is soft and springy to touch (about 10 minutes) and return to bowl. Cover the bowl, allowing room for the dough to double in bulk. Let rise in warm area (about 80°–85°) for 1½ hours or until dough has doubled its size. Divide dough in half and let rest 10 minutes. Form into an oblong shape the length of the loaf pan, pinching the dough together tightly at the seams. Lightly oil two 9-by-5-inch loaf pans. Place dough seam side down, in the pans. Cover the pans to protect from draft and let the loaves rise once more until they have doubled in bulk.

Preheat the oven to 350° toward the end of this rising period. When the bread has risen until it is just above the rim, it is ready for baking. Bake for 50 minutes. When you remove it from the pan and tap it on the sides or bottom, it should sound slightly hollow. The color should be a rich golden brown.

Makes 2 loaves (32 slices).

PITA BREAD

Make your own pocket bread—they're great fun and taste terrific!

1 tablespoon active dry yeast
1 tablespoon sugar
½ cup warm water
3 cups white flour
3 cups whole wheat flour
½ teaspoon Lite Salt
½ cup skim milk
1 cup lukewarm water

Dissolve yeast and sugar in the ½ cup of warm water. Let stand 5–10 minutes. Place flours and Lite Salt in large bowl, making a depression in the center. Combine milk, remaining water and dissolved yeast; pour into depression. Begin mixing flour with liquid, making sure all batter on sides of bowl is worked into dough. Knead until a smooth dough results and the sides of the bowl are clean. (Occasionally dip hands in more water while kneading to give a smooth, elastic finish.)

Cover with towel and let the dough rise in a warm place until it doubles in size (2–4 hours). Form into 16 smooth balls. Cover and let rise on a cloth for 30 minutes. Roll into ¼-inch thick circles. Cover and let rise again on cloth for 30 minutes.

Preheat oven to 475°. Place dough directly on racks in oven. As soon as the dough rises into a mound, 2–5 minutes, place under broiler for a few seconds until lightly browned. Cool.

Makes 16 pitas.

SOFT PRETZELS

The hardest part of this recipe is learning how to twist them right but they are really fun to make (and eat!).

2 cups skim milk
2 envelopes active dry yeast
½ cup very warm water
½ cup sugar
¾ teaspoon baking powder
1 teaspoon Lite Salt
¼ cup oil
6¾ cups flour
1 quart water
1 egg white
1 tablespoon water

Scald milk—cool to lukewarm. In large bowl, sprinkle yeast over ½ cup very warm water to dissolve. Add sugar, cooled milk, baking powder, Lite Salt and oil. Add 3 cups flour. Cover and let rise until double in size (about 45 minutes). Stir down batter, add remaining flour and knead for about 10 minutes on lightly floured board. Punch down dough. Cut into 20 pieces and set aside 10 minutes. Roll each piece into a thin, ropelike, 24-inch length, using your hands to roll and stretch dough. Dough will be elastic and will retract somewhat after being stretched.

To form a pretzel, grasp each end of dough, forming a horseshoe with curved part away from you. Twist ends once around each other and press each firmly onto loop of dough beneath them. Set dough aside to rest on a lightly floured work surface, covered, for 10 minutes.

Preheat oven to 450°F. Dust baking sheet with cornmeal. In a large, deep pan, simmer 1 quart water. Poach pretzels 2–3 at a time for about 30 seconds, removing gently with a slotted spoon. Carefully pat dry with paper towels, and put on prepared baking sheet. Mix egg white with 1 tablespoon water. Brush each pretzel with egg white glaze. Bake until golden brown, 12–14 minutes. For crustier pretzels, put under broiler 30 seconds before baking. Serve warm with mustard.

Makes 20 large pretzels.

WHOLE WHEAT FRENCH BREAD

A special "baguette pan" gives this bread a crunchy, crispy crust.

- 1 tablespoon active dry yeast
- 1 tablespoon sugar
- 1 teaspoon Lite Salt
- 2½ cups lukewarm water
- 3 cups white flour
- 2–3 cups whole wheat flour
- 1 egg white mixed with 1 tablespoon cold water

Combine yeast, sugar, Lite Salt and water in a large bowl. Gradually add the flours and mix well (hands work best). At first the dough will be very sticky; add enough flour to transfer it to a lightly floured board. Knead until the dough is no longer sticky (about 10 minutes), adding more flour as necessary. Place in lightly oiled bowl. Cover with a damp cloth and let rise in warm place until doubled in volume (1½–2 hours).

Punch dough down. Transfer to a floured board and cut into four equal parts. Roll and shape each part into a long loaf. Place loaves into lightly oiled, special long-loaf pans (baguette pans). Slash the top of each loaf diagonally in three or four places and brush with the egg white and water mixture. Let dough rise another hour or until doubled in volume.

Preheat oven to 350°. Bake the loaves until browned and hollow-sounding when thumped, about 25 minutes.* Halfway through baking, it may be necessary to cover the loaves with foil to prevent scorching the tops. Let cool on rack.

Makes 4 loaves, about 18 inches long.

* If planning to freeze bread, underbake, i.e., bake in oven only 15 minutes. Wrap in foil when cool. When ready to serve remove from freezer. Leave wrapped in foil. Place in 350° oven for 10 minutes. Remove foil and continue to bake for 5 minutes, until crisp.

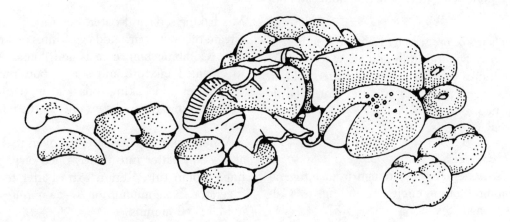

WHOLE WHEAT REFRIGERATOR ROLL DOUGH

So handy to have in the refrigerator, with only a short rising time remaining. This versatile dough can be used for rolls one night and pizza the next evening.

>   1 package active dry yeast
>   1⅓ cups lukewarm water
>   ⅓ cup dried instant potatoes
>   1 tablespoon brown sugar
>   ½ teaspoon Lite Salt
>   1 tablespoon oil
>   1 egg white
>   1½–2 cups white flour
>   2 cups whole wheat flour

To prepare dough for refrigeration: Dissolve yeast in warm water and combine with dried potatoes and brown sugar. Add Lite Salt, oil and egg white. Stir in 1 cup white flour and 2 cups whole wheat flour. Mix in enough additional white flour (½ to 1 cup) to make the dough easy to handle.

Knead on floured board until dough is smooth and elastic. Place in lightly oiled bowl (large enough for dough to double). Cover tightly and refrigerate at least 8 hours and not more than 5 days.

Two hours before serving: Remove from refrigerator. Shape into rolls and allow to rise 30–45 minutes or until doubled in size. Bake in 350° oven for 20–25 minutes until lightly browned.

Makes 18 rolls.

OTHER USES
For Calzones: Remove dough from refrigerator and roll out in circles. For filling, see Calzones, page 289.

For Pizza Crust: Divide in half. Pat onto two lightly oiled baking sheets. Let rise 15 minutes. Cover with pizza sauce, vegetables and grated low-fat cheese and bake in 350° oven 25 minutes.

Makes 2 crusts.

Muffins

A BARREL OF MUFFINS

This recipe makes a large amount—the batter can be stored in the refrigerator for up to 4 weeks and the muffins freshly baked when you are ready for them.

>   5 teaspoons baking soda
>   2 cups boiling water
>   1 cup oil
>   1 cup sugar
>   6 egg whites
>   4 cups All-Bran cereal
>   2 cups Bran flakes
>   5 cups white flour (or part whole wheat)
>   1 quart buttermilk

Mix baking soda and water. Set aside to cool. Cream oil and sugar. Add egg whites and mix well. Combine bran cereals and flours. Add to creamed mixture and stir in buttermilk. Add water and baking soda and mix. Store the batter in a covered container in the refrigerator.

When ready to bake, preheat oven to 375° and spoon batter into lightly oiled or paper-lined muffin tins. Return extra batter to refrigerator. Bake muffins for 20–25 minutes.

Makes 60 muffins.

BLUEBERRY BRAN MUFFINS

These muffins contain no fat at all and are surprisingly good!

2⅔ cups All-Bran cereal
1½ cups skim milk
4 egg whites
1 tablespoon vanilla
2 cups flour
⅔ cup brown sugar
2 tablespoons baking powder
¾ teaspoon baking soda
1½ teaspoons cinnamon
2 cups blueberries, fresh or frozen

Preheat oven to 325°. Combine bran cereal, milk, egg whites and vanilla—let stand 5 minutes. Stir together flour, brown sugar, baking powder, baking soda and cinnamon in large bowl. Add cereal-milk mixture and mix. Add blueberries and stir carefully. Spoon into lightly oiled or paper-lined muffin tins. Bake for 30 minutes.
Makes 16 muffins.

CARROT AND BRAN MUFFINS

These are dense, chewy muffins.

1½ cups raw bran
¼ cup wheat germ
1 cup whole wheat flour
1 teaspoon baking powder
1 teaspoon baking soda
½ teaspoon Lite Salt or less
1 cup shredded carrots
1 cup mixed dried fruit (raisins, chopped prunes or apricots)

½ cup chopped walnuts or almonds
2 egg whites
¾ cup skim milk
½ cup molasses
3 tablespoons oil

Preheat oven to 400°. In bowl mix the first 6 ingredients. Add carrots, fruit and nuts, and distribute evenly. Make a well in the center. In another bowl beat egg whites lightly and mix in milk, molasses and oil. Pour all at once into the dry ingredients and stir just to moisten.
Pour into lightly oiled or paper-lined muffin tins about ¾ full. Bake for 15–20 minutes.
Makes 18 muffins.

CEREAL BRAN MUFFINS

A breakfast staple or coffee break treat.

1½ cups Bran Buds or All-Bran cereal
1¼ cups skim milk
2 egg whites
3 tablespoons oil
½ cup white flour
¾ cup whole wheat flour
1 tablespoon baking powder
1 tablespoon sugar

Preheat oven to 400°. Measure cereal and milk into mixing bowl. Stir to combine. Add egg whites and oil. Let stand 1 to 2 minutes to soften cereal. Mix flours, baking powder and sugar. Beat liquid-cereal mixture with wire whisk. Add dry ingredients to cereal mixture, stirring *only until combined*. Spoon batter gently into lightly oiled or paper-lined muffin tins. Bake for 25 minutes.
Makes 12 muffins.

FRUIT AND NUT MUFFINS

This is a family favorite of many.

1 cup sugar
1 cup applesauce
¼ cup oil
3 egg whites
3 tablespoons skim milk *or* buttermilk
1 cup whole wheat flour
1 cup white flour
1 teaspoon baking soda
1 teaspoon baking powder
½ teaspoon cinnamon
¼ teaspoon nutmeg
¼ cup chopped walnuts
½ cup raisins
½ cup chopped dates

Preheat oven to 350°. In a large bowl combine sugars, applesauce, oil, egg whites and milk. Mix thoroughly. Add flours, baking soda, baking powder and spices. Combine until well mixed. Stir in nuts, raisins and dates. Spoon into lightly oiled or paper-lined muffin tins and bake for 20–30 minutes.

Makes 36 muffins.

NATURAL BRAN MUFFINS

Excellent for breakfast!

3 cups raw bran
1 cup boiling water
3 egg whites
¾ cup sugar
2 cups buttermilk
⅓ cup oil
½ cup raisins *or* dates (optional)
1½ cups whole wheat flour
1 cup white flour
2½ teaspoons baking soda

Preheat oven to 375°. Mix raw bran and boiling water in a large bowl and set aside. Combine egg whites, sugar, buttermilk, oil and dried fruit (if used) in a medium bowl. Add to bran in the large bowl. In a medium bowl, mix the flours and baking soda. Add to bran mixture and mix until just blended. Spoon into lightly oiled or paper-lined muffin tins. Bake for 15–20 minutes. Batter can be kept in the refrigerator in a covered jar for several weeks and baked as needed.

Makes 30 muffins.

WHOLE WHEAT MUFFINS

A basic muffin recipe—vary with blueberries, apples, raisins or dates. Very nice when served warm.

1 cup white flour
1 cup whole wheat flour
¼ cup sugar
2 teaspoons baking powder
½ teaspoon baking soda
2 egg whites
1 cup buttermilk
¼ cup oil

Preheat oven to 400°. Thoroughly mix flours, sugar, baking powder and baking soda. Form a well and add egg whites, buttermilk and oil. Stir only until dry ingredients are moistened. Fill lightly oiled or paper-lined muffin tins about ⅔ full. Bake for 25 minutes or until done.

Makes 12 muffins.

Specialty Items

BAKING MIX

Homemade "Bisquick"—more fiber, less salt

4 cups whole wheat flour
4 cups white flour
1 cup powdered nonfat milk
2 teaspoons cream of tartar
¼ cup baking powder
2½ teaspoons Lite Salt or less
¾ cup shortening

Measure dry ingredients into bowl. Sift together 3 times. Put into large bowl; cut in shortening with pastry blender (or two knives) until size of small peas. Store in tightly covered container. (Recipe may be easily doubled.)
Makes 11 cups.

FOR PANCAKES

2 egg whites
1½ cups water
2 cups Baking Mix

Combine egg whites and water; stir into Baking Mix until well blended. Spoon onto a lightly oiled grill and cook, turning when bubbles appear.
Makes 12–15 medium pancakes.

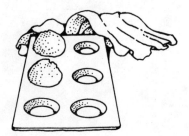

FOR BISCUITS

2 cups Baking mix
⅔ cup water

Preheat oven to 425°. Measure mix into bowl and add water; stir just to blend. Turn onto lightly floured board; knead a few times. Roll to ¾-inch thickness. Cut into circles or squares, place on unoiled baking sheet. Bake for 12–15 minutes.
Makes 12 2-inch biscuits.

OLD-STYLE WHEAT BISCUITS

1 cup white flour
1 cup whole wheat flour
2 teaspoons baking powder
¼ teaspoon Lite Salt or less
¼ teaspoon baking soda
¼ cup oil
2 tablespoons vinegar
1 cup skim milk

Preheat oven to 475°. Sift together flours, baking powder, Lite Salt and baking soda. Cut in oil until mixture looks like coarse cornmeal. Put vinegar and milk together in a cup and stir. Stir enough milk into flour mixture until soft dough is formed. Sprinkle flour on countertop and knead dough. Roll out dough to 1-inch thick. Cut with biscuit cutter or glass. Place on baking sheet. Bake about 12 minutes.
Makes 16 2-inch biscuits.

PIZZA CRUSTS

Choose a thin yeast crust or a quicker thick crust and create your own masterpiece.

THIN PIZZA CRUST
(Makes enough for two crusts.)

  1½ tablespoons yeast
  1¾ cups warm water
  1 tablespoon honey or sugar
  1 tablespoon oil
  2 cups whole wheat flour
  2 cups white flour

Dissolve yeast in warm water and add honey or sugar. Blend in oil and flours. Knead on lightly floured surface, adding more flour if needed. Spread and pat dough out onto two 17-by-11-inch jelly roll pans. Roll edge slightly. Top with pizza sauce, vegetables, and grated imitation mozzarella cheese. Bake at 425° for 25–30 minutes.
  Makes 30 pieces (3½ by 3½ inches each).

THICK PIZZA CRUST
Very quickly made. No rising necessary.

  2 cups white flour
  1 cup whole wheat flour
  1 tablespoon baking powder
  12 ounces beer

Mix all ingredients and spread in a 9-by-13-inch baking pan. Top with pizza sauce, vegetables and grated imitation mozzarella cheese. Bake at 425° for 25–30 minutes.
  Makes 12 pieces (3 by 3 inches each)

READY-TO-BAKE CRUST
See page 234 for Whole Wheat Refrigerator Roll dough which works well for pizza, too. Follow directions given above for toppings.

WHOLE WHEAT TORTILLAS

A wonderful treat to serve with any Mexican food. They can be used to make soft shell tacos—see Your Basic Bean Burrito for topping ideas.

  1½ cups white flour
  1½ cups whole wheat flour, *not* stone-ground
  1 cup water

Stir together flours and water. Turn onto floured board and knead until smooth. Dough will be stiffer than a bread dough. Divide dough into 12 equal balls for large thin tortillas. (For smaller, 7-inch tortillas, make into 16 balls.) Work each ball until smooth and pliable. Roll as thin as possible on lightly floured board. Add flour to board as needed.
  Drop onto a very hot ungreased griddle. Cook until freckled on one side. Turn and cook on second side. Place between folds of towel to keep pliable and hot until serving.
  Makes 12 large tortillas.

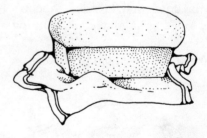

BREAKFASTS AND BRUNCHES

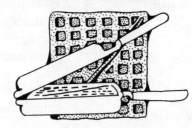

Breakfast is a great opportunity to have low-fat fare and to include fiber in the diet. Whole-grain cereal, either hot or cold, with skim milk is a quick, easy way to start the day. Bran muffins, rolls, or other whole-grain baked products make fine breakfasts as well. We've collected some favorite recipes for brunches, as well as other ideas for daily fare.

Apple Dumplings
Breakfast Volcanos
Crepe Blintzes
German Oven Pancake
Homemade Egg Substitute
Morning Rice
Muesli
Mushroom Strata
Oatmeal Buttermilk Pancakes
Orange Pancakes with Orange Sauce
Our Granola
Spanish Omelet
Sunrise Cake
Vegetable Frittata
Waffles

Quick Breakfast Ideas

Fruited Low-fat Yogurt and Our Granola

Warm muffins and applesauce or jam

Corn Bread and jam or jelly

Hot cereal with fruit (oatmeal, other whole-grain cereal mixes)

Low-fat Yogurt with Grape-Nuts

Potatoes—reheat leftovers (try boiled potatoes with low-fat yogurt or Mock Sour Cream)

Shredded Wheat with skim milk and fresh berries

Leftover Waffles (which were frozen) reheated in toaster with applesauce over top

Whole-grain toast or English muffins with jam

Toast with peanut butter and jelly

APPLE DUMPLINGS

Especially nice for camping, with fresh huckleberries folded into the dumpling dough—makes for a real treat! Don't forget Saturday mornings at home, too!

    3 cups diced apples (dried fruit works
      well or use other diced fresh fruit)
    1 teaspoon cinnamon
    ⅓ cup brown sugar
    ¼ cup raisins
    4 cups water

    2 cups whole wheat baking mix
      (commercial or Baking Mix, page 237)
    1 cup water
    2 tablespoons chopped nuts

Combine first 5 ingredients in large pan. Bring to a boil. Mix together last 3 ingredients and carefully drop by spoonfuls onto boiling fruit mixture, to cover it with a mass of dough. Simmer, partially covered, for about 5 minutes, then remove lid and continue simmering until dough is cooked, about another 8–10 minutes. Serve in bowls with a dollop of plain yogurt, if desired.
    Makes about 4 servings.

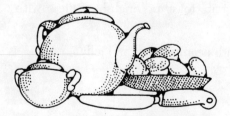

BREAKFAST VOLCANOS

Similar to Eggs Benedict. For a meatless and lower-salt version, serve a tomato slice in place of the Canadian bacon.

    1 cup Mock Hollandaise Sauce, page 376
    2 tablespoons chopped onion (optional)
    2 tablespoons chopped green pepper
      (optional)
    1 cup egg substitute (commercial or
      Homemade Egg Substitute, page 241)
    2 English muffins
    4 slices Canadian bacon or turkey ham or
      4 thick slices tomato

Make 1 cup Mock Hollandaise Sauce and set aside. Steam onions and green pepper in a little water until soft, add egg substitute to make "scrambled eggs." Split and toast English muffins, heat thin slices of Canadian bacon and place one slice of meat on each muffin. Top with scrambled egg mixture and 4 tablespoons of Mock Hollandaise Sauce.
    Makes 4 servings.

CREPE BLINTZES

Nice weekend breakfast idea. Crepes with a cheese filling which are lightly browned and served warm with fresh fruit or other toppings.

    1½ cups low-fat cottage cheese
    3 ounces Neufchâtel cheese (lower- fat
      cream cheese)
    ⅓ cup sugar
    1 teaspoon vanilla
    1 tablespoon freshly squeezed lemon juice
    ½ teaspoon grated lemon rind
    1 tablespoon oil
    1 cup plain low-fat yogurt

4 cups sliced fruit *or* berries
2 tablespoons powdered sugar

Prepare Crepes, page 368.

Mix cottage cheese, Neufchâtel cheese, sugar, vanilla, lemon juice, and lemon rind. Fill each crepe. Fold. Sauté in oil until slightly browned.

Serve with low-fat yogurt, fresh berries or fruit and sprinkle with powdered sugar.

Makes filling for 8 crepes.

GERMAN OVEN PANCAKE

A puff pancake which is very simple to make and so attractive!

½ cup flour
¾ cup egg substitute (commercial *or* Homemade Egg Substitute)
½ cup skim milk
5 teaspoons margarine, melted
2 cups sliced fruit *
2 tablespoons powdered sugar
Lemon wedges

Preheat oven to 450°. Gradually add flour to egg substitute, beating with rotary beater or in blender. Stir in milk and melted margarine. Lightly oil or spray with nonstick spray a 9-inch or 10-inch ovenproof skillet. (Round cake pan works well.) Bake for 20 minutes. (Pancake will form a well in the center and sides will puff up.) Spoon fruit into the center of the pancake.

Loosen pancake from pan with wide spatula and cut into wedges with sharp knife. Serve immediately with powdered sugar and lemon wedges.

Makes 2 servings.

* Any fresh fruit works well (berries, bananas or peaches).

HOMEMADE EGG SUBSTITUTE
(¼ cup = 1 whole egg)

Can be used in place of commercial egg substitute and is considerably cheaper!

6 egg whites
¼ cup powdered nonfat milk
1 tablespoon oil

Combine all ingredients in a mixing bowl and blend until smooth. Store in jar in refrigerator up to 1 week. Also freezes well.

To prepare as scrambled egg: Fry slowly over low heat in a nonstick fry pan.

Makes 1 cup.

MORNING RICE

Breakfast can be unusual, too. This is a good use for leftover rice. It can be mixed in advance and kept in the refrigerator for 2 or 3 days. Serve hot or cold.

2 cups cooked brown rice
1 cup plain low-fat yogurt
2 teaspoons honey or brown sugar
1 apple, chopped (or other fruit)
1 teaspoon cinnamon
2 tablespoons raisins

Mix all ingredients together in medium bowl. This has *lots* of options. Jam could be used in place of sugar and any fruit or combination of fruit could be used.

Makes about 4 cups.

MUESLI

An unusual cold cereal—you can also be creative and add other ingredients you have on hand. Serve with toast or muffins.

   2 cups uncooked oatmeal
   1 cup skim milk
   2 large apples, chopped
   ¼ cup chopped nuts
   ½ cup raisins
   ¼ cup sugar
   1 tablespoon freshly squeezed lemon juice
   ¾ cup plain low-fat yogurt
   2 tablespoons wheat germ
   Dash of cinnamon

Combine milk and oatmeal and let set at least 30 minutes (or overnight in refrigerator). Chop or grate apples and combine all ingredients, adding cinnamon to taste.

   Makes about 6 cups.

NOTE: Other fruits could be added, and water or orange juice could be substituted for milk.

MUSHROOM STRATA

Similar to a soufflé, but really a lovely mushroom casserole. Our version of a quiche—good brunch item. Serve with tiny muffins and fresh fruit.

   1 pound fresh mushrooms, sliced
   ½ cup chopped onion
   ½ cup chopped celery
   ½ cup chopped green pepper (optional)
   1 tablespoon margarine
   ¼ cup plain low-fat yogurt
   ¼ cup imitation mayonnaise
   12 slices bread, quartered with crusts
     removed

   ¾ cup egg substitute (commercial or
     Homemade Egg Substitute, page 241)
   ½ cup skim milk

TOPPING
   Homemade "Cream" Soup Mix, page
     261, to equal 1 can of condensed soup
     or 1 can (10¾ ounces) cream of
     mushroom soup
   ½ cup skim milk
   ¼ cup grated low-fat cheese
   Chopped parsley and paprika to garnish

Earlier in the day or the day before: Sauté mushrooms, onions, celery and green pepper in margarine until tender. Drain off excess liquid. Remove from heat and add yogurt and imitation mayonnaise. Lightly oil a 9-by-13-inch baking dish. Line bottom with quartered bread (use half the quarters). Pour vegetable/yogurt mixture over bread. Add remaining bread to form another layer. Mix egg substitute and milk and pour over bread. Cover and refrigerate at least 1 hour or longer. Overnight is fine.

One hour before serving: Preheat oven to 300°. Combine soup and milk and spread over casserole. Top with grated cheese and bake 1 hour. Garnish with parsley and paprika. Allow to set for a few minutes before cutting into squares. Serve warm.

   Makes 9 servings (about 3 by 4 inches).

OATMEAL BUTTERMILK PANCAKES

If you have time, premix part of batter and refrigerate overnight. These are truly a breakfast treat, especially with fresh fruit or warm syrup.

1½ cups uncooked oatmeal
2 cups buttermilk
3 egg whites
1 cup whole wheat flour
2 teaspoons baking soda
2 tablespoons brown sugar

Combine oatmeal, buttermilk and egg whites and let stand for at least ½ hour or refrigerate up to 24 hours. Add remaining ingredients, and stir the batter just until the dry ingredients are moistened. Bake on a hot, lightly oiled griddle.

Makes 16 pancakes (4 inches each).

ORANGE PANCAKES WITH ORANGE SAUCE

These are a real treat for a leisurely weekend breakfast—beautiful and very tasty. Four pancakes are stacked with layers of ricotta cheese between them. A warm sauce with fresh orange sections is poured overall. The pancake stack is served in wedges.

1½ cups whole wheat flour
2 teaspoons baking powder
2 teaspoons grated orange rind
1 egg white
3 tablespoons honey
¼ cup skim milk
¾ cup orange juice
1 tablespoon oil
1½ cups part-skim ricotta cheese

ORANGE SAUCE

1 tablespoon cornstarch
2 tablespoons grated orange rind
1 cup orange juice
¼–½ cup honey
1 tablespoon margarine
1 fresh orange, divided into sections

To make the sauce: Mix the cornstarch, orange rind, orange juice and honey in a small sauce pan. Bring the mixture to a boil over medium heat, stirring constantly until thickened. Remove from heat and stir in the margarine until it melts. Add the orange sections to the sauce or use as a garnish. Serve warm over the pancakes.

To make the pancakes: Combine flour, baking powder and orange rind. In a separate bowl combine egg white, honey, milk, orange juice and oil. Stir the wet ingredients into the dry ingredients just enough to moisten. Bake four large pancakes on a lightly oiled griddle.

To assemble: Spread ⅓–½ cup ricotta cheese between each pancake and pour half the orange sauce over the top. Cut into wedges and pour sauce over individual wedges.

Makes 6 servings.

OUR GRANOLA

Most commercial granolas are high-fat items —this one is low-fat and is very tasty.

⅓ cup oil
½ cup honey
¼ cup water
1 teaspoon vanilla
4½ cups uncooked rolled wheat
1 cup uncooked oatmeal
2 cups ready-to-eat cereals (Wheaties, Bran Flakes, etc.)
¼ cup shelled sunflower seeds
¼ cup chopped walnuts
½ cup powdered nonfat milk
1 cup raisins or other dried fruit

Preheat oven to 350°. In a saucepan, heat oil, honey, water and vanilla until blended. In a large bowl, combine cereals, nuts and powdered milk. Pour liquid ingredients over dry and mix well. Spread mixture on two jelly-roll pans. Bake for 10 minutes, stirring occasionally. Remove from oven; add raisins. Let cool until crisp before storing in airtight container.

Makes about 10 cups.

SPANISH OMELET

Yes, you can have an omelet!

1 teaspoon oil
¾ cup chopped onion
1½ cups chopped fresh tomatoes
1½ cups frozen peas
¼ teaspoon pepper
1½ cups egg whites (about 12)
⅔ cup egg substitute (commercial *or* Homemade Egg Substitute, page 241)

Sauté onions in oil. Stir in tomatoes and simmer uncovered for 4 to 5 minutes. Add peas and pepper to the tomato mixture and simmer until done.

Combine the egg whites and egg substitute in a mixing bowl. Beat on high speed with an electric mixer until foamy.

Heat a nonstick fry pan over low heat. Pour in egg mixture and cook slowly until mixture begins to set. Loosen the edges from pan. Pour tomato filling in the center of the omelet. Fold one half over the other and tip onto a plate. Serve hot with whole-grain toast.

Makes 6 servings.

SUNRISE CAKE

One of the few low-fat coffee cakes we've found. The texture seems to be best when baked in a tube pan.

¼ cup margarine
2 egg whites
Grated rind of 1 small lemon
2 teaspoons freshly squeezed lemon juice
¾ cup brown sugar
1 cup whole wheat flour
1 cup white flour
1 teaspoon baking soda
¼ teaspoon Lite Salt or less
1 cup plain low-fat yogurt
2 cups chopped fruit*

TOPPING
1 tablespoon margarine
1 tablespoon wheat germ
¼ cup white flour
¼ cup brown sugar
1 teaspoon cinnamon
½ teaspoon allspice

Preheat oven to 350°. Cream margarine, egg whites, lemon rind, juice and brown sugar until smooth. Sift together dry ingredients and add alternately with yogurt to egg white mixture. Fold in fruit, and spread into a tube pan which has been sprayed with nonstick spray.

Combine all topping ingredients (it works well to use the same bowl and incorporate the "scrapings" from the batter) and sprinkle over coffee cake. Bake for about 35 minutes until wooden pick inserted in center comes out clean. Serve topped with yogurt, if desired.

Makes 16 servings.

* Apples, peaches, blueberries, rhubarb, etc. (a combination is nice); if canned fruit is used, drain well.

VEGETABLE FRITTATA

An Italian version of the omelet. Makes a nice brunch or luncheon dish for two.

1 clove garlic
2 teaspoons oil
1–1½ cups leftover, cooked vegetables
½ teaspoon dried thyme leaves
½ teaspoon dried basil leaves
½ teaspoon dried rosemary leaves
Freshly ground black pepper to taste
¾ cup egg substitute (commercial *or* Homemade Egg Substitute, page 241)
2 egg whites
2 tablespoons grated Parmesan cheese

Mince garlic and sauté in oil in a 7-inch skillet until softened. Add vegetables and seasonings and cook very briefly, just to heat. Beat egg substitute and egg whites together; stir in Parmesan cheese. Pour over vegetable mixture and cook until golden on the bottom.

Turn over with a broad spatula and cook until other side is golden, or, without turning, place under broiler until top is set and very lightly browned. Serve from skillet.

Makes 2 servings.

WAFFLES

3 egg whites
2 cups buttermilk
2 cups white flour *or* 1 cup white flour and 1 cup whole wheat flour
2 teaspoons baking powder
1 teaspoon baking soda
¼ cup oil

Heat waffle iron. Lightly beat egg whites until frothy; fold in remaining ingredients until smooth.

Pour ½ cup batter onto center of hot waffle iron. Bake about 5 minutes or until steaming stops. Remove waffle carefully.

Makes 8 waffles (7 inches each).

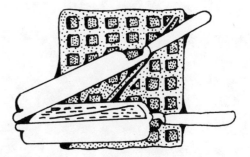

SALADS

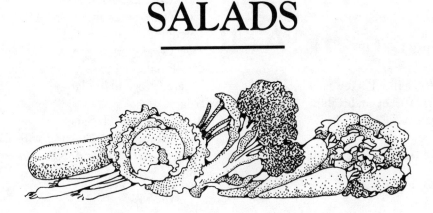

We were looking for new and different salads for this section to help increase variety as well as to help keep the fat to less than 1 teaspoon for each serving. We have also included a few old favorites that are usually made with lots of high-fat mayonnaise or Miracle Whip. Such recipes are Potato Salad and Alphabet Seafood Salad (a macaroni salad), which show that these types of recipes can be prepared in a delicious, yet lower-fat way.

The Hearty Salads include several made with pasta, as well as those with rice, beans, bulgur and potatoes. These have more calories, are obviously more filling, and could even be used as lighter main dishes if you wish. Our Lighter Salads are lower in calories and are to be used as typical dinner salads.

Sunshine Spinach Salad and Vinaigrette Salad Dressing with Greens are our only salad recipes which use greens. We assume that you already have lots of ideas for making a variety of tossed green salads. These can be nearly fat-free if low-fat salad dressings are selected (also if you do not add commercially made croutons or avocados). Look for salad dressing recipes in the "Sauces, Gravies and Salad Dressings" section.

HEARTY SALADS

Alphabet Seafood Salad (see "Fish and
 Shellfish" section)
Basic Pasta Salads
 Party Pasta Salad
 Pasta Salad Italiano
 Picnic Salad
 South of the Border Salad

Chicken Salad with Yogurt-Chive Dressing
(see "Chicken, Turkey and Rabbit"
section)
Chili Bean Salad
Crunchy Rice Salad
Four Star Pasta Salad with Green Sauce
Lentil Salad
Montana Pasta Salad
Potato Salad
Simply Wonderful Turkey Salad (see
"Chicken, Turkey and Rabbit" section)
Spicy Soybean Salad
Tabouli
Taco Salad (see "Beef, Veal and Pork"
section)
Wild Broccoli Salad

LIGHTER SALADS

Carrot-Raisin Salad
Chinese Cucumber Salad
Chinese Salad Rich Style
Confetti Appleslaw
Cucumber Cumin Salad
Five Veggie Salad
Greek Salad
Layered Vegetable Platter
Salata
Sunshine Spinach Salad
Vinaigrette Salad Dressing with Greens (see
"Sauces, Gravies and Salad Dressings" sec-
tion)
Waldorf Salad

Hearty Salads

BASIC PASTA SALADS

Cold pasta and a yogurt-mayonnaise dressing create lovely salads. Here are several variations on this theme—they can be varied to suit *your* tastes. Serve these pasta salads as side dishes with chicken or fish or as light main dish entrées with whole wheat dinner rolls and fruit.

Basic salad (to be used with one of the suggested variations)

> **16-ounce package of pasta. The best kinds to use are elbow macaroni, salad macaroni, large or small seashells, corkscrew, trombette, or mostaccioli. (Use something that can hold its shape.)**
> **1 cup plain low-fat yogurt**
> **¼ cup imitation mayonnaise**

> **2 tablespoons freshly squeezed lemon juice**
> **½ teaspoon pepper**
> **1 clove garlic, minced**
> **1 tablespoon basil leaves, crushed**
> **1 tablespoon finely chopped parsley (save a little for garnish)**

Blend the yogurt, mayonnaise, lemon juice and spices together until creamy. Cook the pasta, according to package directions, until just tender. It is wise to undercook pasta *slightly* for a salad. Drain the pasta and rinse under cold water until completely cool. Transfer to a large bowl. Add the ingredients for any one of the following variations and mix gently. *Shortly before serving,* add the yogurt mixture to the pasta and gently fold until each piece is coated. It is especially important not to add the dressing too early, or the noodles will absorb the low-fat dressing and the salad will not be creamy. If you have any left-over salad, more dressing will need to be added to it. After stirring well, garnish the salad with parsley and serve.

Makes 12–14 servings (1 cup each).

VARIATIONS

PARTY PASTA SALAD

Add 1 package (10 ounces) frozen peas, un-cooked, ¼ cup chopped green onions, 1 small can (4¼ ounces) drained shrimp, ¼ teaspoon Lite Salt or less and a dash of Tabasco sauce. This is beautiful with seashell pasta. Decorate with parsley and lemon wedges.

PASTA SALAD ITALIANO

Add 1 cup finely chopped steamed broccoli, a small can (2.2 ounces) sliced black olives, and 1 cup chopped fresh red tomatoes (add the tomatoes just before serving). Use a pasta shaped like a corkscrew for this one.

PICNIC SALAD

Add 1 can (6½ ounces) water-packed light tuna fish (drained), ¼ cup chopped green on-ions, 2 teaspoons Dijon mustard and a dash of Worcestershire sauce. This is great with elbow macaroni, seashells or trombette.

SOUTH OF THE BORDER SALAD

Add 1 package (10 ounces) frozen corn, un-cooked, ¼ cup chopped green pepper, ¼ cup chopped red pepper, 1 cup grated carrots, 2 chopped green onions, and ½ teaspoon chili powder. This is great for barbecues. Use a classic salad macaroni.

CHILI BEAN SALAD

Colorful and unusual salad. This is a great main dish sandwich when served in pocket bread. Try it for a brown bag lunch (assemble at eating time).

1 can (16 ounces) kidney beans *
1 can (16 ounces) pinto beans *
1 can (16 ounces) garbanzo beans *
1 can (16 ounces) unsalted whole kernel
  corn
½ cup chopped green onions
¼ cup chopped parsley
1 cup sliced celery
1 can (4 ounces) diced green chiles,
  drained

Drain and rinse beans and corn. Combine all ingredients.

DRESSING

2 tablespoons oil
¼ cup vinegar
1–2 cloves garlic, minced
1 teaspoon chili powder
1 teaspoon oregano leaves
¼ teaspoon ground cumin
⅛–½ teaspoon pepper or taco sauce (to
  taste)

Mix all ingredients together. Pour dressing over salad, mix well, and chill 6 hours or overnight (stirring several times).

Makes 10 servings (1 cup each).

* Use low-sodium beans if available.

CRUNCHY RICE SALAD

Nice idea for leftover brown rice. Works well for lunches. Add garlic and curry powder to suit your taste.

2 cups cooked brown rice
2 stalks celery, chopped
2 green onions, chopped
1 tablespoon blanched almonds, slivered
1 clove garlic, minced
Parsley for garnish

DRESSING
½ cup plain low-fat yogurt
¼ cup imitation mayonnaise
1 teaspoon freshly squeezed lemon juice
¼ teaspoon Lite Salt or less
½ teaspoon curry powder
½ teaspoon pepper

Cool rice well. Mix with celery, onions, almonds, garlic and refrigerate. Mix dressing ingredients together. For best results, add dressing to rice ingredients shortly before serving. Garnish with parsley.

Makes 4 cups.

FOUR STAR PASTA SALAD WITH GREEN SAUCE

A beautiful and unusual salad which really deserves ten stars! It is served with a pungent Green Sauce. Some preparation is needed the day before serving.

1 package (16 ounces) pasta (curled, short pasta works well)
¼ pound shrimp meat (optional)

MARINADE
2 tablespoons oil
¼ cup white vinegar
½ teaspoon Lite Salt or less
⅛ teaspoon pepper
1 tablespoon sherry (optional)
1 clove garlic, minced

GREEN SAUCE
(Double this sauce if you wish to have lots of dressing—also it keeps well, and can be used on other salads.)

¼ cup white vinegar *or* lemon juice
1–2 tablespoons Dijon mustard
½ cup tightly packed fresh basil *or* 2 teaspoons dried basil leaves
¾ cup chopped parsley
1–3 cloves garlic, minced
2 tablespoons oil
1 cup plain low-fat yogurt
Pepper

SALAD INGREDIENTS
1 cup frozen peas, uncooked
1 cup broccoli (cut into small pieces)
2 cups halved cherry tomatoes
1 cup sliced mushrooms
1 cup sliced zucchini
6 green onions, chopped
2 cups fresh spinach leaves (torn into bite-size pieces)

On the day before: Cook pasta in unsalted water. Drain and cool. Combine ingredients for marinade and mix with shrimp and cooked pasta. Refrigerate overnight. Place Green Sauce ingredients in food processor or blender and mix until smooth. Refrigerate for several hours; it will thicken.

Just before serving: Combine marinated pasta and shrimp with salad ingredients and toss. Add a small amount of the Green Sauce to the salad when you toss it and serve the rest on the side or toss the salad with the sauce as for other salads.

Makes 10 servings as a main dish (about 20 cups).

LENTIL SALAD

Lentils have made a name for themselves in soup; they also make a very nice salad. This one complements a lamb dish or try it as stuffing for tomatoes.

1½ cups uncooked lentils
4 cups water
2 onions, sliced
8 whole cloves
2 bay leaves
2 cloves garlic, crushed
½ teaspoon Lite Salt or less
½ teaspoon Tabasco sauce

⅓ cup oil
½ cup red wine vinegar
½ teaspoon Tabasco sauce
2 cups chopped celery
½ cup chopped parsley
½ cup chopped onion
2 tomatoes, cut in wedges
Salad greens

In a large saucepan combine lentils, water, onion slices, cloves, bay leaves, garlic, Lite Salt and ½ teaspoon Tabasco sauce. Bring to boil, reduce heat and simmer, covered, 30 minutes, until lentils are tender. Drain. Add oil, vinegar and remaining ½ teaspoon Tabasco sauce. Mix well and cool. After chilling, add celery, parsley and onions. Cover and chill several hours. Turn into bowl lined with cold greens or onto individual serving plates lined with lettuce. Garnish each serving with tomato wedges.
Makes 14 servings (½ cup each)

MONTANA PASTA SALAD

A very pretty salad—the pineapple gives it a little sweetness.

1 can (15 ounces) chunk pineapple, unsweetened
2 cups broccoli or asparagus tips
4 cups cooked pasta, shaped like a corkscrew
1 cup frozen peas, uncooked
1 cup sliced celery
½ cup chopped parsley
⅓ cup chopped green onion
⅓ cup diced pimiento *or* sweet red pepper

Drain pineapple, reserving 2 tablespoons juice for dressing. Wash broccoli or asparagus and cut in bite-size pieces. Combine all ingredients and toss with Spring Dressing. Chill at least 1 hour.

SPRING DRESSING
2 tablespoons juice from canned pineapple
1 clove garlic, crushed
2 tablespoons olive oil
⅓ cup white wine vinegar
2 tablespoons freshly squeezed lemon juice
2 tablespoons Dijon mustard
2 teaspoons basil leaves
½ teaspoon Lite Salt or less

Combine ingredients in jar and shake well.
Makes 6 servings (1½ cups each).

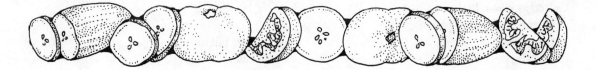

POTATO SALAD

Tastes like the all-American favorite and is much lower in fat. Remember, low-fat dressings need to be added just before serving or the salad will be dry.

6 medium potatoes
3 hard-cooked egg whites
½ cup finely chopped sweet pickles
¼ cup finely chopped onion
⅛ teaspoon pepper

Cook unpeeled potatoes until tender (about 45 minutes). Drain and peel while hot. Stir with fork to break up into very small pieces. Add chopped egg whites, pickles, onion and pepper. Refrigerate in covered container until serving time.

DRESSING
1 cup plain low-fat yogurt
¼ cup imitation mayonnaise
6 tablespoons sweet pickle juice
1 tablespoon prepared mustard

Mix together and refrigerate.
Just before serving: Mix dressing with potato mixture. Garnish with paprika. Leftover salad will become dry and need more dressing before it is served.

Makes 4–6 servings (about 1 cup each).

SPICY SOYBEAN SALAD

A delicious way to sample soybeans if they're new to your family—also, a great potluck dish.

2 cups uncooked soybeans
½ cup each, chopped
  Onions
  Celery
  Carrots
  Green pepper
  Red cabbage
  Cucumber
  Mushrooms
¼ cup vinegar
3 tablespoons oil
1 teaspoon lower-sodium soy sauce
½ teaspoon Lite Salt or less
¼ teaspoon pepper
1 teaspoon dill weed

Prepare soybeans: Soak overnight, then boil in a large amount of water for 2 hours or until tender. Soybeans sometimes take a long time to cook; they may take up to 3 hours. They should not be crisp, but they will never be soft and mushy. Drain soybeans.

Combine all ingredients and chill for 1 hour or more before serving.

Makes 8 cups.

TABOULI

This salad keeps very well and can be made ahead of time. Serve with Tandoori Fish to make a big hit!

1 cup uncooked bulgur
2 cups boiling water
2 tomatoes, finely diced
1 bunch green onions with tops, sliced
3 tablespoons chopped fresh mint *or* 2 teaspoons dried mint
1 cup finely chopped parsley
3 tablespoons olive oil
½ cup freshly squeezed lemon juice
Pepper to taste

Three to 4 hours before serving time, place uncooked bulgur in a large bowl. Pour boiling water over the bulgur and let soak for 1 hour.

Stir occasionally. Drain well in fine strainer. Return bulgur to bowl and stir in other ingredients. Chill for about 2 hours.

Makes 6 cups.

WILD BROCCOLI SALAD

Peanuts and wild rice create an interesting combination for this salad.

- 1 box (6 ounces) rice and wild rice mix
- 1 carrot, chopped
- 2 green onions, chopped
- 2 stalks celery, chopped
- 1 cup chopped broccoli
- 1 cup chopped cauliflower
- ¼ cup unsalted peanuts
- ½ cup plain low-fat yogurt
- ¼ cup buttermilk

Prepare rice according to package directions except use ½ of seasoning packet and omit the margarine. When rice is cooked, combine with chopped vegetables and peanuts. Combine yogurt with buttermilk and mix with rest of salad. Chill until serving time.

Makes 6 servings (1 cup each).

Lighter Salads

CARROT-RAISIN SALAD

An old standby and colorful lunchtime treat. Add a grated unpeeled green apple for an unusual change.

- 4 cups shredded raw carrots
- 1 cup raisins
- ¾ cup plain low-fat yogurt
- 1 tablespoon imitation mayonnaise

Combine carrots and raisins. Toss with yogurt and imitation mayonnaise.

Makes 8 servings (⅔ cup each).

CHINESE CUCUMBER SALAD

While searching for a salad to have with Chinese dishes we found this one, and it has been very popular. Quick and easy to prepare.

- 2 cups sliced cucumbers
- 2 tablespoons rice-wine vinegar *
- 1 tablespoon dark brown sugar
- 1 tablespoon lower-sodium soy sauce
- 1 teaspoon sesame oil
- Tomato slices (for garnish)

Cut cucumbers into matchstick-size pieces. Combine with remaining ingredients. Toss the salad well and chill it for at least 2 hours. Garnish with tomato slices.

VARIATION:

A tasty variation for this salad is to use asparagus instead of cucumber. Cook 15–20 asparagus spears for 5 minutes or just until tender and cut spears into 2-inch pieces; then mix with the above sauce and chill.

Makes 4 servings (2 cups).

* Available in most supermarkets in the Oriental section.

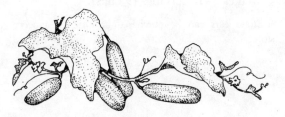

CHINESE SALAD RICH STYLE

Unusual salad which is delicious with a turkey dinner.

1½ cups slivered carrots
1½ cups slivered jicama *or* turnips
½ cup slivered black fungus (cloud ears) *
1 cup cellophane noodles (bean thread)
1½ cups slivered celery (cut 1 inch long)
2 cups bean sprouts
½ cup shredded cooked chicken (optional), *but* omit chicken if served with other poultry, fish or meat

SEASONING SAUCE
3 tablespoons lower-sodium soy sauce
1 tablespoon vinegar
2 tablespoons sesame oil
1 teaspoon sugar
2 teaspoons dry mustard

Cut the carrot and jicama into 1-inch-long shreds. Soften the fungus and cellophane noodles in warm water (soak separately), then cut into 1-inch-long shreds. Boil the celery and bean sprouts separately in water for 10 seconds. Remove and rinse with cold water, then squeeze dry. Mix Seasoning Sauce ingredients together in a small bowl. Lightly toss the ingredients together and arrange on a large platter. Pour the Seasoning Sauce over the ingredients and mix well just before eating.

Makes 8–10 servings (9 cups).

* Cloud ears can be purchased at Oriental grocery stores.

CONFETTI APPLESLAW

2 tablespoons undiluted orange juice concentrate
1½ cups diced unpeeled red apple
4 cups finely shredded cabbage
½ cup finely chopped red onions
1¼ cups thinly sliced red (or green) pepper
3 tablespoons raisins
1 tablespoon imitation mayonnaise
½ cup plain low-fat yogurt
½ teaspoon dry mustard
Paprika
Pepper to taste

Stir orange juice concentrate and diced apple together. Combine with remaining ingredients in a large mixing bowl and toss well. Refrigerate until serving time.

Makes 8 servings (1 cup each).

CUCUMBER CUMIN SALAD

The special flavor of cumin makes this salad unique.

1 teaspoon cumin seeds
½ cup low-fat cottage cheese
½ cup plain low-fat yogurt
¼ teaspoon Lite Salt or less
1 medium cucumber, chopped
1 small onion, finely chopped
1 tomato, chopped
1 tablespoon chopped parsley

Toast cumin seeds in a dry frying pan until brittle (a few minutes). Blend cottage cheese and yogurt in blender, add cumin seeds and Lite Salt. Combine vegetables in bowl, pour dressing over and toss. Refrigerate about ½ hour before serving.

Makes 4 cups.

FIVE VEGGIE SALAD

2 large tomatoes, sliced
2 small zucchini, sliced (unpeeled and scored with a fork)
½ pound fresh mushrooms, sliced
2 leeks, sliced (white part only)
¼ avocado, sliced

Combine first 4 ingredients. Toss with dressing. Add avocado before serving.

OIL AND VINEGAR DRESSING
2 tablespoons oil
¼ cup vinegar
1 tablespoon brown sugar (to taste)
Pepper
Pinch tarragon leaves

Combine dressing ingredients and mix well. Makes 6 servings (1 cup each).

GREEK SALAD

1 large green pepper
1 can (2.2 ounces) sliced black olives, drained
1 small head cauliflower, separated into flowerets
1 clove garlic, minced
1 cup plain low-fat yogurt
1 tablespoon olive oil
2 tablespoons freshly squeezed lemon juice
Pepper

Toss green pepper, olives and cauliflower together. Combine garlic, yogurt, olive oil and lemon juice. Pour over vegetables and stir. Season with pepper and chill.
Makes 12 servings (1 cup each).

LAYERED VEGETABLE PLATTER

An unusual salad with a small amount of feta cheese for those who love it! Nice to serve with Moussaka (an eggplant dish) for a Greek dinner.

1 pound fresh green beans
2 tomatoes, sliced
1 medium red onion, sliced
1 cup artichoke hearts, halved
1½ cups fresh mushrooms, sliced
1 can (2.2 ounces) sliced black olives, drained
1 tablespoon feta cheese

Snap beans into 2-inch lengths and cook only until blanched, less than 5 minutes, drain. Plunge in cold water, drain again. Layer vegetables on platter beginning with sliced tomatoes, onions, artichokes, mushrooms, olives and lastly the beans. Pour dressing over top and chill 4 hours. Baste several times with dressing which has run to sides of platter. Top with crumbled cheese at serving time.

DRESSING
½ cup red wine vinegar
3 tablespoons olive oil
2 cloves garlic, minced
1 teaspoon basil leaves
½ teaspoon oregano leaves
Pepper

Combine dressing ingredients and mix well. Makes 10 cups.

SALATA

A spicy marinated cauliflower salad—good with chicken. This should be prepared several hours before serving—it improves with age.

    1 medium cauliflower
    1 tablespoon olive oil
    4 small onions, sliced into rings
    2 cups sliced carrots
    1 clove garlic, minced
    1 cup dry white wine
    1 cup water
    ¼ cup freshly squeezed lemon juice
    ½ cup unsalted tomato paste
    1 bay leaf
    ¼ teaspoon ground coriander
    ¼ teaspoon pepper
    Fresh parsley *or* fresh basil (optional for garnish)

Separate cauliflower into flowerets and wash well. Drain and set aside. Heat oil in large pan over low heat. Add onions, carrots and garlic. Cook 5 minutes, stirring occasionally. Add wine, water, lemon juice, tomato paste, bay leaf, coriander and pepper. Bring to a boil. Add cauliflower. Simmer 10 to 15 minutes or until cauliflower is *just* tender. Transfer vegetable mixture to serving dish with slotted spoon. Heat remaining liquid until the volume is reduced to about 1½ cups. Remove bay leaf. Pour liquid over cauliflower and other vegetables in serving dish. Chill several hours. When ready to serve, garnish with parsley or fresh basil.

Makes 10 cups.

SUNSHINE SPINACH SALAD

Beautiful *and* tasty!

    4 cups torn lettuce or other salad greens
    4 cups torn fresh spinach
    1 fresh orange, sliced *or* 1 can (11 ounces) mandarin orange sections, drained
    1 can (8 ounces) sliced water chestnuts, drained
    1 cup sliced fresh mushrooms
    1 small red onion, sliced and separated into rings
    ½ cup low-calorie Italian dressing

In large bowl, combine all ingredients except dressing. Chill until serving time. Toss with dressing.

Makes 6 servings (2 cups each).

WALDORF SALAD

A low-fat version of an old standby.

    1 cup diced celery
    1 cup diced unpeeled apple
    ⅓ cup chopped walnuts
    ⅓ cup raisins
    ½ cup low-fat yogurt (can use plain *or* combination of vanilla or orange and plain)

Combine diced celery, apples, chopped nuts and raisins. Blend yogurt into the mixture.

Makes 6 servings (½ cup each).

SOUPS AND SANDWICHES

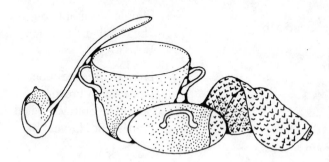

We're often asked "What shall I have for lunch?" The soup and sandwich recipes in this section are all meatless, except for the Tuna Salad Sandwich spread. By having meatless lunches, you can then have a small serving of meat, fish or poultry for dinner. Or, if you have meat for lunch, you could choose from these recipes to have a light supper.

A tasty soup can be the first course of an elaborate meal or a satisfying meal by itself. Bean soups are especially hearty, very low in fat and, with an interesting salad or filling side dish, create a delicious meal. Always serve soup with a good bread, be it corn, rye or wheat.

If you're trying nonmeat soups for the first time, you may be struck by the lack of saltiness of our recipes. Liberal use of herbs and spices, and careful use of Lite Salt, will ensure a flavorful soup.

We have also included two cold soups which may be foreign to you (and your guests) at first—but what conversation pieces!

Soups also make wonderful sack lunches. Use a wide-mouth thermos to keep it hot, pack along some fruit and a roll, and you've got a heartwarming winter lunch.

The meatless, cheeseless sandwich recipes are among the most unusual in this book. Be adventuresome and try them even if you are not sure. We believe you will find at least one or two winners.

Even though peanut butter sandwiches are not included among the recipes, we do recommend them. The goal is to use no more than 1–2 tablespoons for two slices of bread. Omit the margarine. Use jams and jelly, if desired, to make more filling for the sandwich.

SOUPS

Bean and Basil Soup
French Onion Soup
Gazpacho (cold)
Greek Lentil Soup
Greek-Style Garbanzo Soup
Hearty Fish Soup (see "Fish and Shellfish"
    section)
Homemade "Cream" Soup Mix
Hot and Sour Soup
Icy Olive Soup (cold)
Minestrone Soup
Navy Bean Soup
Potato Leek Soup
Red Root Soup
Simple Vegetable Soup
Split Pea Soup
Tomato Soup
Turkey-Vegetable Chowder (see "Chicken,
    Turkey and Rabbit" section)
Vegetable-Beef Soup (see "Beef, Veal and
    Pork" section)
Zucchini and Basil Soup

SANDWICHES

Baked Bean Special Sandwich
"Egg" Salad Sandwich Spread
Falafel
    Tahini Dressing
    Yogurt Dressing
Fruit-Nut Sandwich Spread
Pita Pizza
Tofu "Egg" Salad Sandwich
Tuna Salad Sandwich Spread
Vegetable-Cottage Cheese Sandwich Spread
Your Basic Bean Burrito

SOME MENU IDEAS FOR SOUP DINNERS

Bean and Basil Soup
French bread
Tossed salad
Hot Fudge Pudding Cake

Simple Vegetable Soup
"Egg" Salad Sandwich
Baked Apple

French Onion Soup
Hot French bread
Sunshine Spinach Salad
Northwest Harvest Bar

Navy Bean Soup
Corn Bread
Tossed salad
Sliced apples

Potato Leek Soup
Carrot-Raisin Salad
Whole Wheat Muffin
Mixed fruit cup

SOUP AS A FIRST COURSE

Hot and Sour Soup
Cashew Chicken
Steamed rice
Fortune cookies

Gazpacho
Fillet of Sole Oregon
Red potatoes
Fruit Salad Alaska

A NICE SUMMER MENU

Icy Olive Soup
Super Stuffed Potato
Whole Wheat Rolls
Strawberry Yogurt Pie

Soups

BEAN AND BASIL SOUP

A hearty soup from Southern France.

1 cup chopped potatoes
2 cups chopped carrots
2 cups chopped onions
3 quarts water
2 cups fresh green beans
1 cup uncooked macaroni
½ teaspoon Lite Salt or less
¼ cup unsalted tomato paste
3 cloves garlic, minced
2 tablespoons fresh basil or 2 tablespoons
  dried basil leaves
¼ cup grated Parmesan cheese
1 tablespoon oil
1 can (16 ounces) white beans, drained *

Boil potatoes, carrots and onions in 3 quarts water until almost cooked. Add green beans, macaroni and Lite Salt. Cook until tender. In separate bowl combine tomato paste, garlic, basil and cheese; very slowly beat in the oil. Add about 2 cups of hot soup (prepared above) slowly, beating vigorously.

Pour mixture back into soup pot and mix well. Add cooked white beans. Serve hot.

Makes 10 cups.

* Use low-sodium beans if available.

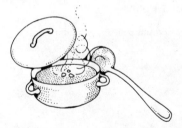

FRENCH ONION SOUP

An elegant soup for onion lovers.

SOUP
1 tablespoon oil
6 cups sliced onions
¼ teaspoon sugar or less
2 tablespoons flour
3 cups water
1 can (10½ ounces) beef broth
½ cup dry white wine or vermouth
Pepper

Heat oil in 3-quart pan. Add onions and sugar and sauté slowly until golden brown. Use medium-low heat and stir often (takes 30 minutes or more). Stir in flour and cook 2 minutes longer. Remove from heat and stir in water, broth and wine. Simmer partially covered for 15 minutes. Season to taste with pepper. Can be refrigerated at this point to serve later, if desired. The flavor is enhanced by refrigerating overnight and reheating.

BREAD
6 slices French bread (with small
  diameter) cut ½ inch thick
3 tablespoons grated part-skim mozzarella
  cheese
3 tablespoons grated Parmesan cheese

Toast bread in 325° oven for 20 minutes. Save cheese to add at serving time. Store bread in an airtight container to keep bread crisp until ready to serve.

To serve: Heat soup slowly until very hot. Sprinkle cheese on toasted bread and brown under broiler. Float 1 piece bread in each bowl of soup.

Makes 6 servings (1⅓ cups each).

GAZPACHO (a cold soup)

This is a cold tomato soup made with small chunks of your favorite vegetables. Prepare early on a hot day so it will be nicely chilled. This soup travels very well to concerts in the park.

2 cans (16 ounces each) unsalted
  tomatoes
¼ cup wine vinegar
½ teaspoon garlic powder or less
Cayenne pepper to taste
1 can (14½ ounces) chicken broth
1 small avocado, cut in half, peeled and
  sliced
1 tomato, chopped
12 ripe olives, cut into wedges
½ cup thinly sliced and chopped
  cucumber
2 tablespoons sliced green onions
2 limes, cut into wedges (optional)

Mix first 4 ingredients in a blender. Add chicken broth, vegetables and olives. Chill at least 4 hours. Serve very cold and with lime wedges, if desired.
Makes 7 cups.

GREEK LENTIL SOUP—Easy

Lentil soup and baked potatoes are a natural combination. Serve the potatoes with Mock Sour Cream or low-fat yogurt.

2 cups uncooked lentils
8 cups water
½ cup chopped onions
¾ cup chopped carrots
1 cup chopped celery
1 cup chopped potatoes
2 bay leaves
½ teaspoon ground cumin

½ teaspoon Lite Salt or less *or* garlic
  powder
2 teaspoons freshly squeezed lemon juice

Cook all ingredients except lemon juice in a large pot until lentils are soft, about 45 minutes. Add lemon juice and serve.
Makes about 10 cups.

GREEK-STYLE GARBANZO SOUP—Quick

Very quick to prepare and delicious! Serve with whole wheat rolls.

2 tablespoons olive oil
2 medium onions, chopped
1 clove garlic, minced
2 stalks celery, chopped
1 or 2 carrots, sliced
1 large potato, diced
1 sprig parsley, finely chopped
1 green pepper, chopped
1 can (6 ounces) unsalted tomato paste
¼ teaspoon black pepper
2 cans (16 ounces each) garbanzo beans,
  drained *
5 cups water
1 chicken bouillon cube

Heat oil in a kettle and sauté onions, garlic and celery for about 5 minutes. Add the remaining vegetables, tomato paste, and pepper. Add garbanzo beans, water and bouillon cube. Bring to boil and simmer for 10 minutes. Stir well before serving.
Makes 14 cups.

* Use low-sodium beans if available.

HOMEMADE "CREAM" SOUP MIX

To use in place of canned cream soups in casseroles or as a base for your own soups. Much lower in fat and salt than the canned versions. The trick is to have it made up ready to use!

2 cups powdered nonfat milk
¾ cup cornstarch
¼ cup (or less) instant chicken bouillon
2 tablespoons dried onion flakes
1 teaspoon basil leaves
1 teaspoon thyme leaves
½ teaspoon pepper

Combine all ingredients, mixing well. Store in an airtight container until ready to use.
To substitute for one can of condensed soup: Combine ⅓ cup of dry mix with 1¼ cups of cold water in a saucepan. Cook and stir until thickened. Add to casserole as you would the canned product.

Makes equivalent of 9 cans of soup.

HOT AND SOUR SOUP

3 or 4 dried black mushrooms
1 cup boiling water
12 ounces tofu (bean curd)
2 tablespoons cornstarch
¼ cup water
5 cups chicken broth
1 tablespoon sherry
2 tablespoons white vinegar
1 teaspoon lower-sodium soy sauce
¼ teaspoon white pepper
2 tablespoons egg substitute, beaten (commercial *or* Homemade Egg Substitute, page 241)
½ cup frozen peas
Few drops sesame oil
1 green onion, minced

Soak dried mushrooms in 1 cup boiling water for 30 minutes, reserving soaking liquid for later use. Sliver mushrooms and bean curd. Blend cornstarch and ¼ cup water to a paste. Bring broth and mushroom-soaking liquid to a boil. Add mushrooms and simmer, covered, 10 minutes. Stir in sherry, white vinegar, soy sauce and pepper. Thicken with cornstarch paste. Slowly add egg substitute, stirring gently once or twice. This may be prepared in advance and refrigerated until serving time. When ready to serve, heat the soup, add the bean curd and frozen peas and heat for 1 minute or until peas are thawed. Remove from heat. Sprinkle with sesame oil and green onion.

VARIATIONS
In place of white vinegar, substitute wine vinegar or lemon juice. For the sesame oil, substitute Tabasco sauce. Omit vinegar and pepper—it's then called "Mandarin Soup."

Makes 9 cups.

ICY OLIVE SOUP—Easy

An unusual cold soup, great on hot summer evenings.

2 cups plain low-fat yogurt
2 cans (10¾ ounces each) chicken broth
1 cup sliced black olives
½ cup chopped green onions
½ cup chopped green pepper
1 cup chopped cucumber (bite-size pieces)

Stir yogurt until smooth. Add chicken broth and stir until blended. Add remaining ingredients and stir to distribute vegetables. Cover and refrigerate for 4 hours.

Makes 7½ cups.

MINESTRONE SOUP

This hearty soup needs only some crusty French bread and fruit to make a fine meal.

½ cup uncooked navy beans
1 can (10¾ ounces) chicken broth
1 quart water
2 medium carrots, cut in small strips
½ small head cabbage, shredded
1 medium potato, diced
1 can (16 ounces) unsalted tomatoes
1 medium onion, sliced
1½ tablespoons olive oil
1 stalk celery, sliced diagonally
1 zucchini, sliced
2 cloves garlic, minced
⅛ teaspoon pepper
¼ teaspoon Lite Salt or less
½ teaspoon basil leaves
¼ teaspoon marjoram leaves *or*
** ⅛ teaspoon ground marjoram**
2 tablespoons chopped parsley
1 can (8 ounces) unsalted tomato sauce
** (optional)**
½ cup broken uncooked spaghetti*

In a very large kettle (6–8 quart) add navy beans to chicken broth and water. Cover and cook together for 1 hour. Add carrots, cabbage, potatoes and tomatoes. Cook another 30 minutes. Sauté onions in oil until translucent. Add celery, zucchini, garlic, pepper, Lite Salt, basil and marjoram. Continue to sauté until tender. Add to beans and vegetable mixture. Add parsley and tomato sauce. Cook 20 minutes. Add more water if too thick. Add spaghetti and cook for 10 additional minutes.
  Makes 14 cups.

* If you are going to freeze leftover soup, do not add spaghetti as it does not freeze well.

NAVY BEAN SOUP

The Senate's famous bean soup without the meat! The ground cloves add an unusual flavor.

2 cups uncooked white beans
8 cups water
½ teaspoon Lite Salt or less
⅛ teaspoon pepper
1 bay leaf
2 cups chopped celery
1 cup chopped carrots
1 cup chopped onion
1 can (8 ounces) unsalted tomato sauce
¼ cup chopped parsley
Dash of ground cloves

Soak beans at least 3 hours in cold water. Drain. Add 8 cups water, Lite Salt, pepper and bay leaf. Bring to a boil, then simmer for 2 hours or until beans are tender. Add celery, carrots, onions, tomato sauce, parsley and cloves. Mash some of the beans to thicken the soup. Simmer for 2 hours.
  Makes 16 cups.

POTATO LEEK SOUP

Chunky potatoes and savory leeks make this soup very tasty. Serve with bread and a tossed green salad.

4 leeks
1 tablespoon margarine
4 cups potatoes, peeled and chopped (3
** large or 4 medium)**
5 cups water
1 cup skim milk
½ teaspoon Lite Salt or less
¼ teaspoon pepper

Wash leeks thoroughly and cut up into small rounds. Use both the white and green parts. Melt the margarine in a large pot. Add cut-up leeks and cook for 5 minutes over medium heat, until leeks are limp. Add potatoes and water and bring to a boil. Boil uncovered for 30 minutes until potatoes are thoroughly cooked. (They should fall apart when prodded with a fork.) Add the skim milk, Lite Salt and pepper. The soup should be thick, creamy, and green from the color of the leeks. Mash some of the potato chunks to thicken the soup or puree in blender if smooth creamy soup is desired.

Makes 10 cups.

RED ROOT SOUP

A good recipe for people who say they don't like beets! It really is delicious.

6 shallots, peeled and chopped
5 carrots, chopped
2 beets, peeled and chopped
2 potatoes, peeled and chopped
4 leeks, chopped
1 cup chopped parsley
5 cups chicken broth
2 cups water
2 cups skim milk
½ teaspoon curry powder

Combine first 6 ingredients in a large kettle. Add chicken broth and water to vegetables and cook for 20–25 minutes, or until vegetables are tender. Blend the vegetable mixture in 4 batches in a blender for a few seconds, or until the vegetables are just minced but not smooth. At this point the mixture can be refrigerated or frozen for future use.

When ready to serve: Combine the blended vegetable mixture, the skim milk and curry powder in a saucepan. Simmer until heated through.

Makes 10 cups.

SIMPLE VEGETABLE SOUP

Low in calories—for larger appetites serve with baked potatoes, rolls and dessert.

1 large potato, diced
1 small onion, chopped
½ green pepper, diced (optional)
2 cups water
½ beef bouillon cube

Simmer above ingredients together for 10 minutes and add:

1 package (10 ounces) frozen mixed vegetables
1 can (16 ounces) unsalted stewed tomatoes
1 tablespoon oil
1 teaspoon oregano leaves

Bring to boil, reduce heat and cook an additional 20–30 minutes, covered.

Makes 7 cups.

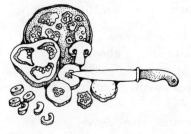

SPLIT PEA SOUP

Hearty enough for a meal—try this with Onion Squares.

- **2 cups uncooked split peas**
- **5 cups water or more**
- **1 bay leaf**
- **¾ teaspoon Lite Salt or less**
- **2 cups chopped carrots**
- **1 cup chopped celery**
- **1 cup chopped onion**
- **½ teaspoon thyme leaves**
- **½ teaspoon pepper**
- **½ teaspoon garlic powder**
- **2 tablespoons vinegar *or* lemon juice**

Combine dried split peas, water, bay leaf, and Lite Salt in a large kettle. Bring to a boil and then reduce heat and simmer for 2 hours. Stir occasionally and check to make sure there is enough water and that the split peas do not stick. Add more water if it becomes too dry. Add carrots, celery, onions and herbs. Continue to simmer for 30 minutes or longer (overcooking cannot hurt this soup, as long as it is stirred to prevent sticking). Just before serving add the vinegar or lemon juice and more pepper, if desired.

Makes about 12 cups.

TOMATO SOUP

A homemade version of an old standby.

- **1 carrot, chopped**
- **2 stalks celery, chopped**
- **¼ cup water**
- **3 cups unsalted canned *or* fresh tomatoes, peeled**
- **½ teaspoon basil leaves**
- **¼ teaspoon oregano leaves**

- **1 cup powdered nonfat milk**
- **2 bouillon cubes**
- **1 quart water**
- **Pepper to taste**

Steam carrots and celery in ¼ cup water until tender. Add tomatoes, basil and oregano. Simmer gently for 5 minutes. Puree tomato mixture in blender or food mill. Blend in powdered milk. Pour back into pan. Dissolve bouillon cubes in 1 quart of water and add to other ingredients. Heat thoroughly but do not boil. Add pepper to taste.

Makes 8 cups.

OPTIONAL
A little wine *or* brandy makes this a very fancy soup.

ZUCCHINI AND BASIL SOUP

- **2 teaspoons margarine**
- **1 large onion, finely chopped**
- **1 clove garlic, minced**
- **4 cups sliced zucchini (¼ inch thick)**
- **4 cups chicken broth**
- **2 cups water**
- **1 teaspoon basil leaves**
- **½ teaspoon pepper**
- **2 cups skim milk**
- **¼ cup water**
- **2 tablespoons cornstarch**

In a 5–6 quart kettle, melt margarine over medium heat. Add onion and garlic to margarine and cook, stirring, until onions are limp (about 5 minutes). Add the zucchini slices, chicken broth, 2 cups of water, basil and pepper. Bring to boiling, then reduce heat, cover and simmer until zucchini is very tender (about 20 minutes).

In a bowl blend skim milk, ¼ cup water

and cornstarch. Increase heat and add the cornstarch mixture to the kettle. Cook, stirring, until soup boils and thickens slightly.

Makes about 9 cups.

Sandwiches

BAKED BEAN SPECIAL SANDWICH

An open-faced sandwich which is served warm.

- 1 can (16 ounces) vegetarian-style baked beans in tomato sauce *
- ½ cup chopped onion
- ¼ cup chopped green pepper
- 3 tablespoons brown sugar
- 1 tablespoon molasses
- 2 teaspoons Worcestershire sauce
- ¼ teaspoon dry mustard
- ¼ teaspoon pepper
- 8 slices rye bread, English muffin halves or hamburger buns
- 8 slices tomato *or* canned pineapple
- Parsley (for garnish)

Preheat oven to 400°. Mix first 8 ingredients together well. Place in ovenproof dish, cover and bake for approximately 45 minutes, stirring occasionally.

Spread ¼ cup of bean mixture on one slice rye bread, half of an English muffin or half of a hamburger bun. Top with tomato or pineapple slice. Broil for a few minutes, if desired. Garnish with parsley.

Makes 4 servings.

* Use low-sodium beans if available.

"EGG" SALAD SANDWICH SPREAD

Use as a sandwich filling or as a salad on crisp lettuce leaves

- 1 cup egg substitute (commercial *or* Homemade Egg Substitute, page 241)
- 2 hard-boiled egg whites, chopped
- 2 tablespoons finely chopped celery
- 2 tablespoons finely chopped green pepper
- 2 tablespoons finely chopped onion
- ¼ cup Miracle Whip Light *or* imitation mayonnaise
- Dash pepper
- ½ teaspoon prepared mustard

Pour egg substitute into an 8-inch nonstick skillet. Cover tightly. Cook over very low heat until just firm to the touch, about 10 minutes. Remove from skillet in large pieces. Cut into small cubes.

Combine cooked egg substitute, egg whites, celery, green peppers, and onions in a mixing bowl. In a separate bowl combine mayonnaise, pepper and mustard; blend well. Lightly toss with egg substitute mixture. Chill before serving.

Makes filling for 4 sandwiches (2 cups spread).

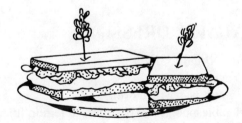

FALAFEL—Quick

Traditional filling for pocket or pita bread in the Middle East.

To make a falafel "sandwich" all you need to do is cut a pita bread in half and put 2 or 3 cooked falafel balls or patties into the open half. Add lettuce, alfalfa sprouts, sliced tomatoes, chopped green onions and Yogurt Dressing or Tahini Dressing (see recipes below).

Falafel is not difficult to make, particularly if you use falafel mix found in many supermarkets or delicatessens. Most mixes list the traditional garbanzo beans and yellow peas, wheat germ, onion, parsley, herbs, spices, salt and baking soda as ingredients.

Instructions on preparation and serving are on the back of the package. We edited them as follows:

1 cup falafel mix
¾ cup water

Mix instant falafel and water. Let stand for 10 minutes. Make into tablespoon-sized patties or balls. Preheat oven to 350°. Place on nonstick cookie sheets and bake for 10 minutes on each side for patties or for 20 minutes if shaped into balls.

Makes 4 servings (one 10-ounce package contains 2 cups dry mix).

FALAFEL DRESSINGS

TAHINI DRESSING
¼ cup tahini*
½ cup water or more
1 tablespoon freshly squeezed lemon juice
⅛ teaspoon Lite Salt or less
1 clove garlic (optional)

Mix and serve. Should be the consistency of a creamy salad dressing. Add more water if necessary. Use about 2 tablespoons as a sauce for a falafel sandwich.

Makes ¾ cup.

* Tahini is sometimes labeled "sesame seed butter" and is usually available in supermarkets in the specialty food section.

YOGURT DRESSING
1 cup plain low-fat yogurt
1 tablespoon freshly squeezed lemon juice
¼ teaspoon Lite Salt or less
1 tablespoon chopped parsley

Combine and serve.
Makes 1 cup.

FRUIT-NUT SANDWICH SPREAD

Looking for variety in lunches? Use wheatberry rolls or graham crackers with this filling.

1½ cups low-fat cottage cheese
1 teaspoon freshly squeezed lemon juice
⅓ cup chopped pecans or walnuts
⅓ cup raisins
⅓ cup canned crushed pineapple, drained

Place the cottage cheese and lemon juice in a blender and blend until smooth. Scrape mixture out of the blender and into bowl. Stir in pecans *or* walnuts, raisins and pineapple. Spread ½ cup of mixture on 2 slices of bread to make a sandwich.

Makes filling for 5 sandwiches (2½ cups spread).

PITA PIZZA—Quick

A quickie! The amounts are to make one pita pizza. Make as many as you need.

1 whole wheat pita bread
2 tablespoons no salt added spaghetti sauce
2 tablespoons finely chopped green pepper
2 tablespoons finely chopped mushrooms
2 tablespoons finely chopped onion
2 black olives, sliced (optional)
2 tablespoons shredded imitation mozzarella cheese

Preheat oven to 425°. Spread sauce on one side of unsliced pita bread. Sprinkle green peppers, mushrooms, onions, and black olives over sauce. Sprinkle cheese over vegetables. Place on ungreased pizza pan or cookie sheet. Bake 5–10 minutes or until done.
Makes 1 pita pizza.

TOFU "EGG" SALAD SANDWICH

Some say this sandwich spread is even better than the real thing!

4 ounces firm tofu, drained
1½ teaspoons tahini *
1 dill pickle, chopped (about two tablespoons)
¼ teaspoon minced onion
½ teaspoon prepared mustard
½ teaspoon oil
¼ teaspoon turmeric
Pinch basil and celery seed

Crumble tofu into small pieces with a fork. Combine with other ingredients.
Makes 1 cup spread (filling for 2 sandwiches).

* Tahini is sometimes labeled "sesame seed butter" and is usually available in supermarkets in the specialty food section.

TUNA SALAD SANDWICH SPREAD

Yogurt and a small amount of imitation mayonnaise with tuna makes a nice sandwich filling.

1 can (6½ ounces) water-packed tuna
¼ cup diced celery
¼ cup chopped onion
¼ cup plain low-fat yogurt
1 tablespoon imitation mayonnaise

Drain tuna. Combine with celery, onions, yogurt and mayonnaise and stir to blend well.
Makes 1½ cups spread.

VARIATION
For a hot sandwich—spread on English muffin halves and place under broiler 2–3 minutes.

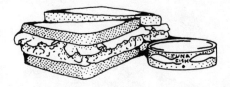

VEGETABLE-COTTAGE CHEESE SANDWICH SPREAD

Who says sandwiches must have meat?

1½ cups low-fat cottage cheese
½ teaspoon sugar
1 teaspoon freshly squeezed lemon juice
1 tablespoon chopped onion
⅓ cup chopped carrot
¼ cup chopped celery
Dash of Worcestershire sauce

Place the cottage cheese, sugar, and lemon juice in a blender and blend until smooth. Scrape mixture out of the blender and into bowl. Stir in vegetables and Worcestershire sauce.

Makes 2½ cups of spread.

SERVING IDEAS
Serve on whole wheat, pumpernickel, Vienna, rye or French bread. For a sack lunch, make a poor-boy sandwich of the vegetable spread, lettuce and tomato slices.

YOUR BASIC BEAN BURRITO

Perfect for a quick meal. This recipe is for 1 burrito and is very low-fat.

½ cup Refried Beans, page 281, or ½ cup canned vegetarian refried beans *
1 tablespoon canned, chopped green chiles (optional)
1 flour tortilla (8-inch diameter)
2 tablespoons chopped tomato
1 tablespoon chopped green onion
¼ cup shredded lettuce
2 tablespoons plain low-fat yogurt

Heat refried beans in a small saucepan. Add green chiles if used. Soften tortilla by warming in oven or microwave, *or* by placing in an unoiled heated skillet for 1 minute on each side. Place hot beans on warm tortilla and sprinkle chopped tomatoes, onions, lettuce and yogurt over beans. Fold tortilla over, and eat quickly—before it cools.

Makes 1 serving.

* Use low-sodium beans if available.

SIDE DISHES

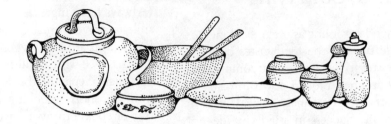

By side dishes we mean that extra special vegetable or grain dish which accentuates poultry, lean red meat or fish entrees—and even those which are meatless. All these dishes are winners!

Because each serving generally contains less than a teaspoon of fat, these dishes make excellent lunches, so make large amounts and plan to have leftovers!

GUIDE TO STIR FRYING

VEGETABLE DISHES

Basic Stir-Fried Vegetables
Corn Bake
Cottage Spinach
"Creamed" Vegetables
Eggplant Parmesan
Eggplant Szechuan Style
Garden Peas
Mexican Corn Medley
Onion Squares
Ratatouille Provençale
Stir-Fried Mushrooms and Broccoli
Stuffed Acorn Squash
Stuffed Zucchini Boats

Tomatoes "Provençale"
Zucchini Mexicali

POTATO DISHES

Homemade Tatertots
Mashed Potatoes
Potato Puff
Scalloped Potatoes
Skinny "French Fries"
Super Stuffed Potatoes
Twice-Baked Potatoes, Cottage Style

GRAIN DISHES

Bulgur Pilaf
Curried Rice
Gourmet Pasta Pilaf
Millet Vegetable Casserole
Mushroom Barley Pilaf
Spanish Rice
Spinach and Rice Casserole

BEAN DISHES

Classic Baked Beans
Refried Beans

Guide to Stir Frying

We recommend stir frying as it can be done with very little oil and the food tastes delicious. At first stir frying may seem complex and baffling, but when broken down into its component parts, it's extremely logical and not at all difficult. Success in stir frying depends on two things: understanding the underlying principles of this cooking method and getting organized before you begin.

PRINCIPLES OF STIR FRYING

Stir frying consists of the following steps: heating the pan (3-quart saucepan, at least a 10-inch skillet or a wok) and oil; adding the first seasonings (garlic, ginger root, etc.); then the meat; liquid seasonings; vegetables; stock and a cornstarch paste.

PREPARATION—GETTING ORGANIZED

The following suggestions on getting organized should help prevent frayed nerves and frazzled tempers.

1. Read the recipe well in advance to see what ingredients are needed and what preparation they require.
2. If dried ingredients are called for, allow 30 minutes for soaking.
3. Slice and stack the meat, poultry or seafood. (These may be sliced several hours in advance, wrapped and refrigerated until needed.) If they are to be marinated, allow time for this.
4. Wash, drain and cut the vegetables. (Always have ingredients as dry as possible to prevent splattering.)
5. If more than one vegetable is used, check to see which will be added to the pan first. Separate the longer-cooking from the shorter-cooking vegetables. A tray or cookie tin works well for this.
6. Mix the liquid seasonings (soy sauce, sherry, etc.) in a separate container.
7. If a cornstarch paste is called for, mix and set this aside.
8. Get out all the other ingredients such as oil, garlic, ginger, green onions, stock, garnish, etc.
9. Set out the cooking pans, utensils and serving dishes . . . and you're off.

Vegetable Dishes

BASIC STIR-FRIED VEGETABLES

1 pound vegetables—see combinations which follow
3 slices fresh ginger root, peeled and chopped
1 clove garlic, minced
¼–½ cup chicken broth or water
1 tablespoon low-sodium soy sauce or less
½ teaspoon sugar
1 tablespoon oil
1 teaspoon cornstarch
2 tablespoons water

Prepare vegetables as indicated in the instructions below. The individual vegetables are added to the pan according to their specific cooking time. Remember: The toughest vegetables are added first, the more tender ones last.

Combine chicken broth *or* water, soy sauce and sugar.

Heat oil. Add ginger root and garlic, and stir-fry a few times. Add vegetables (adjust heat to prevent scorching). Stir-fry to coat with oil and heat through.

Add broth/soy mixture and heat quickly. Then simmer, covered, over medium heat until vegetables are done. The aim is to have vegetables that are tender but still crunchy.

When vegetables are tender, thicken the sauce with a cornstarch paste made of 1 teaspoon cornstarch and 2 tablespoons cold water.

Makes 4 cups

VARIATION
To make Sweet and Sour Vegetables omit ginger root and chicken broth. Add 2 tablespoons sugar or honey and 3 tablespoons vinegar. Thicken with cornstarch and water.

SUGGESTED COMBINATIONS FOR BASIC STIR-FRIED VEGETABLES:
—Cabbage, onions, green pepper, fresh mushrooms, carrots and snow peas.
—Chinese cabbage and 2–3 dried black mushrooms (soaked and sliced).
—Broccoli, fresh mushrooms and carrots.
—Zucchini, green pepper, mushrooms, onions and tomatoes.
—Bean sprouts and onions.
—Cauliflower and fresh mushrooms.

CORN BAKE-Easy

A nice dish to accompany enchiladas for a Mexican dinner. So easy it's hard to realize it's so good!

1 small onion, finely chopped
1 small green pepper, finely chopped
1 can (16 ounces) unsalted cream-style corn
½ teaspoon Lite Salt or less
Pepper to taste
½ cup bread crumbs

Preheat oven to 350°. Mix chopped onions and green peppers with corn, Lite Salt and pepper. Place in baking dish. Sprinkle with bread crumbs. Bake for 45 minutes.

Makes 4 servings.

COTTAGE SPINACH

Try this with Cornish Game Hens à la Crock or Orange Baked Chicken.

2 packages (10 ounces each) frozen chopped spinach
4 egg whites *or* ½ cup egg substitute (commercial *or* Homemade Egg Substitute, page 241)
1½ cups low-fat cottage cheese
⅓ cup grated Parmesan cheese

Preheat oven to 350°. Defrost spinach or cook briefly and drain very well; use a colander or paper towels. When most of the liquid is gone, combine spinach with the remaining ingredients and bake uncovered in a lightly oiled casserole dish (1½ quarts) for 30 minutes.

Makes 6 servings.

"CREAMED" VEGETABLES

Any vegetable can be prepared "creamed" and still be lower in fat. Here are a few ideas.

4 cups vegetables (e.g., broccoli, carrots, cauliflower, onions, potatoes or turnips)
1½ tablespoons margarine
1½ tablespoons flour
¼ teaspoon Lite Salt or less
¼ teaspoon pepper
½ teaspoon nutmeg (optional)
1½ cups skim milk

Cut vegetables into serving sizes and cook until barely tender by steaming, cooking in small amount of water or in microwave. Drain vegetables well.

While vegetables are cooking, melt margarine in a medium-size saucepan over low heat. Add flour, Lite Salt, pepper and nutmeg. Stir over low heat until mixture is smooth. Remove from heat. Add milk. Heat to boiling, stirring constantly until mixture thickens, about 1 minute. Add cooked, drained vegetables. Heat through.

Makes 4 servings.

EGGPLANT PARMESAN

Simple, elegant and delicious.

3 cups Marinara Sauce, page 376
1 eggplant, sliced ½ inch thick
½ cup grated Parmesan cheese

Preheat oven to 350°. Steam eggplant slices *or* roll in flour and broil for 3 minutes on each side. Place in a casserole dish and cover with Marinara Sauce. Sprinkle with Parmesan cheese. Heat in oven for about 20 minutes until bubbly.

Makes 6 servings.

EGGPLANT SZECHUAN STYLE

A spicy side dish to serve with Parmesan Yogurt Chicken. This is a low-fat version of a popular eggplant dish served in Northern Chinese restaurants.

4–6 Japanese eggplants (about 12 ounces total)
1 tablespoon oil
2 cloves garlic, minced
½ tablespoon chopped fresh ginger
1 teaspoon black bean sauce with chili*
2 tablespoons lower-sodium soy sauce
1 teaspoon sugar
½ cup chicken broth
½ tablespoon vinegar
½ teaspoon sesame oil
1 tablespoon chopped green onion

Choose firm purple eggplants and remove stalk. Without peeling, cut into thumb-size pieces. Brush skillet with oil or treat with nonstick spray. Stir-fry eggplant over medium heat until soft (about 10 minutes). Remove from pan and set aside.

Into the frying pan, place 1 tablespoon oil, and sauté garlic, ginger and black bean sauce quickly. Add soy sauce, sugar and chicken broth and bring to a boil. Add eggplant, cook about 1 minute until sauce is done. Add vinegar and sesame oil, stir until heated through. Thicken with cornstarch if desired. Sprinkle with chopped green onion. Mix carefully and serve.

Makes 4 servings.

* Available in Oriental groceries.

GARDEN PEAS

Simple and unusual.

2 teaspoons margarine
10–12 lettuce leaves, shredded into
**   ¼-inch strips**
¼ cup finely chopped onion
2 packages (10 ounces each) frozen peas,
**   thawed *or* 3 cups shelled, fresh peas**
½ teaspoon sugar
¼ cup water
¼ teaspoon pepper

In a saucepan melt margarine. Add lettuce, onions, peas, sugar and water; cover. Bring to a boil—then simmer for 5 minutes or until peas are tender. Sprinkle with pepper.

Makes 4 servings.

MEXICAN CORN MEDLEY

A brightly colored vegetable dish! Good to serve with bean casseroles such as Spanish Beans or Mexican Bean Pot.

2½ pounds zucchini, cut into ½-inch
**   cubes**
1 package (10 ounces) frozen corn,
**   thawed**
1 red or green pepper, chopped
1 medium onion, chopped
2 cloves garlic, minced
Pepper

Place all ingredients (except pepper) in a large pot over medium-high heat. Stir mixture frequently until most vegetable liquid has evaporated and vegetables are tender-crisp (about 5 minutes). Add pepper to taste.

Makes 6 to 8 servings.

ONION SQUARES

We can't decide if this is a side dish or a corn bread—it came to us from Eastern Oregon and goes very well with chili or a bean soup. If cut in small squares it makes a great appetizer.

1 onion, sliced
½ cup low-fat yogurt
¼ teaspoon dill weed
¼ teaspoon Lite Salt or less
½ cup flour
½ cup cornmeal
1 teaspoon sugar
1½ teaspoons baking powder
3 tablespoons oil
½ cup skim milk
1 egg white
1 package (10 ounces) frozen corn,
**   thawed**
2 drops Tabasco sauce
2 tablespoons grated Parmesan cheese

Preheat oven to 450°. Sauté onion slices in nonstick fry pan until soft and slightly browned. Add yogurt, dill weed and Lite Salt. In a separate bowl combine flour, cornmeal, sugar, baking powder, oil, skim milk and egg white. Mix well. Add corn and Tabasco sauce. Pour batter into lightly oiled 9-inch-square pan. Spread onion mixture over batter. Sprinkle Parmesan cheese over onions. Bake for 25–30 minutes. Cut into squares to serve.

Makes 9 servings.

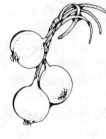

RATATOUILLE PROVENÇALE

2½ cups diced eggplant
¾ cup thinly sliced onion
2 cloves garlic, minced
1 tablespoon olive oil
4 green peppers, sliced
2 cups quartered tomatoes
3 cups sliced zucchini (½ inch thick)
1 teaspoon oregano leaves
Pepper to taste
1 cup plain low-fat yogurt *or* Mock Sour
  Cream, page 224

Dice eggplant in ½-inch cubes. Sauté onions and garlic in olive oil. Add green peppers, tomatoes and zucchini; sauté until heated. Add eggplant, oregano and pepper. Cook very slowly in covered dish for about an hour. Uncover and cook about 15 minutes longer. Serve with dollop of plain yogurt *or* Mock Sour Cream; may be served hot or cold in small bowls.

Makes 8 servings.

STIR-FRIED MUSHROOMS AND BROCCOLI

Great over fresh pasta, too.

1 tablespoon margarine
½ cup chopped onion
½ pound fresh mushrooms, sliced
1 tablespoon oil
1 bunch broccoli, cut into flowerets
1 clove garlic, minced
1 can (8 ounces) sliced water chestnuts,
  drained
1 tablespoon cornstarch
1 teaspoon sugar

¼ teaspoon ground ginger
1 teaspoon lower-sodium soy sauce
½ bouillon cube
¾ cup boiling water

Melt margarine and add onions. Sauté 2 minutes. Add mushrooms and stir for 5 minutes. Remove and set aside. Heat oil. Add broccoli and garlic, cooking for 3 minutes. Add water chestnuts and cook 2 minutes longer. Blend cornstarch, sugar and ginger with soy sauce. Dissolve bouillon in water and pour into pan. Add cornstarch mixture. Cook and stir until thickened. Reduce heat and simmer, covered, 5 minutes, or until broccoli is just crisp-tender. Add mushrooms. Serve over rice, if desired.

Makes 8 servings.

STUFFED ACORN SQUASH

This goes well with chicken and salad.

1½ cups cooked brown rice
2 tablespoons chopped walnuts
¾ cup cracker crumbs
1 medium onion, finely chopped
2 egg whites, slightly beaten
½ teaspoon sage
2 teaspoons chopped parsley
½ teaspoon Lite Salt or less
¼ teaspoon pepper
3 acorn squash, cut in half and cleaned

Preheat oven to 350°. Combine all ingredients except squash. Place mixture loosely in squash halves. Bake stuffed squash in a pan covered with foil for 1 hour or until squash is tender.

Makes 6 servings.

STUFFED ZUCCHINI BOATS

This recipe is excellent with Italian dishes.

2 medium zucchini (8 inches long)
2 teaspoons olive oil
1 clove garlic, minced
¼ cup minced onion
¼ cup chopped green pepper
4 large fresh mushrooms, chopped
1 tomato, chopped
½ teaspoon oregano leaves (see variations)
3 tablespoons grated Parmesan cheese

Preheat oven to 350°. Cut zucchini in half. Scoop out pulp and dice. Place scooped-out zucchini shells cut side down in a baking dish with a small amount of water. Bake or heat in a microwave oven until crisp-tender. Heat olive oil in a skillet and stir-fry garlic, onion, green pepper and mushrooms until crisp-tender. Add a little water if vegetables stick. Add diced zucchini and stir-fry for 1 minute. Add tomato and oregano. Cool slightly. Add 1 tablespoon Parmesan cheese. Mix well. Spoon mixture into zucchini boats. Top with remaining Parmesan cheese. Broil for a few minutes to brown cheese or cover and heat in a microwave oven. Do not overcook.

Makes 4 servings.

VARIATION
Substitute ¼ to ½ teaspoon turmeric for the oregano as an accompaniment for Indian food, use ¼ to ½ teaspoon ground cumin when serving Mexican food or ¼ teaspoon pepper for a less spicy dish.

TOMATOES "PROVENÇALE"

Stuffed tomatoes can be easily served at home, too—not just in restaurants.

6 firm tomatoes
¼ teaspoon thyme leaves
¼ teaspoon rosemary leaves
¼ teaspoon ground coriander
¼ teaspoon garlic powder
Pepper
½ cup soft bread crumbs
¼ cup chopped onion
1 tablespoon oil

Preheat oven to 400°. Cut tomatoes in half crosswise. Press out juice and seeds. Turn upside down on a paper towel to remove excess moisture. Mix spices, bread crumbs, onions and oil in a bowl. Place the tomatoes side by side in a lightly oiled baking dish. Fill each with spice mixture. Place in upper third of oven. Bake for 20 minutes, until the tomatoes are tender and the filling browned.

Makes 6 servings.

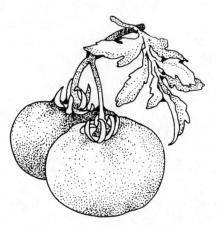

ZUCCHINI MEXICALI

An excellent way to serve zucchini with chicken or fish—or try it over rice for a light meatless main dish.

1 tablespoon oil
4 cups thinly sliced zucchini
1 cup coarsely shredded carrots
1 cup chopped onion
¾ cup chopped celery
½ green pepper, cut into thin strips
½ teaspoon garlic powder
¼ teaspoon basil leaves
Dash pepper
⅓ cup taco sauce
2 teaspoons prepared mustard
2 medium tomatoes, cut into wedges
⅓ cup grated low-fat cheese

Heat oil in a 10-inch skillet. Add zucchini, carrots, onions, celery, green pepper, garlic powder, basil and pepper. Toss to mix well. Cook, covered, over medium-high heat for about 4 minutes, stirring occasionally.

Combine taco sauce and mustard; stir into vegetables. Add tomato wedges; cook, uncovered, 3 to 5 minutes or until heated through. Transfer to serving dish and top with grated cheese.

Makes 6 servings.

Potato Dishes

HOMEMADE TATERTOTS

A good way to use leftover mashed potatoes and cooked rice.

⅓ cup chopped onion
1 tablespoon margarine
½ cup cooked mashed potatoes

1 cup cooked brown rice
1 tablespoon unsalted tomato paste
½ teaspoon Lite Salt or less
½ cup whole grain bread crumbs
3 tablespoons grated Parmesan cheese

Preheat oven to 350°. Sauté onions in margarine. Combine all ingredients and form into 1½-inch balls. Bake until delicately browned, approximately 15–20 minutes.

Makes 4 servings.

MASHED POTATOES

Simple and always good.

6 medium potatoes
⅓–½ cup skim milk
½ teaspoon Lite Salt or less
Pepper

Scrub potatoes and peel if desired. Cube and boil until tender. Mash well, adding milk, Lite Salt and pepper. Serve piping hot.

Makes 6 servings (1 cup each).

POTATO PUFF

Easy fancy mashed potatoes. A very pretty dish.

6 potatoes, cooked and drained
¾ cup skim milk
¾ teaspoon Lite Salt or less
⅓ cup grated low-fat cheese
2 teaspoons Dijon mustard
¼ cup chopped green onions
2 egg whites

Add the skim milk and Lite Salt to potatoes and mash until smooth. Add cheese, mustard and green onions to the mashed potatoes. Mix well. Place in a lightly oiled 1½-quart baking dish. May be prepared ahead to this point and refrigerated.

Just prior to baking, preheat oven to 375°. Beat egg whites until very stiff and spread over potatoes. Bake 50–60 minutes and serve immediately.

Makes 4–6 servings.

SCALLOPED POTATOES

The secret of these scalloped potatoes is long, slow cooking—well worth the time and effort.

  6 medium potatoes
  ¼ cup finely chopped onion
  3 tablespoons flour
  ½ teaspoon Lite Salt or less
  ¼ teaspoon pepper
  1 tablespoon margarine
  2½ cups skim milk

Heat oven to 350°. Wash potatoes and remove eyes. Cut potatoes into thin slices—no need to peel them.

In a lightly oiled 2-quart casserole, arrange potatoes in 4 layers, sprinkling each of the first 3 layers with 1 tablespoon onion, 1 tablespoon flour, ⅛ teaspoon Lite Salt and a dash pepper. Dot each layer with 1 teaspoon margarine. Sprinkle top with remaining onion, Lite Salt and pepper. Heat milk just to scalding (bubbles around edge) and pour over potatoes. Cover and bake 30 minutes. Uncover and bake 60–70 minutes until potatoes are tender. Let stand 5–10 minutes before serving.

Makes 4–6 servings.

SKINNY "FRENCH FRIES"

The taste and texture of French fries—without the fat!

  4 medium potatoes, cut in strips or
    lengthwise, about ½ inch thick
  1 tablespoon oil
  Paprika
  ½ teaspoon Lite Salt or less

Preheat oven to 450°. While cutting potatoes, keep strips in bowl of ice water to crisp. Drain and pat dry on paper towels. Return to bowl and sprinkle with oil. Mix with hands to distribute oil evenly over potatoes. Bake on a jelly-roll pan until golden brown and tender, about 30 to 40 minutes, turning frequently. Sprinkle generously with paprika, and sparingly with Lite Salt.

Makes 4 servings.

SUPER STUFFED POTATOES

Very versatile! These stuffed potatoes can be made ahead since they freeze very well. The "stuffing" can be served in a casserole dish when time is limited.

  6 medium potatoes
  1½ cups broccoli
  ¾ cup grated low-fat cheese, divided
  1 tablespoon margarine
  ¼ cup skim milk
  ⅛ teaspoon pepper
  ½ teaspoon Lite Salt or less

Preheat oven to 400°. Scrub potatoes. Make shallow slits around the middle as if you were cutting the potatoes in half lengthwise. Bake until done, 30–60 minutes.

Steam broccoli until just tender and finely chop.

Carefully slice the potatoes in half and scoop the insides into a bowl with the broccoli. Add ½ cup of the cheese and the margarine, milk, Lite Salt and pepper. Mash all together until mixture is pale green with dark flecks. Heap into the potato jackets and sprinkle with remaining cheese. Return to the oven to heat through.

Makes 12 servings (½ potato each).

TWICE-BAKED POTATOES, COTTAGE STYLE

Try these with Greek Lentil Soup and a salad.

4 medium potatoes
1 cup low-fat cottage cheese
½ cup skim milk or buttermilk
1 tablespoon minced onion
½ teaspoon Lite Salt or less
Dash pepper
Paprika
Chopped parsley

Preheat oven to 400°. Scrub potatoes. Make shallow slits around the middle as if you were cutting the potatoes in half lengthwise. Bake until done, 30–60 minutes, depending on size.

Cut hot potatoes in half lengthwise. Scoop out potatoes, leaving skins intact for stuffing. With wire whisk, beat potato with remaining ingredients, except paprika and parsley, until fluffy.

Pile mixture back into skins. Sprinkle with paprika and parsley. Bake 10 minutes more or until just golden.

Makes 8 servings (½ potato each).

Grain Dishes

BULGUR PILAF

1 teaspoon margarine
1 cup uncooked bulgur
1 teaspoon minced onion
1 cup chicken broth
1 cup water
¼ teaspoon oregano leaves
Few grains pepper

Melt margarine in skillet. Add bulgur and onion. Stir and cook until golden. Add broth, water and seasonings. Cover and bring to boil. Reduce heat and simmer for 15 minutes.

Makes 4 servings.

CURRIED RICE

1½ cups uncooked brown rice
3 cups water
1 clove garlic, minced
½ cup chopped onion
½ cup chopped green pepper
1 tablespoon oil
½ cup raisins
¼ teaspoon curry powder or more to taste
1 cup water

Cook rice in 3 cups water for 45 minutes. Sauté garlic, onions, and green peppers in oil. Add raisins, curry powder and water. Simmer 10 minutes. Combine with rice and cook together 15 minutes.

Makes 6 servings.

GOURMET PASTA PILAF

From a popular local restaurant we found a light and elegant side dish, well suited for Baked Snapper with Wine and Veggies or Fish Almondine with Dilly Sauce.

 1 cup uncooked acini *or* orzo (small, rice-shaped macaroni products)
 2 quarts boiling water
 1 tablespoon margarine
 1–2 cloves garlic, minced
 ½ cup sliced mushrooms
 3 green onions, chopped
 ¼ teaspoon white pepper

Add acini *or* orzo to boiling water and continue boiling, stirring occasionally for 5–8 minutes. (Do not overcook, as this is a two-part cooking process.) Drain well, removing all excess water.

In nonstick frying pan, melt margarine and sauté garlic. Add mushrooms and green onions; cook for 2 minutes. Add cooked acini or orzo and stir-fry until hot. Season with white pepper and serve.

Makes 4 servings.

MILLET VEGETABLE CASSEROLE

A basic grain recipe, other vegetables or herbs can be added to vary the flavor and texture.

 1 tablespoon oil
 1 cup uncooked millet
 1 large onion, chopped
 1 large carrot, sliced
 1 cup sliced mushrooms
 2 cups water
 2 cups chicken broth
 1 cup plain low-fat yogurt

Preheat oven to 350°. Brown millet in oil. Add onions, carrots, mushrooms, water and chicken broth. Bake in 2-quart casserole for 1 hour or until most of the liquid is absorbed. Stir once or twice to blend the vegetables and grain. Top with yogurt and serve.

Makes 9 servings.

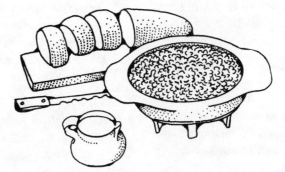

MUSHROOM BARLEY PILAF

A hearty casserole that is especially good when served with chicken or fish.

1 pound fresh mushrooms
1 cup chopped onion
1 tablespoon margarine
1½ cups uncooked pearl barley
1 jar (4 ounces) pimiento, chopped (optional)
2 cups chicken broth
¼ teaspoon pepper

Preheat oven to 350°. Wash, dry and slice mushrooms. Sauté onions and mushrooms in the margarine in a large skillet for 4 or 5 minutes. Transfer to a large casserole. Add barley and pimiento, if used, to the casserole dish. Stir in broth and pepper. Cover and bake for 50–60 minutes or until barley is tender and liquid is absorbed. Additional water may be needed during cooking if mixture seems dry.

This pilaf can also be cooked on stove top in a large kettle. Cook on low heat for 45 minutes.

Makes 8 servings.

SPANISH RICE

This rice dish is a natural with Mexican food. Try it with Acapulco Enchiladas and Chocolate Zucchini Cake for a feast.

1 cup uncooked, long-grain white rice
1 clove garlic, minced
1 tablespoon oil
1 medium onion, sliced
1 green pepper, chopped
1 can (16 ounces) unsalted tomatoes, drained (use liquid as part of the 2 cups of water)

2 cups water
¾ teaspoon chili powder
¼ teaspoon marjoram leaves
½ teaspoon Lite Salt or less

Brown the rice and garlic in the oil in a 10-inch skillet. Add all the other ingredients and bring to a boil. Reduce heat to low, cover and continue cooking for about 15 minutes or until rice has absorbed all the liquid. Remove from heat. Let stand covered 10 minutes before serving.

Makes 6 servings (1 cup each).

SPINACH AND RICE CASSEROLE

1 pound fresh spinach or 1 package (10 ounces) frozen chopped spinach
½ cup chopped onion
¼ cup sliced mushrooms
1 tablespoon oil
3 tablespoons whole wheat flour
2 cups low-fat cottage cheese
2 egg whites
¼ cup egg substitute (commercial or Homemade Egg Substitute, page 241)
3 cups cooked brown rice
¼ teaspoon pepper
½ teaspoon thyme leaves or more
½ teaspoon garlic powder
½ teaspoon Lite Salt or less
1 tablespoon sesame seeds
1 tablespoon grated Parmesan cheese

Preheat oven to 350°. Wash and tear up fresh spinach or defrost frozen spinach, if used.

Sauté onions and mushrooms in the oil. Combine with flour, cottage cheese, egg whites, egg substitute, uncooked spinach, cooked brown rice and seasonings. Pat into a shallow 9-by-12-inch baking dish and top with sesame seeds and Parmesan cheese. Bake for 40–50 minutes until bubbling hot.

Makes 8 servings.

Bean Dishes

CLASSIC BAKED BEANS

Dark, sweet and flavorful—these beans have the aroma of a country picnic. Let them bake for several hours.

> **1 pound uncooked navy beans**
> **3 tablespoons brown sugar**
> **¾ teaspoon Lite Salt or less**
> **1 teaspoon dry mustard**
> **⅓ cup dark molasses**
> **½ cup low-sodium ketchup**
> **2 onions, cut in quarters**

Wash the beans and soak overnight in enough water to cover them. Drain. Place in a saucepan and cover with water. Simmer, covered, 1–2 hours.

Mix with beans and remaining liquid the brown sugar, Lite Salt, mustard, molasses and ketchup. Preheat oven to 325°. Place onion quarters in the bottom of a 2-quart casserole. Pour in the beans. Add enough boiling water to cover beans. Cover casserole; place in oven, and bake for 5–6 hours, adding more water, if needed.

Makes 8 cups.

REFRIED BEANS

Make your own! Contains less salt than the canned ones. If this is below your salt threshold, add a little Lite Salt.

> **1½ cups uncooked pinto beans**
> **¼ cup chopped onion**
> **2 cloves garlic, minced**
> **1 tablespoon oil**
> **1 teaspoon ground cumin**

Soak beans overnight in water. The next day boil beans in 6 cups fresh water until tender (2–3 hours). Drain and save some liquid.

Sauté onions and garlic in oil until clear. Add a little water if vegetables stick. Mash half of the beans, and add to onion and garlic. Continue to sauté for 10 minutes, stirring frequently. Allow some of the mashed beans to brown. Add cumin. Add remaining beans and continue cooking until they are warmed through. Water or liquid from beans may be added to keep the beans soft and mushy.

Makes 4 cups.

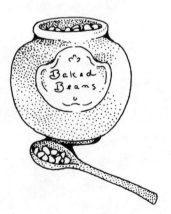

MAIN DISHES FEATURING VEGETABLES, GRAINS AND BEANS

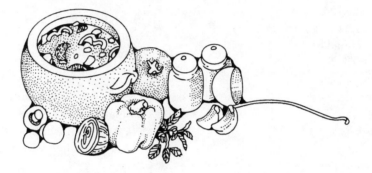

Whole grains and beans, staples for much of the world's population, add variety and nourishment to a low-fat diet as they are high in fiber, vitamins and minerals. In this country we have access to an exotic variety of grains and beans, but all too often we limit ourselves to a familiar one or two.

Each of the main dishes or entrées in this section contains grains, beans or vegetables as a major ingredient. Although some (labeled Easy or Quick) are not much trouble to prepare, others may take some time. In the latter case, try using canned beans instead of dry as a shortcut or cook a large batch of grains in advance—they'll keep in the refrigerator up to a week.

Since these entrées are meatless and very low-fat, portion sizes may appear larger than those you are accustomed to; they tend to be about 2 cups each. Keep in mind that as the fat content goes down, calories are removed, and serving sizes need to go up. Combining one serving of a grain or bean dish with a salad, vegetable side dish and/or bread will result in a meal that is about 500 Calories per person, with about 3 teaspoons of fat and virtually no cholesterol. Thus, the CSI will be low.

If meatless fare on occasional days is a style of eating unfamiliar to your family, serve lean meat as a main course and a grain or bean recipe as a *side dish* until you are comfortable using these dishes as meatless main courses. Also leftover meatless entrées make great lunches.

MENU IDEAS

Acapulco Bean Casserole
Bean Lasagna
Bean Stroganoff
Brazilian Black Beans and Rice
Broccoli Lasagna Rolls
Broccoli with Rice
Bryani
Cabbage Rolls
Calzones
Cauliflower Curry
Cheese-Stuffed Manicotti
Chile Relleno Casserole
Creamy Enchiladas
Curried Lentils
Garbanzo Goulash
Herbed Lentil Casserole
Kidney Bean Gumbo
Lentils over Rice
Macaroni Bake
Mexican Bean Pot
Moroccan Vegetable Stew
Moussaka
No-Meat Enchiladas
Pasta Primavera
Pinto Bean Chow Mein
Plymouth-Style Baked Beans
Rick's Chili
Romano Rice and Beans
Spanish Beans
Spicy Cheese Pizza
Spinach Lasagna
Summer Squash Delight
Sweet and Sour Vegetables with Tofu
Tostadas
Vegetable Creole
Vegetable Crepes
Zucchini Pie
Zucchini Spaghetti Dinner

Menu Ideas

As for menus—salad and bread served with any of the casseroles make a hearty meal. For those who'd like some tried-and-true combinations, here are some other menu ideas using recipes found in this book.

Bean Stroganoff
Fettuccine
Tossed salad with Red French Salad Dressing
Chocolate Zucchini cake

Acapulco Bean Casserole
Cucumber Cumin Salad
Dinner rolls
Baked Apples

Herbed Lentil Casserole
Tomatoes "Provençale"
Natural Bran Muffins
Vanilla Pudding with fruit

Cabbage Rolls
Mashed potatoes
Tossed salad with Thousand Island Salad
  Dressing
Pinto Fiesta Cake

No-Meat Enchiladas
Refried Beans
Fruit salad
Tortillas
Strawberry Ice

Rick's Chili
Corn on the cob
Confetti Appleslaw
Cocoa Cake

Plymouth-Style Baked Beans
Tossed salad
Broccoli spears
Grandma Kirschner's Date Nut Bread
Fresh fruit

ACAPULCO BEAN CASSEROLE—Easy

Tortillas and beans combined for a great dish! The use of canned products makes it very quickly prepared.

1 cup chopped onion
1 cup chopped celery
2 teaspoons margarine
2 cans (16 ounces each) chili with beans *
1 can (16 ounces) refried beans *
1 can (16 ounces) unsalted whole kernel corn, drained
½ cup taco sauce
8 corn tortillas, torn up
1 cup grated low-fat cheese
Fresh whole chile peppers (optional for garnish)

Preheat oven to 350°. In frying pan sauté onions and celery in margarine until tender but not brown, about 10 minutes. Stir in chili, refried beans, corn and taco sauce. Arrange half the tortilla pieces in a 10-inch-square baking dish; top with half the chili mixture. Repeat layer. Bake, covered, for 45–50 minutes. Sprinkle cheese atop. Bake, uncovered, 2–3 minutes more or until cheese is melted. Garnish with fresh whole chile peppers, if desired.

Makes 8 servings (1½ cups each).

* Use low-sodium beans if available.

BEAN LASAGNA

A great meatless dish! Make a double batch and freeze one for a later time.

2 medium onions, chopped
4 cloves garlic, minced
½–¾ pound mushrooms, sliced
2 teaspoons oil
2 teaspoons oregano leaves
1 teaspoon basil leaves
¼ cup chopped fresh parsley
½ teaspoon Lite Salt or less
1 can (16 ounces) kidney or pinto beans *
½ cup liquid from beans
1 can (16 ounces) unsalted tomatoes

8 ounces uncooked lasagna noodles

3 cups low-fat cottage cheese
4 ounces part-skim mozzarella cheese, grated
2 tablespoons freshly grated Parmesan cheese

Prepare the sauce: Sauté onions, garlic, and mushrooms in oil with oregano, basil, parsley and Lite Salt, stirring constantly. Drain beans and reserve the liquid. Add this liquid to the sautéed vegetables and herbs; simmer for 5–10 minutes. When onions look clear, stir in beans and tomatoes. Cover pan and simmer sauce for about ½ hour, until slightly thickened. Break up the tomatoes with a fork and stir sauce occasionally while simmering.

Cook lasagna noodles in large pot of boiling water until tender. Rinse in cold water to prevent sticking together. Drain well.

Preheat oven to 375°.

Assemble lasagna in a 9-by-13-inch baking dish using a third of each ingredient to layer in this order:

* Use low-sodium beans if available.

Noodles
Tomato-bean sauce
Cottage cheese
Mozzarella cheese
Repeat above twice more

Top with grated Parmesan cheese. Bake 20–30 minutes.

Makes 6 generous servings about 4 by 4 inches.

BEAN STROGANOFF—Quick

Yogurt has replaced the sour cream and this dish remains a favorite.

3 cups chopped mushrooms
2 medium onions, sliced
1 teaspoon oil
¼ cup flour
¾ cup beef or chicken bouillon
¼ cup sherry
4 teaspoons Worcestershire sauce
⅛ teaspoon marjoram leaves
⅛ teaspoon chili powder
⅛ teaspoon thyme leaves
Dash nutmeg
½ teaspoon garlic powder
3 cups cooked pinto beans *or* 2 cans (16 ounces each) beans *
1½ cups plain low-fat yogurt
1 teaspoon freshly squeezed lemon juice

Sauté mushrooms and onions in oil until tender in a large skillet. Mix flour, bouillon, sherry, Worcestershire sauce and spices; add to skillet and cook until thick. Stir in cooked drained beans and stir over low heat until heated through. Remove from heat and stir in yogurt and lemon juice. Serve over cooked bulgur, rice or eggless noodles.

Makes 6 servings.

* Use low-sodium beans if available.

BRAZILIAN BLACK BEANS AND RICE

One of our favorite bean recipes. The black beans, white rice and red sauce look beautiful on a serving platter. Salad, bread and any fruit for dessert would make this a real feast.

BEANS
1¼ cups uncooked black beans
4 cups water
1 clove garlic, minced
1 small onion, peeled and stuck with 3 whole cloves
½ teaspoon Lite Salt or less
1 tablespoon oil
1 cup chopped onion
1 green pepper, chopped

RICE
4 cups cooked rice (1½ cups uncooked)

SALSA
1 can (16 ounces) unsalted tomatoes, drained
¾ cup diced red or white onion
2 cloves garlic, chopped
1 tablespoon wine vinegar
1 teaspoon oil
3 dashes Tabasco sauce

To prepare salsa: In a small bowl, break up tomatoes with a spoon. Mix in remaining ingredients, cover and refrigerate to let flavors blend.

Soak beans overnight. The next day, bring beans to a boil and then reduce heat to moderate. Cook for 1 hour. Add garlic and clove-studded onion and Lite Salt and cook for 1 hour longer. *Or if using a pressure cooker,* cook beans, garlic and onion and Lite Salt (without prior soaking) for 15 minutes. Reduce pressure slowly. Beans should be tender but not mushy.

Sauté chopped onions and green peppers in oil briefly. Remove whole onion with cloves from beans and discard. Add the sautéed onions and green peppers to the beans. Stir and cook a few minutes to blend flavors.

Serve black beans over cooked rice and top with salsa.

Makes 4–6 servings (2 cups each).

BROCCOLI LASAGNA ROLLS

A lovely meatless dinner. Lasagna noodles are cooked and rolled around a spicy broccoli filling. Can be served with fruit salad, French bread, and Hot Fudge Pudding Cake.

SAUCE
    1 teaspoon olive oil
    ¼ cup chopped green pepper
    1 teaspoon finely chopped fresh parsley
    ½ teaspoon marjoram leaves
    ½ teaspoon thyme leaves
    1 teaspoon oregano leaves
    1 teaspoon basil leaves
    1 bay leaf
    2 cans (8 ounces each) unsalted tomato
      sauce
    ¼ cup water

    6 spinach or plain lasagna noodles

FILLING
    3 cups finely chopped cooked broccoli
    ¼ cup freshly grated Parmesan cheese
    ½ cup low-fat cottage cheese
    ½ cup part-skim ricotta cheese
    ½ teaspoon nutmeg
    1 teaspoon cayenne pepper (or to taste)

To make sauce: Heat olive oil in medium-sized

pan. Add green peppers, parsley, spices and bay leaf. Sauté over very low heat, being careful not to burn spices. Add tomato sauce and water. Simmer 2–3 hours. Remove bay leaf.

About ½ hour before sauce will be finished, cook lasagna noodles according to package directions in unsalted water. Set aside.

To make filling: Finely chop cooked broccoli and place in a medium-sized bowl. Add Parmesan cheese, cottage cheese, ricotta cheese and seasonings; mix well.

Preheat oven to 350°. Spread cooked noodles evenly with the filling. Carefully roll noodles up. Place in lightly oiled baking dish. Cover with sauce and bake for about 20 minutes.

Makes 6 servings.

BROCCOLI WITH RICE

A true favorite. Very popular for potluck dinners.

    2 onions, chopped
    2 stalks celery, chopped
    1 tablespoon margarine
    3 cups chopped fresh broccoli or 2
      packages (10 ounces each) chopped
      frozen broccoli
    2 cans (10¾ ounces each) cream of
      celery soup or use Homemade "Cream"
      Soup Mix, page 261
    ¼ cup freshly grated Parmesan cheese
    5 cups cooked brown rice
    4 drops Tabasco sauce
    1 can (8 ounces) sliced water chestnuts,
      drained
    4 tablespoons soft bread crumbs

Preheat oven to 350°. In large skillet, sauté the onions and celery in margarine until clear. Cook broccoli until barely tender and drain well. Mix broccoli with soup and cheese. Add to celery and onions. Stir in rice, Tabasco sauce and water chestnuts and mix well. Pour into a lightly oiled casserole dish and top with bread crumbs. Bake for about 20–30 minutes, until bubbly and heated through.

Makes 6 servings as a main dish, 12 servings as a side dish (about 12 cups total).

BRYANI

An Indian dish which is very filling—also spicy hot.

6 cups cooked rice
Juice of 1–2 lemons
¼ teaspoon saffron
6 cups fresh mixed vegetables: peas, broccoli, cauliflower, peppers, carrots, potatoes, green onions
1 tablespoon margarine
2 tablespoons mustard seed
¼ teaspoon ground cumin
½ teaspoon Lite Salt or less
⅛ teaspoon cayenne
¼ cup chopped almonds
¼ cup chopped unroasted, unsalted cashews
½ cup raisins
2 cups plain low-fat yogurt

Cook the rice and drain well. Prepare *saffron rice* by putting lemon juice in a bowl. Crumble in saffron, let it dissolve, then put in half of the cooked rice. Leave remaining half of rice plain.

Chop vegetables into medium-sized chunks. Melt the margarine and add spices. Add vegetables; stir until well coated. Cover and simmer until nearly tender; be careful to not overcook.

Preheat oven to 325°. Layer in an attractive 9-by-13-inch dish in the following order:

Plain cooked white rice
Cooked vegetables
Saffron rice
Nuts and raisins
Yogurt

Bake, covered, for 40 minutes.

When serving, carefully cut the portions, so that the colorful layers can be seen.

Makes 6 generous servings (about 4 by 4 inches).

CABBAGE ROLLS

These are very popular as a main dish, but can also be a delicious side dish with a fish entrée. They are easily made when cooked rice is on hand.

2 small heads cabbage

SAUCE
1 onion, chopped
3 cans (8 ounces each) unsalted tomato sauce
1 bay leaf
½ teaspoon ground ginger
¼ cup honey
¼ cup vinegar
¼ teaspoon thyme leaves
½ teaspoon Lite Salt or less
Pepper to taste

FILLING
1 large onion, chopped
8 ounces tofu, cubed
½ cup chopped fresh parsley
½ cup unsalted tomato paste
2 cups cooked brown rice
½ teaspoon Lite Salt or less
¼ teaspoon garlic powder

Steam cabbage 20 minutes. Cool, then carefully separate leaves from the head.

Prepare sauce: Steam onion until transparent; add remaining ingredients and gently simmer for about 30 minutes.

Preheat oven to 350°.

Prepare filling: Steam the chopped onion, add the tofu and stir to crumble. Add remaining ingredients and heat thoroughly. Place about 1 tablespoon on each cabbage leaf, roll up tightly and secure with a wooden pick.

Assemble dish: Place a small amount of sauce in shallow baking pan and add cabbage rolls. Pour remaining sauce over. Cover pan and bake for 45 minutes to 1 hour, until cabbage is soft.

Makes 16 cabbage rolls, about 4 servings.

CALZONES

Rounds of raised dough filled with a spinach-cheese mixture. Nice to serve warm with Marinara Sauce or excellent, when cold, for lunches.

DOUGH

> 2 teaspoons active dry yeast
> 1 tablespoon honey
> 1¼ cups warm water
> 2 cups whole wheat flour
> 2 cups white flour
> ½ teaspoon Lite Salt or less

FILLING

> 1 pound fresh spinach *or* 1 package (10 ounces) frozen chopped spinach, thawed
> ½ cup minced onion
> ½ cup low-fat cottage cheese
> ½ cup part-skim ricotta cheese
> 8 ounces tofu, cut into small pieces
> 2 cloves garlic, crushed

> 8 ounces part-skim mozzarella cheese, grated
> ¼ cup freshly grated Parmesan cheese
> Pepper to taste

For dough: Dissolve yeast and honey in water. Stir in flours and Lite Salt. Knead dough on floured board for 10–15 minutes. Cover and set in a warm place to rise until doubled in bulk (1 hour). After the dough has doubled, punch it down. Divide into 8 sections and roll out into rounds approximately ¼ inch thick.

For filling (it is easiest to prepare while the dough rises): Wash, stem and finely chop the spinach. (If using frozen spinach, omit this step.) Steam the spinach and onions together quickly. The spinach should be wilted and deep green in color. Combine the onions and spinach with the rest of the ingredients and mix well.

To complete: Preheat oven to 450°. Fill each dough round with about ½ cup filling, placing filling on ½ of circle and leaving a ½-inch rim. Moisten the rim with water, fold the empty side over and crimp the edge with a fork, taking care not to break the crust. Bake on a lightly oiled baking sheet for 15–20 minutes or until crisp and lightly browned.

Makes 6–8 servings.

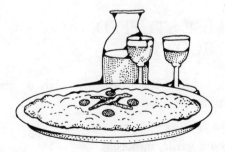

CAULIFLOWER CURRY—Easy

Curry cheese sauce over cauliflower.

1 head cauliflower
1 tablespoon oil
1 medium onion, chopped
4 cloves garlic, crushed
½ teaspoon Lite Salt or less
¼ cup flour
1½ cups water
½ cup skim milk
¼ teaspoon celery seed
½ teaspoon ground ginger
1 teaspoon curry powder
1 cup grated low-fat cheese

Wash and cut cauliflower into flowerets (about 5 cups needed). Steam until barely tender. Heat oil; add onions, garlic and Lite Salt. Cover and sauté until tender. Add flour and stir until blended. Add water and milk; cook and stir until thickened (a wire whisk helps). Add seasonings; mix well. Add cheese and drained cauliflower. Serve over rice or spinach noodles.

Can also be made with stronger curry flavor and served with yogurt.

Makes 4 servings.

CHEESE-STUFFED MANICOTTI

Simple to fix—the manicotti shells do not need to be precooked!

TOMATO SAUCE
1 clove garlic, minced
1 tablespoon olive oil
2 cans (8 ounces each) unsalted tomato sauce
2 cans (16 ounces each) unsalted tomatoes
1½ teaspoons oregano leaves
1 tablespoon chopped parsley

FILLING
2 cups low-fat cottage cheese
1 cup part-skim ricotta cheese
3 tablespoons freshly grated Parmesan cheese
2 egg whites
¼ cup chopped parsley
Dash pepper
8 ounces uncooked manicotti shells (15 pieces)
1 cup water

Preheat oven to 375°.
Prepare sauce: Sauté garlic in olive oil. Add tomato sauce and tomatoes slowly. Stir in oregano and parsley. Bring to boil and simmer covered for 20 minutes to 2 hours, stirring occasionally. Makes 5 cups.

Combine filling ingredients and stuff *uncooked* manicotti shells using small butter knife. Fill bottom of 9-by-13-inch casserole dish with 2 cups tomato sauce. Arrange stuffed manicotti shells in a single layer over sauce side by side. Cover shells with remaining 3 cups sauce and pour *1 cup water* over sauce.

Cover dish with foil and bake for 50 minutes. Remove foil and bake another 10 minutes.

Makes 5–6 servings.

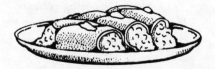

SPINACH VARIATION
To filling add 1 package (10 ounces) frozen chopped spinach (thawed and squeezed dry), 1 tablespoon freshly squeezed lemon juice and 2 cloves garlic, finely minced.

dish. Cover them with th
bean mixture. Mix tomato
chives *or* green onions. Po
for 30 minutes.

Makes 4 servings.

* Use low-sodium beans if available.

CHILE RELLENO CASSEROLE

A spicy, hearty casserole—serve with a crisp salad and Baked Corn Chips.

⅔ cup uncooked brown rice
2 cups Refried Beans, page 281, *or* 1 can (16 ounces) refried beans *
1 can (7 ounces) whole green chiles *or* 8 fresh chiles
4 ounces low-fat cheese
1 can (8 ounces) unsalted tomato sauce
1 teaspoon oregano leaves
¼ teaspoon Lite Salt or less
½ teaspoon garlic powder
2 tablespoons minced chives *or* green onions

Cook rice. Lightly oil a large, deep casserole dish. Mix beans and rice. Place half of this mixture on the bottom of the dish and set aside.

Prepare chile peppers. If you are using fresh chiles, blanch them or hold them over an open gas flame until the skin crackles and burns all around; peel the skins off. Slit the fresh or canned chiles lengthwise and remove all of the seeds and cut off the stem ends. Rinse under cold water if you prefer a less spicy casserole. Cut peppers crosswise into 1-inch-long sections.

Preheat oven to 350°. Cut the low-fat cheese into chunks that will fit into the chiles. Stuff the chile peppers with the cheese chunks and nestle them into the casserole

CREAMY ENCHILADAS

This is quick to assemble as it calls for canned enchilada and tomato sauces.

2 cups low-fat yogurt
2 cups low-fat cottage cheese
5–8 green onions, finely chopped
1 can (16 ounces) enchilada sauce
2 cans (8 ounces each) unsalted tomato sauce
12 corn tortillas
4 ounces low-fat cheese, grated

Preheat oven to 350°. Mix yogurt, cottage cheese and green onions (including tops). Set aside.

Mix enchilada sauce and tomato sauce in saucepan and heat. To make enchiladas, dip corn tortillas into warm sauce in pan to soften or warm for a few seconds in a microwave oven. Spoon generous amount of yogurt mixture into center. Roll up tortillas and place in baking dish. Pour remaining enchilada sauce over the top. Sprinkle with the grated cheese. Bake uncovered for 30 minutes.

Makes 4 servings.

CURRIED LENTILS—Easy

Very simple to prepare—the spicy curry and sweet apple make this dish special. The beauty of this dish is that you may add many other vegetables such as turnips, rutabagas, broccoli, etc.

1 large onion, chopped
1 carrot, chopped
2 stalks celery, chopped with the leaves
1 apple, chopped
2 cloves garlic, minced
Dash anise seed
½ teaspoon Lite Salt or less
1 cup uncooked lentils
1 teaspoon curry powder (more or less to taste)
3 cups water

Combine all ingredients and bring to a boil. Reduce heat and cook until done, about 60 minutes. Serve over generous portions of steamed rice.

Makes 4 main dish servings or 6 side dish servings (about 7 cups).

GARBANZO GOULASH —Quick

A quick macaroni dish. Nice to serve with Old-Style Wheat Biscuits.

1½ cups uncooked small shell macaroni
  or 2 cups uncooked large-sized macaroni
1 medium onion, chopped
2 teaspoons oil
1 can (16 ounces) garbanzo beans, drained *
1 can (16 ounces) unsalted tomatoes
2 tablespoons chopped fresh parsley
1 teaspoon ground cumin

Cook macaroni in unsalted boiling water according to package directions. In the meantime, sauté onions in oil until tender. Add drained beans and canned tomatoes with juice. Cut up canned tomatoes with spatula. Let simmer until macaroni is ready.

Drain macaroni. Add to bean-tomato mixture and mix. Add seasonings. For best flavor, let mixture simmer or boil for a few minutes until macaroni has been slightly colored by the tomato juice.

Makes 3 to 4 servings (about 8 cups).

* Use low-sodium beans if available.

HERBED LENTIL CASSEROLE —Easy

A surprisingly light casserole and very easy to prepare.

¾ cup uncooked lentils
2⅔ cups water
½ cup uncooked brown rice
1 onion, chopped
1¼ cups white wine
½ teaspoon basil leaves
½ teaspoon Lite Salt or less
¼ teaspoon oregano leaves
¼ teaspoon thyme leaves
¼ teaspoon garlic powder or to taste
3 tablespoons grated part-skim mozzarella cheese

Preheat oven to 350°. Combine all ingredients except cheese in an ungreased casserole (1½-quart size). Bake, uncovered, for 1½–2 hours. It should be moist but not runny.

Spread grated cheese over the top and bake for an additional 5 minutes.

Makes 4 servings (about 6 cups).

OPTION

Vegetables, such as tomatoes or green peppers, can be added for more color and variety, if desired.

KIDNEY BEAN GUMBO
—Easy

1½ cups frozen okra
1 cup chopped onion
2–3 cloves garlic, mashed
1 tablespoon oil
½ cup diced celery
1 green pepper, chopped
2 cans (16 ounces each) unsalted
  tomatoes
Pepper
Cayenne to taste
1 teaspoon thyme leaves
1 cup frozen peas
1 can (16 ounces) kidney beans,
  drained *

Cook okra in boiling water until tender. Set aside. Sauté onions and garlic in oil until onion is soft and golden. Add celery and green peppers and cook until tender. Add tomatoes and heat to boiling. Reduce heat. Add pepper, cayenne and thyme and simmer for 45 minutes. Add cooked okra, peas and beans. Cook for a few minutes longer until peas are done. Be sure not to overcook vegetables. Serve over rice.

Makes 6 servings (about 9 cups).

* Use low-sodium beans if available.

LENTILS OVER RICE

Lentils, herbs and tomato sauce served over brown rice make a tasty, easy winter dish. Chopped cooked turkey is a nice addition to this.

1 large onion, chopped
1 carrot, chopped
1 tablespoon olive oil
½ teaspoon thyme leaves
½ teaspoon marjoram leaves
2 cups chicken broth
1 cup water
1 cup uncooked lentils
2 cans (8 ounces each) unsalted tomato
  sauce
1 cup wine, red *or* white
¼ cup chopped parsley

Cooked brown rice (about 6 cups)

In a large pot, sauté onions and carrots in the olive oil for about 3 minutes. Add thyme and marjoram and sauté for 1 minute more. Add chicken broth, water, lentils, tomato sauce, wine and parsley and simmer for 1 hour. Serve over hot cooked brown rice.

Makes 4 servings as a main dish or 6 servings as a side dish.

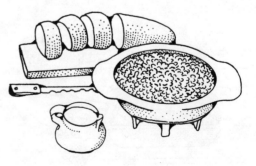

MACARONI BAKE

A light version of macaroni and cheese. It is very low in calories so serve with generous portions of vegetables, salad, and bread, or try it as a side dish with baked chicken.

2 cups uncooked elbow macaroni
1 onion, chopped
2 tablespoons margarine
¼ cup flour
2 cups skim milk
2 teaspoons dill weed
2 teaspoons parsley flakes
⅛ teaspoon garlic powder
½ teaspoon pepper
½ teaspoon Lite Salt or less
2 cups low-fat cottage cheese
⅓ cup bread crumbs
Paprika

Preheat oven to 350°. Cook and drain elbow macaroni. Sauté onions in margarine until tender. Stir in flour. Cook 1 minute, stirring constantly. Blend in milk. Cook and stir over medium heat until thick. Add spices, cottage cheese and cooked macaroni to the sauce. Pour into shallow, 2-quart baking dish. Top with crumbs and paprika. Bake for 45 minutes or until bubbly.

Makes 4 servings (2 cups each).

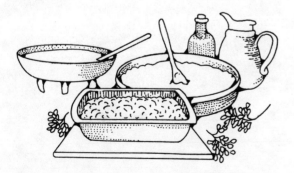

MEXICAN BEAN POT

Spicy baked beans! Serve with Zucchini Mexicali and Hearty Corn Bread.

1½ cups chopped onion
2 large green peppers, chopped
1 tablespoon oil
1 can (16 ounces) kidney beans *
2 cans (16 ounces each) pinto beans *
1 can (16 ounces) unsalted tomatoes
1 teaspoon oregano leaves
½ teaspoon ground cumin
1 teaspoon sage
¾ teaspoon pepper

Preheat oven to 325°. Sauté onions and green peppers in oil. Drain beans, reserving liquid. Combine beans, onions, green peppers, tomatoes, oregano, cumin, sage and pepper in a 3-quart casserole. Add enough reserved liquid to just cover beans (about ½ cup). Bake for 1 hour.

Makes 6 servings (about 10 cups).

* Use low-sodium beans if available.

MOROCCAN VEGETABLE STEW—Easy

1 medium onion, chopped
2 tablespoons water
1 tablespoon oil
2 cups chopped potatoes, in 1-inch-square pieces
2 cups carrots, chopped into large chunks
1 can (16 ounces) unsalted tomatoes *or*
    2 cups fresh tomatoes
¾ teaspoon ground cumin
½–1 cup unsalted tomato juice

2 cups fresh green beans, sliced into
  2-inch pieces
¼ teaspoon black pepper or cayenne, to
  taste

Simmer onions in oil and water until transparent. Add potatoes and carrots and simmer for 15 minutes, stirring occasionally. Add chopped tomatoes and cumin. Cover and simmer for about 1 hour, checking to see if the stew needs more liquid. If so, add tomato juice. Add green beans and cook for 15 minutes more. Check seasoning—add ¼ teaspoon or more black pepper and more cumin, if desired.

Makes 4 servings (about 8 cups).

MOUSSAKA

A Greek casserole with eggplant, tomatoes and a cheese filling. Serve with Layered Vegetable Platter, pita bread and Angel Quickie for dessert.

TOMATO SAUCE
3 onions, chopped
1 clove garlic, crushed
4 medium tomatoes, peeled, coarsely
  chopped (reserve juice)
¼ teaspoon rosemary leaves, crumbled
2 tablespoons minced fresh mint or
  1 tablespoon mint flakes
2 tablespoons chopped parsley
2 teaspoons sugar
¼ teaspoon pepper
1 can (8 ounces) unsalted tomato sauce

CHEESE FILLING
2 cups low-fat cottage cheese
2 egg whites
⅛ teaspoon rosemary leaves, crumbled
⅛ teaspoon mace
⅛ teaspoon pepper

2 large eggplants, sliced ½ inch thick but
  not peeled
1 tablespoon oil
½ cup freshly grated Parmesan cheese

To make tomato sauce: Mix all sauce ingredients in a heavy pan and heat uncovered, stirring occasionally, until tomatoes begin to release juice. Cover, lower heat and simmer 1 hour, stirring occasionally. Remove cover and simmer 15 minutes longer.

To make cheese filling: Mix together all ingredients and refrigerate.

Brush both sides of each eggplant lightly with oil and quickly broil on each side to brown.

To assemble Moussaka: Preheat oven to 375°. Spoon half the tomato sauce over the bottom of a 9-by-13-inch baking pan. Sprinkle with Parmesan cheese and arrange half the browned eggplant on top. Spread with all the cheese filling. Arrange remaining eggplant on top. Finally, cover with remaining tomato sauce and Parmesan cheese.

Bake uncovered for 45–50 minutes until bubbling and brown. Remove from oven and let stand 15 minutes before cutting into squares.

Makes 6 servings (about 4 by 4 inches).

NO-MEAT ENCHILADAS

Bean-filled corn tortillas.

SAUCE (VERY QUICKLY PREPARED)
 1 tablespoon oil
 1 tablespoon chili powder
 1½ tablespoons flour
 1½ cups water
 1 teaspoon vinegar
 ½ teaspoon garlic powder
 ½ teaspoon onion powder
 ½ teaspoon Lite Salt or less
 ¼ teaspoon oregano leaves

FILLING
 ½ cup low-fat cottage cheese
 ¾ cup Refried Beans, page 281, *or* ¾ cup
  canned refried beans *
 1 cup grated low-fat cheese, divided
 1 medium onion, finely chopped

 8 corn tortillas
 1 cup Mock Sour Cream, page 224
 4 tablespoons chopped green onions

To make sauce: Heat oil, chili powder and flour in a small saucepan to make a paste. Add water gradually to make a smooth sauce; add vinegar, garlic powder, onion powder, Lite Salt and oregano. Bring to a boil. Lower heat; simmer uncovered for about 3 minutes.
To assemble dish: Preheat oven to 350°. Reserve a third of the grated cheese for topping. Mix refried beans, remaining cheese, cottage cheese and onions in a bowl. Warm tortillas in the oven or microwave or dip in warm sauce. Place ¼ cup of the bean filling down center of each tortilla. Roll up; place seam side down in shallow baking dish. Pour sauce over filled enchiladas and sprinkle with reserved cheese. Bake for 20 minutes or until bubbly.

Top with Mock Sour Cream and chopped green onions before serving.
 Makes 4 servings (2 enchiladas each).

* Use low-sodium beans if available.

✓ PASTA PRIMAVERA

"Spring pasta" refers to the combination of pasta with lightly cooked fresh vegetables. Let your imagination be the guide to experimenting with other vegetables.

 12 ounces uncooked spaghetti
 1 tablespoon oil
 1½ cups sliced mushrooms
 1 medium onion, cut into very thin
  wedges
 2 cloves garlic, minced
 2 cups broccoli (cut into flowerets)
 2 cups sliced and halved zucchini
 1 cup carrots (cut into thin strips)
 ⅓ cup dry white wine
 ¼ cup chopped parsley
 2 teaspoons basil leaves
 ¼ teaspoon Lite Salt or less
 ⅛ teaspoon pepper
 ½ cup grated Parmesan cheese

Cook spaghetti in boiling water for 10–12 minutes until done. Drain well in colander.

In large skillet or wok heat oil over medium-high heat. Add mushrooms, onions and garlic, stirring frequently. Cook 1–2 minutes. Add broccoli, zucchini and carrots; continue stirring and cook 2–3 minutes more. Add wine, parsley, basil, Lite Salt and pepper. Simmer 4–5 minutes or until vegetables are tender-crisp.

Toss together hot cooked spaghetti, vegetable mixture and cheese. Serve immediately.
 Makes 5 servings (about 12 cups).

PINTO BEAN CHOW MEIN —Quick

An Oriental stir fry with beans. Fruit salad goes well with this.

    3 tablespoons cornstarch
    ¼ cup cold water
    ¼ cup lower-sodium soy sauce
    ½ bouillon cube
    1¼ cups boiling water
    3 cups diagonally sliced celery
    1 cup sliced onions
    ¾ cup sliced mushrooms
    1 tablespoon oil
    1 can (16 ounces) pinto beans, drained *
    1 can (16 ounces) bean sprouts, drained
    1 can (8 ounces) sliced water chestnuts, drained
    1 can (6 ounces) bamboo shoots (optional)

Blend cornstarch in ¼ cup cold water and soy sauce; dissolve ½ bouillon cube in 1¼ cups boiling water. Set aside. Stir-fry celery, onions and mushrooms in oil until crisp-tender. Add cornstarch mixture and bouillon to vegetables.

Add pinto beans, bean sprouts, water chestnuts and bamboo shoots. Cook and stir until thickened. Serve over rice.

Makes 6 servings (about 10 cups).

* Use low-sodium beans if available.

PLYMOUTH-STYLE BAKED BEANS—Easy

Canned beans * can be used, if desired.

    1 onion, chopped
    1 tablespoon oil

    2 apples, grated
    ½ teaspoon Lite Salt or less
    2 teaspoons dry mustard
    1 can (8 ounces) unsalted tomato sauce
    1 cup water
    2 tablespoons molasses
    8 cups cooked beans, drained (Great Northern, navy or small red beans work well)

Preheat oven to 350°. Sauté onions in oil for 3 minutes. Add grated apple and cook over low heat, keeping tightly covered, for 5 minutes. Mix with remaining ingredients. Bake covered for 45 minutes.

Makes 6 servings (about 12 cups).

* Use low-sodium beans if available.

RICK'S CHILI

A meatless version which is simple and delicious. Onion Squares are great with it.

    2 cloves garlic, minced
    1 medium onion, chopped
    2–3 stalks celery, chopped
    ½ pound mushrooms, sliced
    1½ green peppers, chopped
    1 tablespoon oil
    1 tablespoon water
    2 cans (16 ounces each) unsalted tomatoes, cut up
    2 cans (16 ounces each) kidney beans, drained *
    1–3 tablespoons chili powder, or to taste

Lightly sauté fresh vegetables in oil and water until onions are tender. Add tomatoes, beans and chili powder. Cook covered for 1 hour or longer on low heat.

Makes 6 servings (about 10 cups).

* Use low-sodium beans if available.

ROMANO RICE AND BEANS —Quick and Easy

A colorful way to prepare leftover rice and beans—simply toss the ingredients together in a skillet.

2 cloves garlic, minced
1 large onion, chopped
2–3 carrots, chopped
1 green pepper *or* 1 large stalk celery, chopped
1 tablespoon olive oil
2/3 cup chopped fresh parsley
2–3 teaspoons basil leaves
1 teaspoon oregano leaves
3 large tomatoes, chopped coarsely
Pepper to taste
1/2 teaspoon Lite Salt or less
2 cups cooked kidney beans *or use canned* *
5 cups cooked brown rice
1/2 cup grated Parmesan cheese

Sauté garlic, onions, carrots, green peppers or celery in oil until tender. Add parsley, basil and oregano. Combine with tomatoes, pepper, Lite Salt and drained beans. A large cast-iron skillet works well for this. Add cooked rice and Parmesan cheese; toss all together and heat through. Garnish with additional fresh parsley.

Makes 6 servings (about 12 cups).

* Use low-sodium beans if available.

SPANISH BEANS—Quick and Easy

A hearty versatile casserole, very easy to make. Serve with Corn Bread and Zucchini Mexicali.

1 onion, chopped
1 green pepper, chopped
1 tablespoon margarine
1 cup canned unsalted tomatoes, chopped
1 teaspoon Worcestershire sauce
1/4 teaspoon pepper
1/8 teaspoon cayenne pepper
1 can (16 ounces) butter beans or pinto beans,* drained
1 can (16 ounces) kidney beans,* drained
3/4 cup grated mozzarella cheese

Preheat oven to 350°. Sauté onions and green peppers slowly in margarine until onions are transparent. Add tomatoes, simmer 10 minutes. Stir in seasonings and well-drained beans. Alternate layers of bean mixture and cheese in a 1-quart casserole. Bake for 30 minutes.

Makes 6 servings (about 7 cups).

* Use low-sodium beans if available.

SPICY CHEESE PIZZA

Choose a thick or thin crust (see Pizza Crusts, page 238) and add the following toppings:

1 can (6 ounces) unsalted tomato paste
2 cans (8 ounces each) unsalted tomato sauce
2 teaspoons ground anise seed
1/4 teaspoon pepper

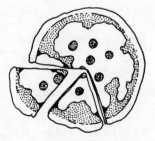

¼ teaspoon garlic powder
1 teaspoon oregano leaves
1 teaspoon Italian seasonings
1 teaspoon chopped parsley
½ cup fresh mushrooms, sliced, *or* 1 can
  (4 ounces) sliced mushrooms, drained
1 green pepper, chopped
1 medium onion, chopped
6 ounces part-skim or imitation
  mozzarella cheese, grated

Preheat oven to 425°. Combine tomato paste, tomato sauce and seasonings. Spread sauce over the dough. Sprinkle pizza with the remaining ingredients. Bake 25–30 minutes.

Makes enough for 1 pizza.

SPINACH LASAGNA

This is a low-fat version of an old favorite. Other vegetables such as zucchini or eggplant may be added for extra appeal.

SAUCE
1 large onion, chopped
3 cloves garlic, minced
1 tablespoon oil
2 cans (16 ounces each) unsalted
  tomatoes, chopped
1 can (6 ounces) unsalted tomato paste
Pinch of basil, oregano, rosemary leaves

NOODLES AND VEGETABLE
12 ounces lasagna noodles
1 pound fresh spinach, lightly steamed
  and chopped, *or* 1 package (10 ounces)
  frozen chopped spinach, thawed

FILLING
½ cup chopped tofu
½ cup part-skim ricotta cheese
2 tablespoons grated Parmesan cheese
½ cup low-fat cottage cheese
½ cup sliced mushrooms (optional)

TOPPING
6 ounces part-skim mozzarella cheese

Make sauce: Sauté onions and garlic in oil. Add tomatoes, tomato paste and herbs. Simmer for ½ hour or longer.

Prepare noodles and vegetables: Cook noodles according to package directions in unsalted water until tender. Drain. Steam spinach and drain, if using fresh, or thaw and drain, if using frozen.

Prepare filling: Mix tofu, ricotta, Parmesan cheese, cottage cheese and mushrooms. Blend well so tofu is thoroughly mixed in.

Complete casserole: Preheat oven to 350°. Assemble ingredients in a 9-by-13-inch baking dish in the following order:

  Small amount of tomato sauce
  Cooked noodles
  ⅓ of cheese/tofu mixture
  ⅓ of drained spinach
  Tomato sauce
  Repeat as above ending with noodles and
    tomato sauce

Place thinly sliced mozzarella cheese on top of casserole and bake for about 40 minutes until bubbly. Let stand about 15 minutes before serving.

Makes 6 generous servings about 4 by 4 inches.

SUMMER SQUASH DELIGHT

You might use zucchini, yellow crooked neck, or pale-green scalloped summer squash or mix all three types for this beautiful casserole.

1½ cups uncooked brown rice
1 teaspoon paprika
5 cups summer squash, sliced into bite-sized pieces
2 cups plain low-fat yogurt
1 teaspoon oil
⅓ cup grated low-fat cheese
¼ teaspoon Lite Salt or less
2 egg whites
¼ cup chopped fresh chives *or* green onions
2 tablespoons sesame seeds
⅓ cup bread crumbs

Cook the rice in 3 cups water with paprika. Prepare the squash and set it aside. Stir the yogurt, oil, grated cheese and Lite Salt together in a small saucepan; heat at a low temperature until the cheese melts. Remove from heat and stir in the egg whites and chives *or* green onions. Preheat oven to 350°.

To assemble the dish: Stir the cooked rice and sesame seeds together and spread on the bottom of a 7-by-11-inch shallow baking dish. Arrange the squash pieces over the rice, pour the yogurt sauce over, and top with a layer of bread crumbs. Bake the casserole about 30 minutes until the crumbs are browned and the squash is tender but still firm.

Makes 4–6 servings (about 10 cups).

SWEET AND SOUR VEGETABLES WITH TOFU

A well-liked Cantonese recipe. Serve over generous portions of brown rice. This is a good way to introduce someone to tofu.

2 tablespoons cornstarch
½ cup vinegar
½ cup brown sugar
2 tablespoons lower-sodium soy sauce
¼–½ teaspoon ground ginger
1 can (16 ounces) crushed pineapple, with juice

1 tablespoon oil
1–2 cloves garlic, crushed
1 onion, diced
1 large green pepper, sliced
6 large mushrooms, sliced
1 can (8 ounces) sliced water chestnuts, drained
1 package frozen pea pods, thawed, *or* 1 cup fresh pea pods
12 ounces firm tofu, cubed
2 fresh tomatoes, quartered

Prepare sauce by making a paste of cornstarch and vinegar. Cook over medium heat, adding brown sugar, soy sauce, ginger and pineapple. Simmer until thick and set aside.

Heat oil and garlic in fry pan or wok. Stir-fry vegetables except tomatoes until done. Gently stir in cubed tofu and sauce. Add the quartered tomatoes. Heat until warmed through.

Makes 6 servings (about 10 cups).

TOSTADAS—Quick

A low-fat convenience food that the whole family will love.

12 corn tortillas
1 teaspoon margarine
2 cups Refried Beans, page 281, *or* 1 can (16 ounces) refried beans *
1 can tomatoes and green chiles *or* 1 can (10 ounces) taco sauce
¾ cup grated low-fat cheese
Chopped lettuce
Chopped tomatoes
Optional: chopped cucumbers, grated carrots, avocado, Mock Sour Cream, page 224

Preheat oven to 350°. Scrape margarine lightly on tortillas. Place on baking sheets to bake for 10–15 minutes. When crisp, spread with refried beans. Spoon 2 tablespoons or more tomato-chili sauce on top. Put back in oven until hot, 5–10 minutes. To serve, top with grated cheese, lettuce and tomatoes. Add other vegetables as desired.
  Makes 6 servings.

* Use low-sodium beans if available.

VEGETABLE CREOLE

An unusual vegetable stew, served over rice. If canned beans are used it is very quickly prepared.

½ cup diced celery
⅓ cup sliced onions
1 tablespoon oil
1 can (16 ounces) unsalted tomatoes
1 teaspoon basil leaves
½ teaspoon rosemary leaves
1 teaspoon celery seed
Pepper to taste
1 package (10 ounces) frozen peas

½ cup cooked kidney beans (canned * and drained work fine)
Cooked brown rice (about 6 cups)

Sauté celery and onions in small amount of water and the oil until tender. Add tomatoes, basil, rosemary, celery seed and pepper. Cook slowly 20 minutes, stirring occasionally. Add peas and cooked or canned kidney beans. Cover; cook 5 minutes longer until thoroughly heated. Serve over hot cooked brown rice.
  Makes 4 servings (about 4 cups).

* Use low-sodium beans if available.

VEGETABLE CREPES

To complete the meal serve with brown rice, peas, rolls and fruit cup.

1 tablespoon oil
¼ cup chopped onion
1 clove garlic, minced
6–8 mushrooms, sliced
¼ cup diced green pepper
2 cups cubed zucchini
¼ cup chopped parsley
2 fresh tomatoes, chopped
¼ teaspoon Lite Salt or less
⅛ teaspoon basil leaves
1 can (8 ounces) unsalted tomato sauce

Prepare Crepes, page 368.
  Preheat oven to 350°. Heat oil in nonstick saucepan. Sauté onions, garlic, mushrooms and green peppers until slightly cooked. Add zucchini, parsley, tomatoes and herbs. Cook until tender, about 5 minutes. Drain off excess liquid. Fill crepes, then roll. Place in baking dish and cover with tomato sauce. Bake 10 minutes.
  Makes filling for 12–15 crepes (about 3¾ cups).

ZUCCHINI PIE

Our version of a vegetable quiche.

CRUST
   1 tablespoon active dry yeast
   ½ cup warm water
   ½ cup whole wheat flour
   ¾ cup white flour
   ½ teaspoon Lite Salt

FILLING
   4 cups zucchini, unpeeled, thinly sliced
   1 cup coarsely chopped onion
   1 tablespoon margarine
   2 tablespoons chopped parsley
   ½ teaspoon Lite Salt or less
   ½ teaspoon pepper
   ¼ teaspoon garlic powder
   ¼ teaspoon basil leaves
   ¼ teaspoon oregano leaves
   3 egg whites
   2 cups grated, part-skim mozzarella
      cheese
   2 teaspoons Dijon-style or prepared
      mustard

Dissolve yeast in water. Stir in flours and Lite Salt. Knead dough on floured board for 5 minutes or until smooth and elastic. Let rise for 45 minutes.

Preheat oven to 375°. In large skillet, cook zucchini and onions in margarine until tender, about 10 minutes. Stir in parsley and seasonings. In large bowl, blend egg whites and cheese. Stir into vegetable mixture.

Transfer raised dough to an ungreased 11-inch quiche pan, 10-inch pie pan or 9-by-13-inch baking dish. Press over bottom and up sides to form crust. Spread crust with mustard. Pour vegetable mixture evenly over crust.

Bake for 25–35 minutes or until knife inserted near center comes out clean. If crust becomes too brown, cover with foil during last 10 minutes of baking. Let stand 10 minutes before serving.
Makes 4 servings.

ZUCCHINI SPAGHETTI DINNER—Quick

This is quite low in calories so add rolls or bread to make a filling meal. A baked dessert or cookie is appropriate, also.

   4 cups cooked spaghetti (amount raw
      equal to 1½-inch diameter bunch)
   2 medium zucchini, sliced (about 7 cups)
   1 medium onion, chopped
   1 clove garlic, crushed
   1 teaspoon oregano leaves (optional)
   1¼ teaspoons Lite Salt or less
   ¼ teaspoon pepper
   2 tablespoons chopped chives (optional)
   2 teaspoons oil
   2½ cups no salt added spaghetti sauce

While spaghetti is cooking, sauté zucchini, onions, garlic and other spices in oil until tender. Add sauce. Heat and serve over cooked spaghetti.
Makes 4 servings (about 8 cups).

FISH AND SHELLFISH

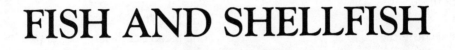

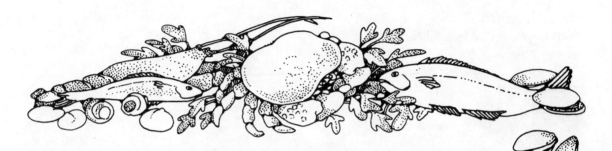

Fish is hard to beat! Extremely low in fat, it's also quick to prepare. Our recipes are low in both fat and calories so that it is important to serve generous portions of filling side dishes and, of course, lots of bread. In addition, when you serve fish dinners, baked desserts like fruit cobbler or cake are appropriate.

SOUPS AND STEWS

Bouillabaisse
Cioppino
Hearty Fish Soup
Pacific Stew Pot

ELEGANT DISHES

Fillet of Fish Florentine
Fillet of Sole Oregon
Salmon and Red Pepper Pasta
Salmon Mousse
Scallops in Creamy Sauce
Sesame Halibut

Shrimp and Asparagus Crepes
Tandoori Fish

BAKED FILLET QUICKIES

Baked Herbed Fish
Cod Curry
Creole Salmon
Fish Hampton
Savory Fish Fillets

FISH WITH SAUCES

Baked Snapper with Spicy Tomato Sauce
Baked Snapper with Wine and Veggies
Fish Almondine with Dilly Sauce
Fish à L'Orange
Medallion of Cod

FISH ROLL-UPS

Fish Fillets with Walnuts
Lively Lemon Roll-Ups
Stuffed Sole

POTPOURRI

Clam Pilaf
Clam Sauce for Pasta
Creole Shrimp
Fish à la Mistral
Portuguese Casserole
Salmon Loaf
Skinny Sole
Tangy Snapper
Vegetable-Topped Fish Fillets

TUNA DISHES

Alphabet Seafood Salad
Bean Sprout Tuna Chow Mein
Sweet 'n' Sour Supper
Tuna Noodle Casserole
Tuna Salad Sandwich Spread (see "Soups and
   Sandwiches" section)

Soups and Stews

BOUILLABAISSE

Serve with French bread to dip in soup so all the sauce can be enjoyed! Great party dish.

2 large onions, thinly sliced
2 leeks, minced
1 tablespoon oil
4 cloves garlic, mashed
3 large tomatoes, peeled, seeded and diced
5 cups water
3 cups clam juice (2 cans, 12 ounces
   each)
2 tablespoons chopped parsley
1 bay leaf
⅛ teaspoon fennel seeds
½ teaspoon thyme *or* basil leaves
⅛ teaspoon saffron
2-inch-piece orange peel
½ teaspoon Lite Salt or less
½ teaspoon pepper
2 pounds lean fish bones, trimmings, etc.
   for stock

2 pounds assorted lean fish and shellfish
   (more than one kind—bass, snapper,
   halibut, turbot, cod, scallops, etc.) cut
   in large pieces

To prepare stock: In a large kettle cook onions and leeks slowly in oil until tender but not browned. Stir in the garlic and tomatoes. Cook 5 minutes. Add water, clam juice, herbs and seasonings. Tie fish bones and trimmings together in a large piece of cheesecloth. Add this bundle to vegetables. Simmer covered for 30 minutes. Discard fish bones and trimmings, strain the stock or puree it through a food mill. Stock can be refrigerated or frozen at this point.

Twenty minutes before serving: Bring the fish stock to a boil. Add fresh fish and shellfish. Bring rapidly back to boiling and cook 5 minutes or until fish flakes easily with a fork. Do not overcook.

   Makes 8 servings (1½ cups each).

CIOPPINO

A fine kettle of fish—serve with lots of crusty bread, salad and a hearty fruit cobbler for dessert.

1 pound red snapper *or* halibut *or* use ½ pound snapper *or* halibut and ½ pound scallops *or* prawns
1 tablespoon oil
1 cup chopped onion
2 cloves garlic, finely minced
1 can (8 ounces) unsalted tomato sauce
2 cans (16 ounces each) unsalted tomatoes
½ cup water *or* dry white wine
1 teaspoon basil leaves
1 teaspoon thyme leaves
1 teaspoon marjoram leaves
1 teaspoon oregano leaves
1 bay leaf
¼ teaspoon pepper
¼ cup chopped parsley *or* 1 tablespoon dried parsley flakes
1 dozen steamer clams (optional)
1 cup shrimp meat

Cut fish into ½-inch chunks and set aside. Heat oil in large kettle and sauté onions and garlic until onions are tender but not brown. Add tomato sauce, tomatoes, liquid and all seasonings. Let simmer 20–30 minutes until as thick as desired, stirring occasionally. Soup base can be refrigerated at this point to serve at later time.

When ready to serve, reheat soup base and add fish chunks and scrubbed steamer clams (in shell). Cook until clams open, about 10 minutes. Just before serving, add shrimp meat. Serve warm in large soup bowls.

Makes 4 servings (2¼ cups each).

HEARTY FISH SOUP—Easy

A very quick meal—especially if you have the soup base prepared ahead of time.

1 large onion, chopped
1 stalk celery with leaves, chopped
1 clove garlic, minced
1 tablespoon oil
2 cans (16 ounces each) unsalted tomatoes, chopped
½ cup white wine
2 tablespoons chopped parsley
½ teaspoon Lite Salt or less
¼ teaspoon thyme leaves
Few grinds of pepper
1 pound red snapper, cut into bite-size pieces

In a large saucepan, sauté onions, celery and garlic in oil until tender. Stir in tomatoes, wine, parsley, Lite Salt, thyme and pepper. Cover and simmer gently about 30 minutes. (Can refrigerate or freeze at this point.)

To finish soup, bring tomato base to a boil. Add fish and lower heat. Simmer gently for 7–10 minutes or until fish is opaque. Do not overcook.

Makes 4 servings (1¾ cups each).

PACIFIC STEW POT

A little messy to eat because the shells are still on the shrimp, but makes for a fun, casual meal. The stew is very low in fat so this is a good time to serve a baked dessert (Apple Crisp, Rhubarb Buckle).

- 1 cup chopped onion
- 1 cup chopped celery
- 1 quart water
- 3 cans (16 ounces each) unsalted tomatoes
- ¼ cup low-sodium ketchup
- ⅛ teaspoon Tabasco sauce
- ½ teaspoon Lite Salt or less
- ¼ teaspoon curry powder
- 1 tablespoon Worcestershire sauce
- ¾ pound snapper *or* cod
- ¾ pound raw shrimp, with shell
- ¾ pound scallops
- ¼ cup sherry (optional)
- ½ lemon, thinly sliced, for garnish

Simmer onions and celery in 2 cups of water for 5 minutes. Add remaining water, tomatoes, ketchup and spices. Cook slowly for 30 minutes. Cut snapper into bite-size pieces and add with shrimp and scallops. Add sherry, if desired, and cook 10 minutes or until fish flakes easily with a fork. Garnish with lemon slices.

Makes 8 servings (2 cups each).

Elegant Dishes

FILLET OF FISH FLORENTINE

Don't be afraid to poach fish—it's quite easy.

SPINACH SAUCE
- 1 package (10 ounces) frozen chopped spinach
- 2 tablespoons margarine
- 1 tablespoon finely chopped onion
- 2 tablespoons flour
- 1 cup skim milk
- ½ teaspoon Lite Salt or less
- ½ teaspoon pepper
- ¼ teaspoon oregano leaves
- ¼ teaspoon thyme leaves

- ½ cup bread crumbs

Cook spinach according to package directions and drain well. Melt margarine in a skillet. Add onion and cook until golden. Stir in flour until blended. Add milk slowly and stir until sauce is smooth and thickened slightly. Add drained, cooked spinach. Season with Lite Salt, pepper, oregano and thyme.

POACHED FISH
- 2 pounds red snapper *or* other white fish
- 4 peppercorns
- ½ bay leaf
- 2 teaspoons freshly squeezed lemon juice

Cut fish fillets into 6 servings and place in large pan. Cover with boiling water. Season with peppercorns, bay leaf and lemon juice. Simmer about 10 minutes or until fish flakes easily with a fork. Remove fish with slotted spoon and place on ovenproof platter.

Assemble dish: Pour creamed spinach over poached fish on serving platter. Sprinkle bread crumbs on top. Place under broiler to heat through until sauce is glazed. Serve immediately.

Makes 6 servings.

FILLET OF SOLE OREGON

Well suited for a guest menu, sole fillets are stuffed with salmon and poached in the oven, then topped with a shrimp sauce. Serve them warm with small red potatoes.

½ pound salmon, boned and skinned
1 tablespoon skim milk
Dash pepper

12 small sole fillets, about 2 ounces each
1 cup frozen peas
1 teaspoon thinly sliced green onion
1 cup dry white wine
1 cup hot water
1½ tablespoons margarine
1½ tablespoons flour
1 tablespoon freshly squeezed lemon juice
¼ cup shrimp meat
2 tablespoons chopped green onion for garnish

Preheat oven to 350°. Make a stuffing with the salmon by chopping it fine or grinding it. Mix in the milk and pepper. Spread about 1½ tablespoons of the mixture over each of the sole fillets, covering only about ¾ of each fillet. Sprinkle 1 teaspoon peas over the top of each fillet and gently roll each one toward the end which does not have filling on it. Secure each roll with a wooden pick and place them side by side in a baking dish. Top with chopped green onions. Add the wine and hot water and cover with foil; place in oven and poach for 20–30 minutes, or until the fish flakes easily with a fork. Remove fish rolls from the baking dish, reserving the liquid. Arrange rolls on a serving platter and keep warm.

Pour the liquid from the baking dish into a saucepan and boil to reduce it by ½. Add margarine and flour and stir with wire whisk until thickened. (If there are lumps, pour through wire strainer.) Add lemon juice, shrimp and remaining peas. Ladle the sauce over each fish roll. Garnish with chopped green onion. The serving platter looks especially attractive when the cooked red potatoes are served alongside the fish rolls.

Makes 6 servings (2 stuffed fillets each).

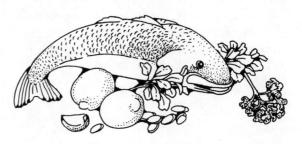

SALMON AND RED PEPPER PASTA—Quick

A gorgeous stir-fry dish to serve over fresh pasta!

½ pound salmon, skinned and boned
3 shallots, diced
2 tablespoons chopped parsley
1 tablespoon olive oil, divided
3 tablespoons freshly squeezed lemon juice, divided
3 sweet red peppers, sliced into thin strips
¼ cup fresh basil leaves *or* 1 teaspoon dried basil leaves
6 green onions, cut into 3-inch strips
Pepper

6 cups cooked fettuccine
2 tablespoons grated Parmesan cheese

Cut salmon into small thin slices. Marinate salmon, shallots and parsley together with 1 teaspoon of olive oil and 2 tablespoons of lemon juice. Toss red pepper strips with basil leaves.

Boil water for pasta. Sauté red peppers and green onions in the other 2 teaspoons of olive oil for 1–2 minutes until onions are softened. Begin cooking fettuccine. Add salmon to the peppers and continue cooking another 1–2 minutes until fish is just done. Do not let salmon overcook and become dry. Season with pepper and the other tablespoon of lemon juice. Add the cooked fettuccine and mix all together in warm serving dish. Sprinkle with Parmesan cheese.

Makes 4 servings.

SALMON MOUSSE

This versatile recipe is quickly prepared in a blender. It can be served in many attractive ways as described below.

1 tablespoon unflavored gelatin
2 tablespoons freshly squeezed lemon juice
¼ small onion, cut in chunks
½ cup boiling water
½ cup imitation mayonnaise
¼ teaspoon paprika
1½ cups low-fat cottage cheese
1 can (16 ounces) salmon, drained, with skin and bones removed *or* 2 cups leftover cooked salmon
½ teaspoon Tabasco sauce
1 tablespoon capers (optional)

Empty gelatin into blender container. Add lemon juice, onion and boiling water. Cover and blend on high speed 40 seconds. Add imitation mayonnaise, paprika and cottage cheese. Cover and blend on high speed for 30 seconds or until well blended. Remove cover and add salmon *or* leftover cooked salmon, Tabasco sauce and capers. Blend well for 30 seconds.

Pour into a lightly oiled 1½-quart mold (use a fish-shaped mold if possible), 8 individual molds or an attractive pottery bowl, depending on how you want to serve it. Refrigerate until set.

SERVING IDEAS
—For an attractive buffet entrée, unmold and decorate with lemon wedges and thin cucumber slices. Serve with Dilly Sauce, page 373. Bring it to a potluck and you will be thanked warmly. Makes 10 servings.
—For individual servings, unmold on lettuce leaves and top with a dollop of Dilly Sauce.

Serve with crusty French bread. It will make an unusual entree. Makes 8 individual servings.
—As an appetizer, serve directly from a pottery dish and sprinkle with dill weed or paprika. It can be offered as a dip with vegetables or low-fat crackers. Makes 12 servings.

excellent! ✓

SCALLOPS IN CREAMY SAUCE

A low-fat version of the famous Coquilles St. Jacques. Lovely when baked in individual scallop shells and served with Twice-Baked Potatoes, Cottage Style. Baba au Rhum for dessert would complete this elegant menu.

1 pound bay scallops (small ones)
½ cup dry sherry
¼ cup water
1 bay leaf
½ pound mushrooms, sliced
1 small onion, chopped
1½ tablespoons margarine
1½ tablespoons flour
1 tablespoon freshly squeezed lemon juice
⅛ teaspoon paprika
Dash ground pepper
1 tablespoon dry bread crumbs
1 tablespoon grated Parmesan cheese

Preheat oven to 325°. Put scallops, sherry, water and bay leaf in skillet. Cover and simmer on stovetop for 5 minutes. Remove scallops, drain and reserve broth. Cook and stir mushrooms and onions in margarine until onions are tender and mushrooms brown. Stir in flour and cook, stirring, for 1 minute or until bubbling. Stir in reserved broth, lemon juice, paprika and pepper. Heat, stirring constantly, until mixture thickens. Add scallops. Pour into casserole dish or divide among individual scallop shells. Sprinkle bread crumbs and cheese on top. Garnish with a sprinkling of paprika for color. Bake until golden brown and heated through, 5–15 minutes.

Makes 4 servings.

SESAME HALIBUT—Easy

A very popular fish dish! The sauce for this grilled halibut is tangy and delicious. Served with rice and salad this dish is perfect for a summer meal.

2 pounds halibut fillets or steaks
¼ cup orange juice
2 tablespoons low-sodium ketchup
1 tablespoon lower-sodium soy sauce
1 tablespoon freshly squeezed lemon juice
¼ teaspoon pepper
¾ teaspoon sesame oil
1 tablespoon brown sugar
1 tablespoon sesame seeds, toasted

Two hours before mealtime rinse fish with cold water. Pat dry with paper towels. Cut fish into 4 portions. Place in single layer in baking dish. In a small bowl combine orange juice, ketchup, soy sauce, lemon juice, pepper, sesame oil and brown sugar. Pour mixture over fish, cover and marinate in refrigerator for 2 hours, turning once. Remove fish, reserving marinade. Fish is best cooked over barbecue grill, or may be broiled in oven. Baste with marinade, turn once during cooking. Fish is done when it flakes easily with a fork. Heat the remaining marinade; pour over fish. Top with toasted sesame seeds.

Makes 4 servings.

SHRIMP AND ASPARAGUS CREPES

A gourmet treat!

2 teaspoons oil, divided
1½ tablespoons minced green onions
1¼ cups shrimp meat
2½ tablespoons flour
1½ cups skim milk
¼ teaspoon Lite Salt or less
¼ teaspoon pepper
⅛ teaspoon nutmeg
⅛ teaspoon paprika
2 tablespoons grated low-fat cheese
24 cooked asparagus spears

Prepare Crepes, page 368.

Preheat oven to 350°. In a nonstick sauce pan heat 1 teaspoon oil. Sauté green onions over low heat until tender. Stir in shrimp, cooking slowly for 2 minutes. Remove from pan. Add remaining 1 teaspoon oil to pan and stir in flour. Mixture will be dry. Add milk slowly and stir until mixture thickens (wire whisk works well). Add Lite Salt, pepper, nutmeg and paprika and continue stirring until thick. Fold in shrimp-onion mixture and grated cheese. Stir until cheese is melted.

Fill each crepe with 2 asparagus spears and 2 tablespoons of shrimp filling. Roll and place in baking dish. Pour remaining sauce over stuffed crepes. Bake 10 minutes and serve immediately.

Makes filling for 12 crepes (about 1½ cups sauce).

VARIATIONS

Any white fish may be substituted for the shrimp.

Or salmon and well-drained spinach.

Or crab, tomatoes and green pepper.

TANDOORI FISH

Halibut is marinated in spicy yogurt sauce, flavored with lime and garlic and then broiled. Tabouli salad is great with this recipe.

1½ pounds halibut steaks
1 cup plain low-fat yogurt
⅓ cup lime juice
2 to 3 cloves garlic, crushed
2 teaspoons fresh ginger root, peeled and chopped
1½ teaspoons ground coriander
½ teaspoon Lite Salt or less
1 teaspoon paprika
½ teaspoon ground cumin
Pinch cayenne pepper
Lime wedges, tomatoes, cilantro (for garnish)

Early in the day or the day before fish is to be cooked, rinse fish under cold water, pat dry. Mix yogurt, lime juice, garlic, ginger root, coriander, Lite Salt, paprika, cumin and cayenne together. Marinate fish for several hours or overnight.

When ready to cook, place fish and sauce in an attractive baking dish. Broil for 10 minutes or until fish flakes easily with a fork. Garnish with lime wedges, fresh tomatoes and chopped cilantro.

Makes 4 servings.

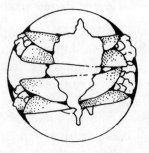

Baked Fillet Quickies

BAKED HERBED FISH ✓
—Quick

Fresh fish is the secret ingredient!

**2 pounds white fish fillets (red snapper,
  halibut, etc.)**
1 tablespoon oil
½ teaspoon Lite Salt or less
½ teaspoon marjoram leaves
⅓ teaspoon thyme leaves
¼ teaspoon garlic powder
⅛ teaspoon white pepper
2 bay leaves
½ cup chopped onion
Paprika
½ cup white wine *or* skim milk
Lime wedges, for garnish

Preheat oven to 350°. Wash fish, pat dry and
put in dish. Combine oil with Lite Salt and
herbs. Dribble over fish. Top with bay leaves
and onions. Sprinkle with paprika. Pour wine
or skim milk over all. Bake uncovered for 20–
30 minutes or until fish flakes easily with a
fork. Serve with lime wedges.
  Makes 4 servings.

COD CURRY—Easy

Fish and curry are a natural combination.
Nice to serve with Bulgur Pilaf, peas and
Pears in Wine.

2 pounds cod fillets
1 cup finely sliced celery
½ cup chopped onion

1 tablespoon oil
½ teaspoon curry powder
½ teaspoon Lite Salt or less
Dash of pepper
⅓ cup skim milk
**Paprika, parsley and lemon slices to
  decorate**

Preheat oven to 350°. Place fillets in a lightly
oiled baking dish. Sauté celery and onions in
oil until soft. Mix celery and onions with seasonings and milk. Spread over fish. Bake for
20–25 minutes or until fish flakes easily with
a fork. Sprinkle with paprika and garnish with
parsley and lemon slices.
  Makes 4 servings.

CREOLE SALMON—Easy

Very colorful way to served baked salmon.

1½ pounds salmon steaks
⅓ cup freshly squeezed lemon juice
3 tomatoes, chopped
1 green pepper, chopped
⅓ cup chopped onion
½ teaspoon pepper
12 drops Tabasco sauce

Preheat oven to 350°. Wash fish, pat dry with
towel and arrange in baking dish. Pour lemon
juice over salmon. Arrange tomatoes, green
peppers and onions around salmon. Sprinkle
with pepper and Tabasco. Cover and bake for
20–30 minutes or until fish flakes easily with
a fork.
  Makes 6 servings.

FISH HAMPTON—Easy

If the fish is on hand, dinner can be ready in 40 minutes.

⅓ cup freshly squeezed lemon juice
2 pounds fish fillets
⅓ cup chopped onion
½ teaspoon pepper
Pinch garlic powder
½ teaspoon dried lemon peel
1 tablespoon chives *or* chopped green
   onion
½ teaspoon dill weed
½ teaspoon chervil
½ teaspoon parsley flakes
½ teaspoon dry mustard

Preheat oven to 350°. Pour lemon juice over fish. Sprinkle remaining ingredients on top of fish. Cover and bake for 20–30 minutes or until fish flakes easily with a fork.
   Makes 4 servings.

SAVORY FISH FILLETS
—Quick

When you have frozen fish fillets on hand, fish can be a great convenience food. This dish cooks fast in a conventional oven, and with a microwave oven, it's very speedy!

2 pounds fresh or frozen fish fillets (red
   snapper, sole, etc.)
¾ cup thinly sliced onion
1 tablespoon oil
1 tablespoon freshly squeezed lemon juice
1 can (2.2 ounces) sliced black olives
Pepper and garlic powder to taste
½ cup soft bread crumbs
2 tablespoons chopped parsley

Separate fish fillets, if frozen, and cut into serving-size pieces. Sauté sliced onions in oil. Place fish fillets in a 12-by-8-inch baking dish and sprinkle lemon juice over top. Top with cooked onions and drained olives. Sprinkle with pepper and garlic powder. Combine bread crumbs and parsley; sprinkle over top of fish.

To bake in conventional oven: Cover with foil and bake at 350° for 20–30 minutes or until fish flakes easily with a fork. For frozen fillets bake 40–45 minutes.

To bake in microwave oven: Cover with plastic wrap and cook on high heat for 6½–8 minutes, or until fish flakes easily with a fork. For frozen fillets cook for 12–15 minutes. Let stand, covered, 2 minutes before serving.
   Makes 4 servings.

Fish With Sauces

BAKED SNAPPER WITH SPICY TOMATO SAUCE

This fish is good with Scalloped Potatoes if you have time to start them baking earlier.

1 tablespoon oil
¼ cup chopped onion
1 cup chopped celery
2 tablespoons chopped green pepper
1 can (16 ounces) unsalted tomatoes,
   drained
¾ teaspoon Worcestershire sauce
1½ teaspoons low-sodium ketchup
½ teaspoon chili powder
½ of 1 lemon, finely sliced
1 bay leaf
1 clove garlic, minced
Few grains cayenne pepper

2 pounds red snapper *or* other white fish fillets
1 tablespoon flour

Heat oil and sauté onions, celery and green peppers. Add tomatoes, Worcestershire sauce, ketchup, chili powder, lemon, bay leaf, garlic and cayenne. Simmer until celery is tender and mixture is thick.

Preheat oven to 350°. Coat fish with flour and place in baking dish. Spread sauce over fish. Cover and bake 20–30 minutes or until fish flakes easily with a fork.

Makes 4 servings.

BAKED SNAPPER WITH WINE AND VEGGIES—Easy

A very popular fish dish!

2 pounds red snappper
½ onion, chopped
1 cup sliced mushrooms
1 tablespoon oil
½ cup unsalted tomato sauce
¼ cup dry white wine or water
½ teaspoon Italian seasoning *or* oregano leaves
1 package (10 ounces) frozen peas (optional)

Preheat oven to 350°. Place fish in an 8-inch-square baking pan. Sauté onions and mushrooms in oil. Add tomato sauce and spoon over snapper. Sprinkle with wine or water and seasoning. Bake about 20–30 minutes until fish flakes easily with a fork. If desired, add frozen peas before baking. (It makes the dish very attractive.)

Makes 4 servings.

FISH ALMONDINE WITH DILLY SAUCE

A meal fit for guests—the almonds add a great finishing touch.

2 pounds white fish
Juice of 2 lemons
2 teaspoons tarragon leaves
1 cup Dilly Sauce (see below)
¼ cup sliced almonds, toasted

Wash fish in cold water and pat dry. Place in a flat baking dish. Squeeze lemon juice over both sides of fish. Cover tightly and place in refrigerator until time to cook (no longer than 24 hours).

Twenty minutes before serving, preheat oven to 350°. Sprinkle tarragon over the fish. Cover the dish and bake for 15 minutes. Prepare Dilly Sauce while fish cooks. Remove the fish from the oven and pour off excess liquid. Spoon Dilly Sauce evenly over the fish. Place under the broiler until sauce starts to bubble, about 1 minute. Sprinkle the sliced almonds on top of each serving.

Makes 4 servings.

DILLY SAUCE
2 tablespoons imitation mayonnaise
1 cup plain low-fat yogurt
¾ teaspoon tarragon leaves
1½ teaspoons dill weed

Put the mayonnaise and yogurt in a mixing bowl. Mix thoroughly with a wire whisk. Add the other ingredients and blend well.

Makes about 1 cup.

FISH À L'ORANGE—Easy

This is good to serve with rice—the orange sauce is delicious.

   2 pounds fish fillets
   2 tablespoons orange juice
   2 teaspoons freshly squeezed lemon juice
   1 tablespoon margarine, melted
   Ground nutmeg
   1 tablespoon snipped parsley or dried
     parsley flakes
   ⅛ teaspoon lemon pepper
   Orange slices

Preheat oven to 375°. Arrange fish in glass baking dish, skin (dark) side down. Combine orange juice, lemon juice and melted margarine. Pour over fish. Sprinkle nutmeg, parsley and lemon pepper on fish. Bake 15–20 minutes, until fish flakes easily with a fork. Garnish with orange slices.

Makes 4 servings.

MEDALLION OF COD
—Quick

The "Ten-Minute Dinner" idea! Broiled fish with a "mock" sour cream sauce on top.

   1 cup low-fat cottage cheese
   2 tablespoons buttermilk
   ½ teaspoon dill weed
   ¼ teaspoon dry mustard
   2 pounds cod

Mix cottage cheese and buttermilk in blender until smooth. Stir in dill weed and dry mustard.

Cut fish into serving sizes. Place on broiling pan and broil 4–5 minutes on each side. Spread sauce over fish and broil only to heat through and brown slightly. The sauce will curdle if heated too long. Serve immediately.

Makes 4 servings.

Fish Roll-Ups

FISH FILLETS WITH WALNUTS

A very elegant and tasty dish. The walnuts make it special.

   2 pounds sole fillets or other white fish
   Freshly ground black pepper
   1 tablespoon oil
   1 tablespoon flour
   1 cup clam juice
   2 tablespoons prepared mustard
   ¼ cup chopped walnuts

Preheat oven to 400°. Season fish with pepper. Heat oil in a saucepan; blend in flour and cook over medium heat about 1 minute, stirring until smooth. Add clam juice and mustard. Cook until thickened, stirring constantly.

Roll fish fillets jelly-roll style and place seam side down in a shallow casserole. Spoon sauce over fish. Sprinkle with nuts. Bake for 15–20 minutes, until fish flakes easily with a fork.

Makes 4 servings.

LIVELY LEMON ROLL-UPS

One of the favorite recipes in this book.

   1 tablespoon margarine
   ½ cup freshly squeezed lemon juice
   ½ chicken bouillon cube
   ½–1 teaspoon Tabasco sauce
   2 cups cooked brown rice
   2 packages (10 ounces each) frozen
     chopped broccoli, thawed, or 1 head
     fresh broccoli, finely chopped

¾ cup chopped green onion
½ cup grated low-fat cheese
3 pounds sole (thin white fish works best)
Paprika

Preheat oven to 375°. In small saucepan, melt the margarine. Add lemon juice, bouillon cube and Tabasco. Heat slowly until bouillon dissolves; set aside. In medium bowl combine cooked rice, broccoli, green onions, cheese and half of the above sauce. Mix well and place half of rice mixture on bottom of shallow baking dish.

Cut fish into 6 fillets and spread flat on work surface. Divide remaining broccoli mixture equally among fillets. Roll fillets up around rice mixture (secure with wooden picks if necessary) and place seam side down on top of rice in baking dish. Pour remaining sauce over roll-ups. Bake 25 minutes or until fish flakes easily with a fork. Garnish with paprika.

Makes 6 servings.

STUFFED SOLE

The stuffing is easily prepared—it's worth the effort!

2½ cups soft bread crumbs
2 pimientos, chopped and drained
2 green onions, minced
2 tablespoons chopped parsley
2 medium carrots, shredded
¼ teaspoon Lite Salt or less
¼ teaspoon pepper
3 pounds sole (6 fillets)
1 tablespoon margarine (to drizzle on top)
Paprika

Preheat oven to 375°. Mix first 7 ingredients and divide into 6 portions. Spread fillets with the stuffing mixture, roll and place in pan. Secure with wooden picks if needed. Drizzle 1 tablespoon of margarine over the top and sprinkle with paprika. Bake for 25–30 minutes or until fish flakes easily with a fork.

Makes 6 servings.

Potpourri

CLAM PILAF—Quick

For the clam lover in your family.

1 tablespoon oil
2 tablespoons minced onion
2 cups diagonally sliced celery
½ clove garlic, minced
½ teaspoon tarragon leaves
½ teaspoon basil leaves
1 teaspoon parsley flakes
Dash pepper
1 cup uncooked long-grain rice
1 chicken bouillon cube
2 cups boiling water
3 cans (6½ ounces each) chopped or minced clams, drained
1 package (10 ounces) frozen peas, thawed

Heat oil in heavy skillet. Add onions, celery, garlic and seasonings; cook a few minutes, stirring often. Reduce heat. Stir in rice and cook 3 minutes more. Dissolve bouillon cube in boiling water, add to rice mixture and bring to a boil. Stir gently with fork. Cover and simmer gently 15 minutes. Add clams and peas. Cover and cook 10 minutes or until rice is tender and liquid absorbed.

Makes 4 servings.

CLAM SAUCE FOR PASTA —Quick

An elegant way to serve pasta—and easy to make as well!

3 cans (6½ ounces each) chopped or
   minced clams
2 cloves garlic, minced
4 teaspoons margarine
2 tablespoons flour
¼ cup finely chopped fresh parsley
¼ teaspoon pepper
¼ teaspoon thyme leaves
¼ cup grated Parmesan cheese for
   topping

Drain clams into a 2-cup measure and add water to make 2 cups. In a saucepan sauté garlic in margarine over medium heat. Add flour and mix well. It will be dry. Add clam juice/water mixture, stirring rapidly with wire whisk to smooth out lumps. Add parsley, pepper and thyme. Stir and simmer for a few minutes. Add clams and heat through. Serve over warm pasta. Sprinkle with Parmesan cheese.

   Makes about 4 cups sauce.

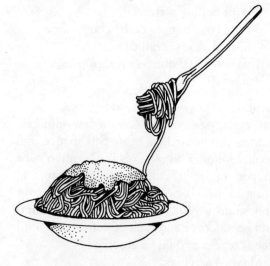

CREOLE SHRIMP—Quick

½ onion, chopped
1 tablespoon oil
1 bay leaf, crushed
¼ cup diced celery
1 teaspoon minced parsley
1 green pepper, chopped
Dash of cayenne pepper
1 can (6 ounces) unsalted tomato paste
2½ cups water
2 cups shrimp meat *

Sauté onions in oil. Add rest of ingredients except shrimp. Cook slowly, stirring occasionally, about 30 minutes. Add shrimp and heat through. Serve over brown rice.

   Makes 6 servings.

* When using uncooked (green) shrimp, do not pre-cook; cook in the sauce only until pink (about 10 minutes).

FISH À LA MISTRAL—Easy

It's worth the effort to have fennel seeds on hand for this delicious dish.

1 onion, finely chopped
1 tablespoon oil
2 tomatoes, peeled and coarsely chopped
½ teaspoon Lite Salt or less
2 pounds fish steaks or fillets (white fish
   or salmon)
4 fresh lemon slices
1 tablespoon chopped parsley
⅛ teaspoon fennel seeds (optional)
½ cup dry white wine

Preheat oven to 350°. Sauté onions in oil in nonstick fry pan until golden brown. Add tomatoes and Lite Salt; cook 3–5 minutes. Pour into baking dish large enough to hold fish. Lay fish on top of vegetable mixture. Add 1 slice of lemon on top of each steak. Sprinkle with parsley, fennel seeds and wine. Bake for 20–30 minutes or until fish flakes easily with a fork. (When serving, spoon vegetable mixture over fish.)

Makes 4 servings.

PORTUGUESE CASSEROLE

Unusual combination of fish, beans and vegetables for a very hearty dish. Add rolls and fresh fruit for a nice meal.

- **6 ounces cod (any white fish can be used)**
- **2 medium potatoes, thinly sliced**
- **1 tablespoon olive oil**
- **2 cloves garlic, crushed**
- **2 medium onions, chopped**
- **2 stalks celery, chopped**
- **1 medium green pepper, chopped**
- **½ teaspoon Lite Salt or less**
- **¼ teaspoon pepper**
- **1 teaspoon oregano leaves**
- **¼ teaspoon turmeric *or* ¼ teaspoon tarragon leaves**
- **2 cans (4 ounces each) mushrooms, drained**
- **1 can (16 ounces) garbanzo beans, drained ***
- **1 can (16 ounces) unsalted tomatoes (save liquid)**
- **10 black olives, pitted**
- **Vinegar (optional)**

Thaw fish, if frozen, and cut into 2-inch chunks. Cook the potatoes in boiling water

until tender, not mushy. (The thin slices cook very quickly.) Drain.

Preheat oven to 350°. Heat olive oil in fry pan. Sauté garlic, onions, celery and half the green peppers. Add spices. Simmer for about 10 minutes, adding liquid from tomatoes as needed. In an ovenproof baking dish, layer the potatoes, mushrooms, garbanzo beans, tomatoes and fish. Top with the sautéed vegetables. Bake for 30 minutes until heated through. Garnish with the rest of the green peppers and olives. Serve with vinegar, if desired.

Makes 6 servings.

* Use low-sodium beans if available.

SALMON LOAF—Easy

Serve slices of this loaf with Super Stuffed Potatoes and a favorite vegetable.

- **2 cups soft bread crumbs**
- **1 onion, chopped**
- **1 tablespoon melted margarine**
- **¼ cup minced celery**
- **1 cup skim milk**
- **2 cups flaked canned salmon**
- **1 tablespoon freshly squeezed lemon juice**
- **Dash pepper**
- **1 tablespoon minced parsley**
- **3 egg whites**
- **½ teaspoon Worcestershire sauce**

Heat oven to 325°. Combine all ingredients and mix thoroughly. Place in lightly oiled 9-by-5-inch loaf pan. Bake for 45 minutes.

Makes 6 servings.

SKINNY SOLE—Quick

Kids love this! Goes very well with Classic Baked Beans.

1½ pounds sole, cut into 4 pieces
½ cup cornmeal
2 tablespoons oil

Coat pieces of fish with cornmeal. Heat oil in skillet. Sauté fish quickly in oil, turning once. Makes 4 servings.

TANGY SNAPPER

Fresh green spinach and fish with a tangy sauce—serve with a baked potato and fruit salad.

1 pound red snapper fillets *or* any firm-textured white fish
Pepper
¾ cup plain low-fat yogurt
2 tablespoons imitation mayonnaise
2 tablespoons flour
2 tablespoons freshly squeezed lemon juice
¼ teaspoon dill weed
2 bunches fresh spinach, stemmed and washed
Paprika

Preheat oven to 350°. Arrange fish fillets in a single layer in a shallow baking pan (about 9 by 13 inches). Sprinkle with pepper. With wire whisk, smoothly blend yogurt, imitation mayonnaise, flour, lemon juice and dill weed. Spread the mixture over fish. Bake fish uncovered until it flakes easily with a fork, about 20–30 minutes. Meanwhile, put spinach and water that clings to leaves in a 10–12-inch frying pan on medium-high heat. Cover and cook, stirring occasionally, until spinach wilts; drain.

To serve, arrange spinach in a layer on a serving platter. Place cooked fish on top. Spoon any extra sauce from baking dish onto fish and sprinkle with paprika.

Makes 4 servings.

VEGETABLE-TOPPED FISH FILLETS

Baked fish served with a vegetable-wine sauce over the top makes a very tasty dish. Good recipe to serve to people learning to "enjoy" fish!

2 pounds red snapper fillets (1 inch thick)
Dash pepper
½ teaspoon tarragon leaves
1 medium onion, chopped
¼ pound mushrooms, sliced
1 tablespoon oil
1 medium tomato, seeded and chopped
¼ cup white wine
¼ cup chili sauce
⅓ cup grated Parmesan cheese

Preheat oven to 350°. Cut fillets into serving-size pieces and remove bones if necessary. Sprinkle lightly with pepper and crumbled tarragon. Place fish in lightly oiled baking dish. Bake 20–30 minutes or until fish flakes easily with a fork. Remove from oven and discard juices.

While fish bakes, sauté onions and mushrooms in oil until onions are limp. Remove from heat and stir in chopped tomato, wine and chili sauce. Spoon mixture evenly over each fillet, then sprinkle with Parmesan cheese. Broil quickly 4 inches from heat, until cheese begins to melt. Do not overcook.

Makes 4 servings.

Tuna Dishes

ALPHABET SEAFOOD SALAD—Easy

A popular cold pasta salad. Excellent for potlucks or picnics—children love this dish.

1 package (12 ounces) alphabet noodles
2 cans (6½ ounces each) water-packed tuna, drained and flaked
1 can (2.2 ounces) black olives, sliced
1 medium onion, finely chopped
¼ cup chopped parsley
¼ teaspoon paprika

DRESSING
1 cup plain low-fat yogurt
¼ cup imitation mayonnaise
1 teaspoon Dijon mustard
2 tablespoons sweet pickle juice

Cook alphabet noodles in unsalted water following package directions. Drain well and combine with tuna, drained olives, onions, parsley and paprika. Cover and chill until serving time.

Meanwhile, mix dressing ingredients together and add to rest of salad *just before serving*. This is especially important in order to keep the salad creamy because the noodles absorb the yogurt dressing.

Makes 12 servings (1 cup each).

BEAN SPROUT TUNA CHOW MEIN—Quick

A tuna stir-fry dish which can be prepared in 20 minutes! Serve with rice, Sunshine Spinach Salad and Cocoa Cake.

½ chicken bouillon cube
1 cup water
1 tablespoon lower-sodium soy sauce
2 tablespoons cornstarch
1 tablespoon oil
6 stalks celery, cut diagonally
2 medium onions, thinly sliced
1 can (6 ounces) bamboo shoots, drained
½ cup sliced fresh mushrooms *or* 1 can (4 ounces) mushrooms, drained
2 cups fresh bean sprouts *or* 1 can (15 ounces) bean sprouts
1 can (6½ ounces) water-packed tuna, drained

Dissolve bouillon in water. Add soy sauce. Stir in cornstarch until dissolved. Heat oil in frying pan or wok over high heat. When hot, toss in celery and onions and stir-fry 1 minute. Add bamboo shoots, mushrooms and bean sprouts. Stir bouillon mixture and add to vegetables. Stir and cook just until sauce is thickened. Add tuna and stir until hot and sauce is clear. Serve immediately over fluffy rice.

Makes 4 servings (1¾ cups each).

SWEET 'N' SOUR SUPPER

A small recipe which can easily be increased. Tuna is always popular.

1 can (8 ounces) chunk pineapple, unsweetened
1 small onion, chopped
1 tablespoon oil
2 tablespoons dry sherry (optional)
2 tablespoons unsalted tomato paste
1 tablespoon cornstarch
1 tablespoon brown sugar
1 tablespoon red wine vinegar
1 tablespoon lower-sodium soy sauce
¼ teaspoon ground ginger
⅛ teaspoon garlic powder
1 green pepper, chunked
1 can (6½ ounces) water-packed tuna, drained
½ cup halved cherry tomatoes

Drain pineapple and reserve juice. In a skillet sauté onions in oil until soft. Combine sherry, tomato paste, cornstarch, brown sugar, vinegar, soy sauce, ginger and garlic powder until blended. Stir into cooked onions along with reserved pineapple juice. Cook until sauce boils and thickens. Add pineapple and green peppers. Cook until green peppers are tender-crisp. Add tuna and cherry tomatoes. Continue cooking until heated through. Remove from heat. Serve over a large helping of fluffy brown rice.

Makes 2 servings (about 4 cups).

TUNA NOODLE CASSEROLE —Easy

The unsalted canned soups and vegetables now readily available make this dish much lower in salt in addition to being lower in fat.

3 cups uncooked eggless noodles
½ small onion, chopped
¼ cup sliced mushrooms
1 can (6½ ounces) water-packed tuna, drained
1 can (10½ ounces) low-sodium cream of mushroom soup *or* use Homemade "Cream" Soup Mix, page 261
½ teaspoon Lite Salt or less
Pepper to taste
1 can (16 ounces) unsalted green beans, drained
½ cup crushed Rice Krispies

Preheat oven to 325°. Cook noodles in unsalted boiling water until tender. Drain well. Steam onions and mushrooms in a small amount of water until onions are transparent. Remove with slotted spoon and combine with the cooked noodles, tuna fish, soup, Lite Salt, pepper and green beans in casserole dish. Bake uncovered for 15–20 minutes or until heated through! Sprinkle crushed cereal over top and serve.

Makes 4 servings (2 cups each).

CHICKEN, TURKEY AND RABBIT

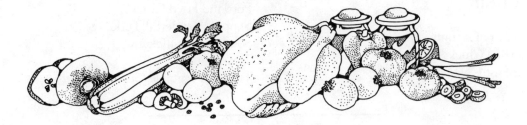

Chicken, turkey and rabbit are excellent choices—they are very low in fat. You'll find some unusual combinations with fruits, vegetables, herbs and spices. Don't forget to accompany these dishes with rice, pasta or potatoes to provide hearty entrées that are filling *and* low in fat and cholesterol.

Turkey is not just for holidays! It is a good alternative to high fat meats for daily fare. In fact, many grocery stores are offering turkey parts (such as hindquarters or breasts) that are good roasted or used in one-pot meals. We particularly like to use ground turkey (usually found in the frozen foods department) in place of higher fat ground beef, especially in dishes that are combined with grains, noodles or vegetables.

We've included a special rabbit dish for you French cooks!

Because these meats are so lean (especially without the skin), they can dry out in the cooking process. For this reason, it's best to cook them with added liquid, much as you would a pot roast.

ORIENTAL DISHES

Basic Stir-Fried Chicken
Cashew Chicken
Chicken and Tomatoes in Black Bean Sauce
Orange Baked Chicken
Spicy Chicken with Spinach
Tangerine Chicken
Turkey Lettuce Stir Fry

MEDITERRANEAN DISHES

Chicken and Mushroom Crepes
Chicken and Vegetables Provençale
Chicken Braised in Wine
Chicken Cacciatore

Chicken Italian
Chicken Madeira
Couscous
Easy Oven Lasagna
Homemade Raviolis
Rabbit Fricassee
Turkey-Mushroom Spaghetti Sauce

CURRIES

Country Captain
Curried Chicken Quickie
Far East Chicken
Chicken Nepal

CHICKEN-TURKEY SPECIALTIES

Acapulco Enchiladas
Chicken Salad with Yogurt-Chive Dressing
Cornish Game Hens à La Crock
Crocked Chicken
Lemony Chicken Kabobs
Parmesan Yogurt Chicken
Pollo Tepehuano
Portland Fried Chicken
Simply Wonderful Turkey Salad
South Seas Chicken
Texas Hash
Turkey-Vegetable Chowder

Oriental Dishes

BASIC STIR-FRIED CHICKEN —Quick

2 chicken breasts
2 slices fresh ginger root, peeled and chopped
1 green onion
1 tablespoon cornstarch
1 tablespoon sherry
2 tablespoons water
1 pound vegetables (see suggestions given below)
1 tablespoon oil
1 tablespoon lower-sodium soy sauce or less
Pinch of sugar
½ cup chicken broth

Skin and bone chicken, then cut into small chunks.

Mince ginger root and green onion, then combine with cornstarch, sherry and water. Add to chicken and toss to coat. Let stand 15 minutes, turning occasionally. Meanwhile, slice vegetables.

Heat oil. Add chicken and stir-fry until it begins to brown (2–3 minutes). Remove from pan.

Add vegetables and stir-fry to coat with oil (1–2 minutes). Sprinkle with soy sauce and sugar.

Stir in chicken broth and heat quickly. Then simmer, covered, until vegetables are nearly done. Return chicken; stir to reheat and blend flavors (about ½ minute). Serve at once.

Makes about 4 servings.

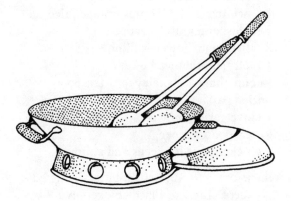

SUGGESTED VEGETABLE COMBINATIONS FOR BASIC STIR-FRIED CHICKEN

Add any of these vegetables, chopped, to previous recipe:

—1 cup onions and 2 tomatoes
—½ pound fresh mushrooms and ½ pound Chinese cabbage
—½ cup asparagus, ½ cup bamboo shoots and 1 cup bean sprouts
—2 green peppers, 3 celery stalks and 8 green onions
—½ cup mushrooms, 1 cup celery, 1 cup peas, ½ cup onion

CASHEW CHICKEN

Be sure to add the nuts as it makes this dish very special! With a small amount of chicken and lots of vegetables, this dish remains low-fat.

> 2 chicken breasts
> ½ pound pea pods *or* 1½ cups broccoli flowerets
> ½ pound mushrooms
> 4 green onions
> 1 can (8 ounces) bamboo shoots, drained
> 1 cup chicken broth
> 1 tablespoon lower-sodium soy sauce
> 2 tablespoons cornstarch
> ½ teaspoon sugar
> 1 teaspoon oil
> ¼ cup cashew nuts, dry roasted

Bone chicken breasts and remove skin. Slice horizontally in ⅛-inch-thick slices, then cut in 1-inch squares. Arrange on a tray. Remove the ends and strings from pea pods or chop broccoli. Wash and slice mushrooms. Cut the green part of the onions into 1-inch lengths and then slash both ends several times making small fans; slice the white part ¼ inch thick. Slice bamboo shoots. Pour chicken broth into small pitcher. Mix together soy sauce, cornstarch and sugar; pour into a small pitcher. Place oil and nuts in containers. Arrange at the table with electric frying pan or wok.

Add oil to pan, add chicken and cook quickly, turning, until it turns opaque. Add peas and mushrooms; pour in broth, cover and simmer 2 minutes. Add bamboo shoots. Stir the soy sauce mixture into the pan juices and cook until sauce is thickened, stirring constantly; then simmer 2 minutes. Mix in the green onions, sprinkle with nuts. Serve with cooked rice.

Makes 4 servings.

CHICKEN AND TOMATOES IN BLACK BEAN SAUCE

Hot and spicy. Serve with a large bowl of steamed rice.

2 chicken breasts, boned and skinned
1 teaspoon lower-sodium soy sauce
2 tablespoons sherry
½ tablespoon fermented black beans *
2 cloves garlic, finely chopped
1 tablespoon cornstarch
2 tablespoons water
2 teaspoons oil
1 teaspoon sugar
¼ cup chicken broth
4 tomatoes, cut in thin wedges

Cut chicken in thin strips and season with soy sauce and sherry. Rinse fermented black beans, then crush them and the garlic with a fork. Mix cornstarch and water until smooth.

Heat oil and sauté quickly the beans and garlic. Add chicken, cook until it just loses pinkness. Sprinkle with sugar and cook 1 minute. Add broth and cook 2 minutes. Add tomatoes and thicken with cornstarch paste. Serve over rice.

Makes 3–4 servings.

* Available in Oriental grocery stores.

ORANGE BAKED CHICKEN
—Easy

Very easy to prepare—the sauce makes a wonderful gravy for potatoes or rice. Some people like to marinate the chicken and sauce 8 hours or overnight.

1 can (6 ounces) frozen orange juice concentrate *or* 1½ cups orange juice
1 tablespoon grated orange rind
2 tablespoons lower-sodium soy sauce
1 tablespoon minced onion
¼ cup chopped parsley *or* 1 teaspoon dried parsley
1 clove garlic, minced
¼ teaspoon pepper
1 chicken, cut in pieces and skinned

Preheat oven to 400°. Combine all ingredients except chicken. Place chicken in a 9-by-12-inch pan. Pour marinade over chicken. Cover pan and bake for 45 minutes. Uncover and continue baking until tender. Baste several times with sauce. If desired, thicken remaining sauce in pan and serve as gravy.

Makes 6 servings.

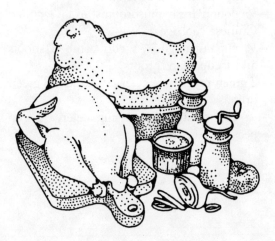

SPICY CHICKEN WITH SPINACH

A special Chinese stir-fry dish.

SAUCE #1
   1 tablespoon lower-sodium soy sauce
   1 teaspoon white wine
   2 tablespoons water
   2 teaspoons cornstarch

SAUCE #2
   1 tablespoon each, finely chopped: green
      onion, ginger root, garlic
   1 teaspoon black bean sauce with chili *

SAUCE #3
   1 teaspoon white wine
   1 tablespoon lower-sodium soy sauce
   2 teaspoons sugar
   ½ teaspoon sesame oil
   1 teaspoon vinegar
   1½ tablespoons water
   1 teaspoon cornstarch

   4 chicken breasts, skinned and boned
   1 tablespoon oil, divided
   3 bunches fresh spinach, stems removed

Prepare 3 sauces in separate bowls. Cut chicken into thin strips. Mix the chicken with Sauce #1 and marinate about 20 minutes. Heat 1 teaspoon oil in a large skillet or wok. Stir-fry the chicken and remove from the skillet or push to sides of skillet. Heat 2 teaspoons oil in the center of the same skillet; add Sauce #2. Heat until mixture is very bubbly. Mix in chicken. Stir in Sauce #3 and cook briefly, then transfer chicken with sauces onto the center of a heated serving platter and keep warm.

Stir-fry the spinach in whatever juices are left in the skillet, until spinach is crisp-tender. Place spinach in 2 portions to either side of chicken on serving platter. Serve with steamed rice.

   Makes 4 servings.

* Available in Oriental grocery stores.

TANGERINE CHICKEN

   6 chicken breasts
   Peel of ½ tangerine, diced finely
   1½ cups water
   1 teaspoon oil
   1 teaspoon sesame oil
   1 cup finely chopped celery
   2 green onions, finely chopped
   1 slice fresh ginger root, peeled and
      chopped *or* ½ teaspoon ground ginger
   Ground pepper to taste
   2 tablespoons white wine
   1 tablespoon lower-sodium soy sauce
   Tangerine slices, cut in half (optional)

Bone and skin chicken and cut into 1-inch cubes. Simmer tangerine peel in 1½ cups water for 15 minutes. Strain. Keep about ¾ cup liquid for later use.

Heat oils in wok or frying pan; add chicken and stir-fry rapidly until opaque. Add tangerine peel, celery, green onions, ginger and pepper. Toss, then pour in the wine, soy sauce and water from simmered tangerine peel. Cook and stir for 5–10 minutes over low heat. Add tangerine slices and serve over rice.

   Makes 6 servings.

TURKEY LETTUCE STIR-FRY

Do you have leftover turkey meat? This makes a cool summertime dish. Serve with rice and end the meal with fresh fruit or sherbet.

6 cups shredded iceberg lettuce
1 tablespoon oil
3½ cups carrots, cut into thin strips (approximately 6 carrots)
1 medium onion, sliced
1 clove garlic, crushed
½ chicken bouillon cube
⅔ cup water
2 tablespoons freshly squeezed lemon juice
1 teaspoon cornstarch
1 teaspoon basil leaves, crumbled
½ teaspoon brown sugar
1 cup cooked turkey, cut into strips (white meat)

Shred lettuce and refrigerate in a plastic bag while preparing the remaining ingredients.

In a wok or large skillet, heat oil. Sauté the carrots with the onions and garlic for 3 minutes, stirring and tossing frequently. Combine bouillon cube, water, lemon juice, cornstarch, basil and brown sugar. Add to the skillet. Add the cooked turkey and heat, stirring constantly, until the sauce boils and thickens. Toss with the crisp shredded lettuce and serve immediately over steamed rice.

Makes 4 servings.

Mediterranean Dishes

CHICKEN AND MUSHROOM CREPES

A very special dish! Good way to use leftover cooked turkey, also.

1 tablespoon oil, divided
1 cup sliced fresh mushrooms
2 cups cooked chicken cubes
¼ teaspoon Lite Salt or less
¼ teaspoon pepper
3 tablespoons flour
2 cups skim milk
2 tablespoons white wine *or* water
¼ teaspoon thyme leaves *or* ½ teaspoon curry powder
2 tablespoons Parmesan cheese

Prepare Crepes, page 368.

In a nonstick saucepan heat 1 teaspoon oil. Sauté mushrooms rapidly. Add to chicken, Lite Salt, and pepper in another dish. Add remaining 2 teaspoons oil to pan and stir in flour. Mixture will be dry. Add milk and stir until mixture thickens (wire whisk works well). Add wine *or* water and thyme *or* curry powder. The sauce should be thick. Remove 1 cup sauce for topping. To remaining sauce, add mushrooms and chicken. Fill each crepe with ¼ cup filling; roll and place in baking dish. Dilute remaining sauce with skim milk, if needed. Pour over stuffed crepes. Sprinkle with Parmesan cheese. Place under broiler until sauce bubbles and is slightly browned.

Makes filling for 12 crepes.

CHICKEN AND VEGETABLES PROVENÇALE

A very colorful dish.

1 small head cauliflower *or* broccoli
2 large ripe tomatoes, sliced
2 medium carrots, pared and thinly sliced
1 large onion, thinly sliced
3 tablespoons chopped fresh parsley, divided
1 tablespoon basil leaves, divided
½ teaspoon Lite Salt or less
¼ teaspoon pepper
½ cup chicken broth
2 cloves garlic, minced
Juice of 1 lemon
4 chicken breasts, skinned

Preheat oven to 350°. Trim outer leaves and tough stalks from cauliflower; break into small pieces. Combine cauliflower, tomatoes, carrots and onions in 2-quart shallow baking dish. Sprinkle with 1 tablespoon parsley, 2 teaspoons basil, Lite Salt and pepper. Pour chicken broth over vegetables.

Make a paste of remaining 2 tablespoons parsley, 1 teaspoon basil, garlic and lemon juice. This can be done by using a mortar and pestle or by chopping parsley and garlic finely and mixing with lemon juice and basil in a small cup or bowl with the back of a spoon. Spread paste over each chicken breast.

Place chicken over vegetables in baking dish; cover with foil. Bake 1½ hours, then uncover and brown. Baste chicken occasionally with pan juice during baking.

Makes 4 servings.

CHICKEN BRAISED IN

A wonderful aroma permeates the kitchen as this dish bakes. Serve with baked potatoes and salad. Skinned pheasant or rabbit works nicely in this dish.

1 chicken, cut in pieces and skinned (for a more elegant version, use 6 skinned and boned chicken breasts)
¼ cup flour
1 tablespoon margarine
1 medium onion, sliced
4 green onions with tops, sliced
1 clove garlic, finely chopped
3 carrots, thinly sliced
1 tablespoon chopped parsley
¼ teaspoon thyme leaves
½ teaspoon oregano leaves
¼ teaspoon Lite Salt or less
2 bay leaves
1 cup white wine
1 can (4 ounces) mushroom stems and pieces, drained

Preheat oven to 350°. Coat chicken pieces thoroughly with flour. Set aside.

Combine margarine, onions, green onions, garlic and carrots in a 3-quart casserole. Place chicken pieces on top. Sprinkle with parsley, thyme, oregano and Lite Salt. Add bay leaves and wine. Cover. Bake for 45 minutes, stirring once. Add mushrooms. Cover and bake for 15 minutes or more, or until chicken and carrots are tender. Remove bay leaves before serving.

Makes 6 servings.

28

CHICKEN CACCIATORE —Easy

Tastes as good as it sounds—traditionally served with pasta, a salad and French bread.

4 chicken breasts
2 tablespoons flour
1 tablespoon oil
2 tablespoons chopped onion
1 can (6 ounces) unsalted tomato paste
½ cup white wine
¼ teaspoon white pepper
¾ cup chicken broth
½ bay leaf
⅛ teaspoon thyme leaves
½ teaspoon basil leaves
⅛ teaspoon marjoram leaves
1 cup sliced fresh mushrooms

Roll skinned chicken breasts in flour. Sauté in the oil until browned. Remove from skillet. Sauté onions in remaining trace of oil. Add remaining ingredients and stir together. Replace chicken breasts in skillet and spoon sauce over top. Simmer the chicken, covered, for 45 minutes or until tender.

Makes 4 servings.

CHICKEN ITALIAN

1 chicken, cut in pieces and skinned
4 cloves garlic, minced
1 teaspoon basil leaves
1 tablespoon oil
2 medium-size onions, cut into large julienne strips
4 carrots, sliced into julienne strips
½ cup chicken broth

Toss the skinned chicken pieces in a bowl with the garlic and basil and coat well. Heat the oil in a nonstick cooking pan and brown the chicken slightly; remove from pan. Toss the vegetables in the drippings and cook until they form a light glaze. Put ½ cup of chicken broth in the bottom of the pan and stir, picking up the cooked juices on the bottom of the pan. Add the chicken and put a tight-fitting lid on pan. Bring the liquid back to a simmer. Cook approximately 30 minutes.

Remove the chicken from the pan and drain the vegetables, leaving some carrots in the sauce. Form a bed on a platter with the drained vegetables, place the chicken on top and then puree the sauce and the remaining carrots in a blender. Pour the sauce over the top of the chicken.

Makes 6 servings.

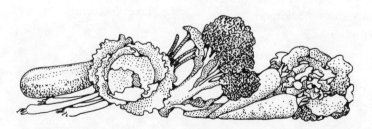

CHICKEN MADEIRA

A recipe from Portugal. To dress this dish up, serve chicken in the center of a large dish encircled by mashed potatoes. Top the potatoes with slivers of orange rind. Serve with green peas and Apple Crisp for a colorful dinner.

½ cup bread crumbs
⅛ teaspoon garlic powder
⅛ teaspoon rosemary leaves
4 chicken breasts, skinned
1 egg white, slightly beaten
2 tablespoons cornstarch
Rind of 2 oranges
1½ cups orange juice *or* juice of 2
    oranges
⅓ cup Madeira *or* dry sherry
8–10 fresh mushrooms, sliced

Mix bread crumbs with garlic powder and rosemary. Dip the chicken in egg white and roll in seasoned bread crumbs. Brown both sides of the chicken under the broiler. Place in shallow baking dish.

Preheat oven to 350°. Combine cornstarch, orange rind, orange juice and Madeira *or* sherry to make a sauce. Pour sauce over browned chicken and bake about 45 minutes (or until done), adding mushrooms during last 5 minutes. Serve chicken with mashed potatoes and pour sauce over both.

Makes 4 servings.

VARIATION
Brown rice with a little wild rice added can be substituted for the mashed potatoes.

CHICKEN NEPAL

This was served by a visitor from Nepal. It's a real gem! Don't be afraid to use these amounts of spices.

1 cup plain low-fat yogurt
1 tablespoon cornstarch
1 tablespoon ground cumin
1 tablespoon ground coriander
1½ teaspoons turmeric
1 teaspoon ground ginger
½ teaspoon pepper
½ teaspoon Lite Salt or less
1 whole chicken, cut up and skinned
1 tablespoon oil
1 clove garlic, crushed
1 large onion, chopped
1 large carrot, chopped
2 cans (16 ounces each) unsalted
    tomatoes, drained
¾ cup frozen peas

Combine yogurt, cornstarch and spices and coat chicken well with the mixture. Chill several hours.

In a large, heavy frying pan, heat oil and add garlic, onions, carrots, marinated chicken and yogurt sauce. Stir often until chicken is browned, then reduce heat and simmer, covered, until chicken is done, stirring occasionally. During last 5 minutes add tomatoes and peas and stir in. Serve over rice.

Makes 6 servings.

COUSCOUS

Couscous is a traditional African dish made with steamed semolina (a fine grain made from hard durum wheat) and a stew of different meats and vegetables. It is a perfect example of a recipe using small amounts of meat as "spice" for a grain and vegetables.

The traditional preparation involves steaming the grain, moistened with water, in the top part of a steamer while meat, vegetables and broth cook in the bottom part. A quicker method, presented here, involves preparing the grain and other food separately and assembling them to be served together. Precooked packaged couscous grain found now in supermarkets makes the preparation of the dish easy and quick.

STEW
    1 tablespoon oil
    2 medium onions, chopped
    1 green pepper, chopped
    2 carrots, cut in 1-inch pieces
    3 tomatoes, chopped *or* 1 can (16
      ounces) unsalted tomatoes, drained
    1 pound squash, turnips or sweet
      potatoes, cut in 1-inch pieces
    1 pound chicken, skinned, boned and
      cubed
    5 cups water or enough to cover
    ½ teaspoon Lite Salt or less
    ½ teaspoon pepper
    ½ teaspoon ground ginger
    ½ teaspoon turmeric
    ½ teaspoon ground cumin
    1 can (16 ounces) garbanzo beans,
      drained *

In a large cooking pot, sauté onions in oil. Add all other listed ingredients together except garbanzo beans. Cook, covered, until chicken and vegetables are tender. Add garbanzo beans. Heat through.

GRAIN
    2 cups dry medium-grain couscous
    1 cup boiling water
    1 cup broth from stew

In a large bowl combine couscous, water and broth. Cover and let stand for 5 minutes. Fluff with fork.
To assemble: Place couscous in serving dish. Top with chicken vegetable stew.

Makes 5 servings.

* Use low-sodium beans if available.

EASY OVEN LASAGNA

An old favorite, prepared an easier way—with *uncooked noodles!*

    ¼ pound ground turkey *or* ground beef
      (10 percent fat)
    ¾ cup water
    4 cups Marinara Sauce, page 376
    8 ounces uncooked lasagna noodles
    1 cup low-fat cottage cheese
    ¾ cup sliced part-skim mozzarella cheese
    ¼ cup grated Parmesan cheese

Preheat oven to 375°. Brown ground turkey in nonstick fry pan and drain well. Add water and Marinara Sauce; bring to boil. Remove from heat. In 2-quart (9-by-13-inch) dish, layer sauce, uncooked lasagna noodles, cottage cheese, mozzarella cheese; repeat layers, ending with sauce and Parmesan cheese. The sauce will be runny. Cover dish with foil and bake for 1 hour. Let stand 5–10 minutes before cutting into squares.

Makes 6–8 generous servings (about 4-by-4 inches).

HOMEMADE RAVIOLIS

Have a party and make these with a group of friends! This recipe is for 12 servings, but it can be easily increased if you wish to put some in the freezer.

SAUCE
12 cups Marinara Sauce, page 376

Prepare sauce and set aside to warm up at serving time.

FILLING
1½ cups cooked chicken (white meat)
1 carrot, chopped
1 stalk celery, chopped
1 small onion, chopped
⅓ package frozen chopped spinach
⅓ cup chopped parsley
2 teaspoons garlic powder
1 teaspoon oregano leaves
1 teaspoon basil leaves
¼ teaspoon pepper
¼ teaspoon Lite Salt or less

Bone and cube chicken. Steam carrots, celery, onions and frozen spinach together in a small amount of water until done. Drain well. Put chicken and vegetables through meat grinder using coarse grind or use a food processor. Add spices to meat/vegetable paste and mix well together. Chill until pasta is prepared. (Unused filling may be frozen.)

Makes filling for 12 dozen raviolis.

PASTA
(These are easier to make if you have a ravioli rolling pin.)

4 cups flour
8 egg whites
4 tablespoons oil
Water

Measure 2 cups of flour into a large bowl; shape deep well in center. Place egg whites and oil in well. Beat egg white/oil mixture with fork until smooth; stir flour from well gradually into egg mixture to make a stiff sticky dough. Knead remaining 2 cups of flour into dough until smooth and elastic on a floured bread board. Sprinkle with water if more moisture is needed. Cover with towel; let stand for 10 minutes.

Roll the dough into a large rectangle on a large flat surface (the kitchen table works well). The dough should be about ⅛ inch thick. Spread ½ of dough with a thin layer of filling (about ⅛ inch thick also). Bring the unfilled half of dough over filled half to cover filling and roll a ravioli rolling pin over it, or mark in squares with a wooden yardstick. Cut the raviolis apart with a pastry cutter. Cook according to directions below or prepare for freezer by placing ravioli in plastic container, separating layers with waxed paper.

Cooking and serving: Place raviolis in unsalted boiling water for 10–12 minutes. Boil gently so they will not split. Drain carefully and arrange on a serving dish. Cover with hot Marinara Sauce and serve with grated Parmesan cheese.

Makes 12 servings (1 dozen raviolis each).

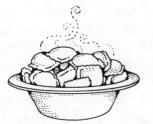

RABBIT FRICASSEE

Anyone ready for a new culinary experience, a hearty French peasant dish? Rabbit can be found or ordered at the meat counter of many supermarkets. It tastes much like chicken, but is sweeter. Serve with brown rice or steamed potatoes; steamed vegetables such as carrots or turnips are the traditional accompaniment to this dish. A piece of crusty French bread (no spread, please!), a green salad and some fruit for dessert complete the meal.

MARINADE
   1 cup wine (full-bodied red is preferable)
   1 tablespoon freshly squeezed lemon juice
   1 small bay leaf
   4 sprigs of fresh thyme *or* ½ teaspoon dried thyme leaves
   ¼ teaspoon marjoram leaves
   ¼ teaspoon Lite Salt or less
   Pepper to taste
   1 whole rabbit, 2½–3 pounds, cut up
   1 tablespoon oil
   1 medium onion, chopped
   1 clove garlic, minced
   1 tablespoon flour or cornstarch

Mix wine, lemon juice, bay leaf, thyme, marjoram, Lite Salt and pepper. Let rabbit pieces marinate in mixture for at least 12 hours in refrigerator. When ready to cook, remove rabbit pieces from marinade; dry well. Strain marinade and set aside.

   Heat oil in a deep saucepan. Cook onions over medium heat until golden brown. Add rabbit pieces. Toss rapidly. Sprinkle with garlic and flour *or* cornstarch. Brown.

   Add the strained marinade. Cover and simmer until tender (1–1½ hours).

   Remove rabbit pieces to a serving dish. Strain sauce, if necessary, and pour over rabbit.

Makes 6 servings.

NOTE: Chicken can be substituted for rabbit. Fricassee can be made ahead of time, cooled or frozen and then reheated when ready to serve. It will taste even better.

TURKEY-MUSHROOM SPAGHETTI SAUCE—Easy

Spaghetti and meat sauce! Only the cook will know that it's low-fat ground turkey.

   ½ cup minced onion
   ½ pound ground turkey
   ½ cup sliced fresh mushrooms *or* 1 can (4 ounces) mushrooms, drained
   ½ cup water
   2 cloves garlic, minced
   1 can (16 ounces) unsalted tomatoes
   1 can (6 ounces) unsalted tomato paste
   1 teaspoon parsley flakes
   1 bay leaf
   ¾ teaspoon basil leaves
   1 teaspoon oregano leaves
   ⅛ teaspoon pepper
   ¼ cup chopped green pepper (optional)

Sauté onions in nonstick pan. Add ground turkey and crumble with a fork. Stir until browned. Mix in mushrooms, water, garlic, tomatoes, tomato paste, parsley, bay leaf, basil, oregano and black pepper. Simmer 1–2 hours, adding green peppers if desired for last 10 minutes of cooking. Serve over cooked spaghetti.

   Makes 4 cups sauce (enough for 8 cups of pasta).

Curries

COUNTRY CAPTAIN

Chicken with a spicy tomato-curry sauce. Serve with brown rice and garnish with a little low-fat yogurt, if desired.

4 chicken breasts, skinned
1 tablespoon oil
1 onion, chopped
1 green pepper, chopped
1 clove garlic, minced
1 teaspoon (or more) curry powder
2 cans (16 ounces each) unsalted tomatoes, chopped
½ cup raisins

Preheat oven to 350°. Brown the chicken breasts in oil. Remove them from the pan and sauté onions, green peppers and garlic in the drippings. (Add a little water if they stick.) Add the curry powder and stir to mix. Stir in the chopped tomatoes, heat mixture and transfer to a baking dish. Place chicken in baking dish; spoon some sauce over the top.

Bake 30 minutes until almost done. Add raisins and bake for 10 minutes more.

Makes 4 servings.

CURRIED CHICKEN QUICKIE—Easy

4 chicken breasts (boned, if desired)
1 can (10½ ounces) low-sodium cream of mushroom soup or use Homemade "Cream" Soup Mix, page 261
2½ cups hot water
2 cups skim milk or chicken broth
2½ cups uncooked white rice*
2 teaspoons curry powder
½ teaspoon Lite Salt or less

Heat oven to 350°. Skin chicken. Combine liquid ingredients in a saucepan. Bring to a boil. Add rice, curry powder and Lite Salt and mix; heat to boiling again.

Lay chicken breasts in a 9-by-13-inch baking dish. Pour soup-rice mixture over the top. Cover tightly with foil and bake for 30 minutes. Remove from oven and let set for 10 minutes.

Makes 6 servings.

* When using brown rice, cook rice in hot soup mixture for 10 minutes before adding to chicken and putting into oven.

FAR EAST CHICKEN—Easy

Unusual ingredients make this dish fun to serve!

1 onion, sliced
1 tablespoon oil
1 or 2 cloves garlic, minced
6 chicken breasts, skinned
¼ cup honey
½ teaspoon Lite Salt or less
1½ cups grapefruit juice
1 teaspoon cinnamon
2 teaspoons curry powder
1 zucchini, sliced
1 green pepper, sliced
1 cup crushed pineapple

Sauté onions in oil in a large skillet. Add garlic and chicken breasts and continue to sauté until chicken breasts are brown. Mix together honey, Lite Salt, grapefruit juice and spices, then pour over the chicken. Simmer for 30 minutes. Add sliced vegetables and pineapple and simmer for 10 minutes until vegetables are crisp-tender. Serve over rice. Sauce can be thickened with a little cornstarch, if needed.

Makes 6 servings.

Chicken-Turkey Specialties

ACAPULCO ENCHILADAS ✓

A favorite recipe—this is great served with Spanish Rice and tossed green salad.

12 corn tortillas
2 cups canned enchilada sauce (mild)
1 can (8 ounces) unsalted tomato sauce
3 cups diced cooked chicken or turkey (white meat)
¼ cup sliced black olives
2 tablespoons slivered almonds
½ cup grated imitation mozzarella cheese
2 cups plain low-fat yogurt *or* 2 cups Mock Sour Cream, page 224
¼ cup chopped green onions

Preheat oven to 350°. Soften tortillas by wrapping in wax paper and microwaving for ½–2 minutes or by wrapping in foil and warming in conventional oven for 10 minutes. Mix enchilada sauce and tomato sauce. Mix chicken, olives, and almonds with about ½ cup sauce to moisten.

Spoon ¼ cup of chicken mixture down center of each warm tortilla. Roll and place seam side down in a 9-by-13-inch baking dish. When all are in place, cover with remaining sauce and grated cheese. Bake uncovered for 15–20 minutes. Before serving, spoon yogurt or Mock Sour Cream down center of dish and sprinkle with green onions.

Makes 6 servings.

CHICKEN SALAD WITH YOGURT-CHIVE DRESSING

6 chicken breasts
2 cans (8 ounces each) sliced water chestnuts, drained
1 can (8 ounces) pineapple chunks, drained
½ cup chopped celery
½ cup chopped green pepper
Leaf lettuce
Cucumber slices for garnish

YOGURT-CHIVE DRESSING
2 cups plain low-fat yogurt
2 tablespoons imitation mayonnaise
2 tablespoons dry white wine
1 tablespoon chopped chives
1 teaspoon freshly squeezed lemon juice
⅛ teaspoon garlic powder
¼ teaspoon curry powder (optional)

Preheat oven to 350°. Skin chicken and arrange in an ovenproof casserole dish. Cover loosely with foil and bake for 25–30 minutes until just tender. Cool. Remove from bones and cube chicken.

Toss in a large bowl water chestnuts, pineapple chunks, celery, green peppers and cooked chicken cubes. Combine dressing ingredients and pour over chicken mixture. Toss. Cover and chill until serving time.

When ready to serve, arrange chicken salad on a bed of leaf lettuce and garnish with cucumber slices.

Makes 6 servings.

CORNISH GAME HENS À LA CROCK—Easy

Using a Crockpot is an easy way to prepare these delicate birds. Serve with bread and tangy Salata.

1 box (6 ounces) wild rice and brown
  rice mix
4½ cups water
1 cup uncooked brown rice
2 Cornish game hens, thawed

Pour contents of wild rice and brown rice mix into Crockpot. Add water plus ½ seasoning packet. Add 1 cup of uncooked brown rice and thawed game hens. Turn Crockpot on high and cook slowly until hens are tender and water is absorbed (3–4 hours). With kitchen shears split cooked hens lengthwise. Remove skin, if possible, and serve on platter with the rice mixture.

Makes 4 servings.

CROCKED CHICKEN—Easy

A Crockpot dish.

1 chicken, cut up and skinned
2 stalks celery, sliced
1 can (8 ounces) bamboo shoots, drained
1 can (4 ounces) mushrooms, drained
1 onion, chopped
1 can (8 ounces) sliced water chestnuts
1 cup chicken broth
1 tablespoon cornstarch
¼ cup water

Place all ingredients except cornstarch and water in Crockpot and cook on low about 8 hours. Remove large pieces of chicken from Crockpot. Make a paste using cornstarch and water. Thicken the sauce with the cornstarch paste, bring to a boil and stir briefly. Remove bones from chicken, if possible, and return chicken to pot to reheat. Serve over rice.

Makes 6 servings.

LEMONY CHICKEN KABOBS

These are for those evenings you wish to use the backyard barbecue. Chicken chunks and vegetables are marinated in lemon juice with a touch of cayenne pepper for zip and laced on skewers with zucchini and mushrooms. They're fun to make as well as to eat!

3 lemons
1 tablespoon oil
1 tablespoon sugar
1 tablespoon vinegar
½ teaspoon Lite Salt or less
¼ teaspoon cayenne pepper
1 clove garlic, minced
4 chicken breasts
3 small zucchini
½ pound medium-sized mushrooms

About 3 hours before serving or earlier: Prepare marinade by grating 1 tablespoon of peel from lemons and squeezing juice from lemons to make ⅓ cup. Mix lemon peel, lemon juice, oil, sugar, vinegar, Lite Salt, cayenne and garlic in small bowl and set aside.

Remove bones and skin from chicken and cut chicken into chunks. Cut zucchini into 1-inch slices. Trim tough stem ends from mushrooms. Add chicken, zucchini and mushrooms to marinade; toss lightly to coat well. Cover and refrigerate at least 2 hours, stirring occasionally.

About 30 minutes before serving: On four 14-inch skewers, alternately thread chicken, zucchini and mushrooms (reserving marinade). Broil 15 minutes or until chicken is fork-tender, brushing frequently with marinade and turning kabobs.

Makes 4 servings.

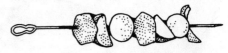

✓ good

PARMESAN YOGURT CHICKEN—Easy

A quickly prepared baked chicken with a zippy sauce. For a company dinner, use thighs and breasts.

1 chicken, cut in pieces and skinned
2 tablespoons freshly squeezed lemon juice
Cayenne pepper or Tabasco sauce, to taste
1 cup plain low-fat yogurt
2 tablespoons flour
¼ cup imitation mayonnaise
2 tablespoons Dijon mustard
¼ teaspoon Worcestershire sauce
½ teaspoon thyme leaves
¼ cup minced green onions
Paprika
2 tablespoons grated Parmesan cheese

Preheat oven to 350°. Arrange chicken in lightly oiled baking dish. Drizzle with lemon juice. Sprinkle lightly with cayenne pepper *or* Tabasco sauce (use more if you like it hot!). In small bowl mix yogurt with flour and add mayonnaise, mustard, Worcestershire and thyme. Spread over chicken. Top with green onions and sprinkle with paprika. Bake uncovered for 60 minutes or until fork tender. Sprinkle chicken evenly with Parmesan cheese. Broil 6 inches from heat until cheese is slightly brown. Serve warm. Sauce is good served over brown rice.

Makes 6 servings.

POLLO TEPEHUANO (pronounced poyo teppawano!)

A chicken and rice dish. This recipe comes from a little town in Mexico. Serve with Sunshine Spinach Salad, warm corn tortillas and a fruit dessert.

2 cans (13½ ounces each) chicken broth plus 2 cans water *or* 6 cups water plus 2 chicken bouillon cubes
2 cans (4 ounces each) diced green chiles
2–3 cloves garlic, chopped
¼–½ teaspoon ground cumin
6 green onions, chopped
2 cups uncooked brown rice
6 chicken breasts
3 medium tomatoes, coarsely chopped
½ cup coarsely chopped cilantro leaves

6 corn tortillas

Combine broth, water, chiles, garlic, cumin and green onions in a large saucepan. Bring to a boil and then add rice and chicken breasts which have been skinned and boned. Cover and reduce heat. Simmer until chicken and rice are just tender, about 60 minutes. When rice is done, gently stir in chopped tomatoes and cilantro. Cover and cook over low heat for about 5 minutes to blend flavors. Serve over corn tortillas, which have been torn up. The dish will have a soupy consistency so serve it in bowls.

Makes 6 servings.

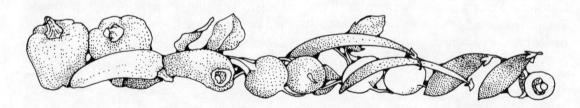

PORTLAND FRIED CHICKEN
—Easy

Our version of fried chicken—much lower in fat and just as good as the traditional recipe.

1 chicken, cut in pieces and skinned
¼ teaspoon pepper
1½ cups crushed Rice Krispies
¼ teaspoon paprika

Preheat oven to 350°. Roll damp chicken in crushed cereal. Place on nonstick baking sheet and sprinkle with pepper and paprika. Bake uncovered for 1 hour. If crispier chicken is preferred, begin baking at 400° for 20 minutes, then lower heat to 350°.

Makes 6 servings.

SIMPLY WONDERFUL TURKEY SALAD

A main dish salad. Fresh spinach and wild rice are a great combination. The dressing is especially delicious.

SALAD
1 package (6 ounces) long-grain and wild rice mix
1 cup cubed cooked turkey (white meat)
¼ pound fresh mushrooms, sliced
2 cups fresh spinach leaves, cut into thin strips
2 green onions with tops, sliced
1 can (8 ounces) sliced water chestnuts, drained
1 cup cooked white rice, cold
10 cherry tomatoes, halved

DRESSING
⅓ cup dry white wine
2 tablespoons oil

2 tablespoons sugar
¼ teaspoon pepper

The day before: Cook wild rice mix with seasoning packet according to package directions, omitting margarine. Cover and chill in refrigerator. Be sure to have 1 cup cooked white rice on hand, also.

Several hours before serving: Add cooked turkey, mushrooms, raw spinach, green onions, water chestnuts and plain cooked white rice to wild rice. Prepare dressing. Add to salad; mix well. Chill in covered container. Add tomatoes just before serving.

Makes 6 servings (1½ cups each).

SOUTH SEAS CHICKEN
—Easy

To serve on a busy day—the tangy marinade on this chicken makes a good sauce for brown rice. Add your favorite vegetable for a nice meal.

⅓ cup vinegar
⅓ cup lower-sodium soy sauce
1 clove garlic, minced
⅛ teaspoon pepper
1 whole chicken, cut in pieces and skinned or 6 chicken breasts

Combine vinegar, soy sauce, garlic and pepper. Marinate chicken in this mixture 30 minutes or longer. Preheat oven to 350°. Bake chicken and marinade in covered dish for 50–60 minutes.

Makes 6 servings.

TEXAS HASH—Easy

Travels well to potlucks or feeds a gang of hungry teenagers. Corn bread and salad are nice additions for a casual meal.

1 tablespoon oil
3 large onions, chopped
1 large green pepper, chopped
½ pound ground turkey
2 cans (16 ounces each) unsalted tomatoes
2 cups uncooked macaroni
1 teaspoon chili powder
½–1 teaspoon pepper
½ teaspoon Lite Salt or less
½ cup water

Preheat oven to 350°. Heat oil in nonstick fry pan. Sauté onions and green peppers, stirring often. Add ground turkey and continue to cook, stirring, until turkey browns slightly. Break up tomatoes with a spoon and add along with uncooked macaroni, seasonings and ½ cup water. Turn into a casserole dish and bake, covered, 30 minutes; remove cover and continue baking 15–20 minutes.

Makes 4 servings (2½ cups each).

TURKEY-VEGETABLE CHOWDER

The meatballs in this hearty soup are delicious and easily prepared by browning in the oven. Whole Wheat Muffins are a great addition.

SOUP BASE
1 medium onion, chopped
1 clove garlic, crushed
1 tablespoon oil
4 cans (16 ounces each) unsalted tomatoes, mashed

2 cans (8 ounces each) unsalted tomato sauce
2 cans (16 ounces each) pinto or kidney beans, drained *
1 teaspoon Worcestershire sauce
½ teaspoon Lite Salt or less
⅛ teaspoon pepper
2 teaspoons basil leaves

MEATBALLS
¼ cup grated Parmesan cheese
½ teaspoon thyme leaves
½ cup cracker crumbs
1 pound ground turkey or chicken

6 cups finely chopped cabbage

Sauté onions and garlic in oil in large soup kettle. Add tomatoes, tomato sauce, beans, Worcestershire sauce, Lite Salt, pepper and basil. Simmer 30 minutes to 2 hours.

Meanwhile prepare meatballs. Combine Parmesan cheese, thyme, cracker crumbs and ground turkey *or* chicken. Shape this mixture into 36 ¾-inch balls and place on nonstick baking sheet. Bake at 375° for 15 minutes to brown. Drain on paper towel. Twenty minutes before serving time add meatballs and chopped cabbage to soup. Simmer approximately 20 minutes.

Makes 10 servings (2 cups each).

* Use low-sodium beans if available.

BEEF,
VEAL AND PORK

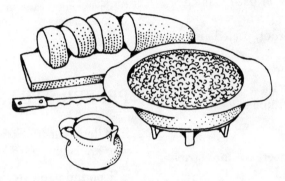

A small amount of lean red meat goes a long way in New American Diet cooking. In keeping with our credo of "meat as a condiment" we've included some favorite beef, veal and pork recipes that provide flavor, while keeping the saturated fat and cholesterol content down. As always, these recipes include plenty of foods from the vegetable realm, and some interesting seasonings.

In recipes that call for round steak, well trimmed chuck may be used. Always use the leanest ground beef, and/or drain off any excess fat from browning. Try ground turkey or turkey sausage for a flavor change—they are low in fat.

CASSEROLES

Bayou Red Beans over Rice
Bean Hot Dish
Beef and Bean Ragout
Beef Barley Skillet
Pizza Rice Casserole
Stay-Abed Stew
Tamale Pie
Veal Stew with Dill

ELEGANT ENTRÉES

Beef Stroganoff
Flank Steak Teriyaki
Moo Shoo Pork
Stuffed Flank Steak Florentine
Veal Roll-Ups

CASUAL MEALS

Beef-Mushroom Spaghetti Sauce
Taco Salad
Vegetable-Beef Soup

STIR-FRIED DISHES

Beef-Tomato Chow Yuk
Pepper Steak

Stir-Fried Dishes

BEEF-TOMATO CHOW YUK

Very attractive stir-fry dish. The fresh ginger makes it special. Good served over steamed rice.

½ **pound flank steak** *or* **use trimmed round steak**
1 **slice fresh ginger root, peeled and minced** *
1 **clove garlic, crushed**
1 **teaspoon cornstarch**
1 **teaspoon lower-sodium soy sauce**
1 **egg white**
1 **tablespoon oil**
1 **medium green pepper, cut into strips**
2 **stalks celery, sliced**
1 **medium onion, cut into strips**
½ **cup water**
¼ **cup low-sodium ketchup**
3 **tablespoons sugar (or less if tomatoes are very ripe)**
1 **tablespoon cornstarch**
2 **tablespoons water**
4 **medium tomatoes, peeled,† seeded and cut into quarters**

Cut the beef into very thin slices (it cuts better if partially frozen). Mix ginger root, garlic, cornstarch, soy sauce and egg white. Add the sliced beef; stir and allow to marinate for 5 minutes.

Put the oil in a preheated skillet or wok; stir-fry the meat until the redness is gone. Remove the meat and set aside. Add the green peppers, celery and onions to the pan along with the water. Cover and cook at medium heat for 3 minutes.

Add the ketchup and sugar; cover and cook for 2 minutes. Meanwhile, mix cornstarch with 2 tablespoons water; stir into the beef mixture and add to pan. Cook until liquid is clear and slightly thickened. Add tomatoes; cover and cook just until heated through. Serve with steamed rice.

Makes 4 servings.

* Chop remaining ginger root and freeze in tightly covered container, ready for the next time you need it.

† Tomatoes peel easily after plunging in boiling water for 30 seconds.

PEPPER STEAK

Excellent stir-fry dish to prepare for people who are beginning a low-fat eating style.

1 **pound flank steak**
1 **tablespoon Chinese rice wine** *or* **pale dry sherry**
3 **tablespoons lower-sodium soy sauce**
1 **teaspoon sugar**
2 **teaspoons cornstarch**
1 **tablespoon oil**
2 **medium green peppers, cut into ½-inch squares**
4 **slices fresh ginger root, peeled and cut ⅛ inch thick** *

Cut the flank steak lengthwise into strips 1½ inches wide, then crosswise into ¼-inch slices.

In a large bowl, mix the wine, soy sauce, sugar and cornstarch. Add the steak slices and toss with a large spoon to coat them thoroughly. The steak may be cooked at once, or marinated for as long as 6 hours.

Heat oil in a wok or large skillet over high heat for about 30 seconds. Reduce the heat to moderate if the oil begins to smoke. Immediately add the pepper squares and stir-fry for 3 minutes, or until they are tender but still crisp. Scoop them out with a slotted spoon and reserve. Add the ginger to the wok, stir for a few seconds, then add the steak mixture. Stir-fry for about 2 minutes, or until the meat shows no sign of pink. Discard the ginger. Add the pepper and cook for a minute, stirring, then transfer the contents of the pan to a heated platter and serve with steamed rice.

Makes 4 servings.

* Chop remaining ginger root and feeeze in tightly covered container, ready for the next time you need it.

Casseroles

BAYOU RED BEANS OVER RICE

A creole favorite—a basic hot bean and rice recipe that can be varied with other spices or more vegetables. Serve Ricotta Cheesecake for dessert.

2½ cups uncooked red kidney beans
4 cups water
Ham bone with 1 cup chopped ham *
1 large onion, chopped
2 stalks celery with leaves, chopped
1–2 teaspoons Tabasco sauce
1 green pepper, chopped (optional)

Soak beans overnight in water. Pour into a large heavy pan or Dutch oven. Add remaining ingredients. Cover and simmer 3 hours or until beans are tender. Remove ham bone, cut off meat and add to beans. Add more water when necessary during cooking. Water should barely cover beans at end of cooking time and beans should be soft, but not mushy. Remove 1 cup of beans at end of cooking time

and mash slightly. Add back to the beans and stir until liquid is thickened. Serve over rice. The addition of green pepper toward the end of cooking adds a little color.

Makes 8 servings (1 cup each).

* Ham flavored TVP may be substituted for ham, making it a meatless dish.

BEAN HOT DISH—Easy

This recipe freezes well. Any combination of beans can be used. It also works well in a Crockpot.

½ cup diced onion
½ pound ground beef (10 percent fat)
¼ cup brown sugar
½ cup low-sodium ketchup
2 tablespoons vinegar
1 tablespoon prepared mustard
1 can (16 ounces) lima beans *
1 can (16 ounces) small red beans *
1 can (16 ounces) kidney beans *
1 can (16 ounces) butter beans *

Preheat oven to 300°. In a nonstick fry pan brown diced onions and lean ground beef. Drain off fat. Drain beans and mix remaining ingredients together. Add to meat and onions and bake 1½ hours in a covered baking dish.

Makes 6 servings (1½ cups each).

* Use low-sodium beans if available.

BEEF AND BEAN RAGOUT

A hearty stew with beans and beef—well liked even by people who thought they didn't like beans.

1 cup uncooked or 2½ cups canned
   kidney beans *or* red beans *
3 cups water (omit if using canned beans)
1 pound trimmed round steak, cut in
   1-inch cubes
1 tablespoon oil
3 cans (16 ounces each) unsalted
   tomatoes, undrained, cut up
¾ cup dry red wine
1 teaspoon sugar
2 cloves garlic, minced
½ teaspoon Lite Salt or less
½ teaspoon thyme leaves
⅛ teaspoon pepper
3 bay leaves
3 potatoes, cubed (about 3 cups)
2 medium onions, cut in wedges
1 green pepper, chopped

Rinse dried beans. Place in 3-quart saucepan with the water; soak overnight. (Or bring to boiling; reduce heat and simmer 2 minutes. Remove from heat; cover and let stand 1 hour.) Do not drain. Bring beans to boiling; reduce heat. Cover and simmer 45 minutes. Drain.

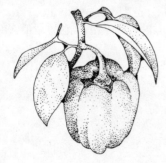

In 4-quart Dutch oven, brown meat in 1 tablespoon oil; drain. Add drained beans, the undrained tomatoes, wine, sugar, garlic, Lite Salt, thyme, pepper and bay leaves to the meat. Bring to boiling; reduce heat. Cover and simmer 1 hour or until meat is nearly tender. Add potatoes, onions and green peppers. Cook 30 minutes more or until meat and vegetables are tender. (The longer the mixture is simmered, the better it tastes!) Remove bay leaves before serving.

Makes 8 servings (about 18 cups).

* Use low-sodium beans if available.

BEEF BARLEY SKILLET

¾ pound ground beef (10 percent fat)
½ cup chopped onion
¼ cup chopped green pepper
¼ cup chopped celery
Pepper to taste
½ teaspoon marjoram leaves
1 teaspoon sugar
1 teaspoon Worcestershire sauce
½ cup chili sauce
1 can (16 ounces) unsalted tomatoes,
   broken up
1½ cups water
¾ cup uncooked barley

Sauté in nonstick fry pan meat, onions, green peppers and celery. Drain off excess fat; stir in remaining ingredients. Bring to a boil. Reduce heat to simmer, cover and cook about 1 hour (35 minutes for quick-cooking barley).

Makes 4 servings (about 7 cups).

PIZZA RICE CASSEROLE

This is an all-family favorite. Great with hot French bread.

- ⅔ cups uncooked brown rice
- 1⅓ cup water
  (*or* use 2 cups leftover cooked rice)
- ½ pound ground beef (10 percent fat)
- 1 onion, chopped
- 2 cans (8 ounces each) unsalted tomato sauce
- ¼ teaspoon garlic powder
- 1 teaspoon sugar
- Dash pepper
- ¼ teaspoon oregano leaves
- 1 teaspoon parsley flakes
- 1½ cups low-fat cottage cheese
- ½ cup grated low-fat cheese

Preheat oven to 325°. Cook rice in water or have leftover rice ready. Brown ground beef and onion in a nonstick fry pan. Drain fat. Add tomato sauce and spices to beef-onion mixture. Cover and simmer for 15 minutes. Combine cottage cheese and rice. Put a third of rice mixture in lightly oiled casserole dish. Top with a third of meat-tomato sauce. Continue to alternate layers, ending with tomato sauce. Sprinkle grated low-fat cheese on top. Bake for 30 minutes or until hot and bubbly.

Makes 6 servings (about 10 cups).

STAY-ABED STEW

This goes in a very low oven ea̶ morning to cook all day. Great wit̶ or add dumplings on top.

- 1 pound trimmed round steak
- 1 onion, chopped
- 1 can (16 ounces) unsalted green beans, undrained
- 1 can (4 ounces) mushrooms, undrained
- 1 green pepper, chopped
- 2 medium potatoes, chunked
- 3 carrots, chunked
- ½ teaspoon Lite Salt or less
- 1 tablespoon parsley flakes
- ½ cup instant tapioca
- 1 can (13 ounces) tomato juice
- 1 cup water

Preheat oven to 250°. Trim and cube round steak and place in bottom of casserole pan. Mix vegetables, seasonings and dry tapioca and spread over meat. Pour tomato juice and water over all. (Add more water if you want thin stew.) Bake for 6–8 hours, stirring occasionally.

Makes 4–6 servings (about 12 cups).

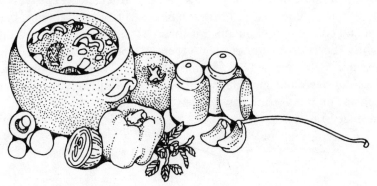

TAMALE PIE

A grain and bean staple with just a bit of beef for flavor. All that's needed to round out a meal is a salad and some fruit.

½ pound ground beef (10 percent fat)
¾ cup chopped onion
1 clove garlic, minced
½ cup chopped green pepper
1 can (16 ounces) unsalted whole kernel corn, drained
1 can (16 ounces) pinto, red or kidney beans, drained *
2 cans (8 ounces each) unsalted tomato sauce
¼ cup sliced black olives, drained
2–3 tablespoons taco sauce or salsa
2 teaspoons chili powder

TOPPING
1 cup yellow cornmeal
2½ cups water
¼ teaspoon Lite Salt or less
½ cup grated part-skim mozzarella cheese

Preheat oven to 375°. In nonstick fry pan brown ground beef with onions and garlic. Drain off fat. Add green peppers, corn, beans, tomato sauce, olives, taco sauce or salsa, and chili powder. Pour into 10-by-10-inch baking pan.

In saucepan combine cornmeal, water and Lite Salt. Stirring constantly, bring mixture to a boil and continue cooking until it thickens slightly. Spoon over top of meat/vegetable mixture. Bake for about 45 minutes. Remove from oven and sprinkle grated mozzarella cheese on top. Return pan to oven and bake another 15 minutes.

Makes 6 servings (about 9 cups).

* Use low-sodium beans if available.

VEAL STEW WITH DILL

2 pounds boneless stewing veal, well trimmed
1 large onion, chopped
6 peppercorns
3 whole cloves
½ teaspoon Lite Salt or less
1 cup chopped carrot
1 cup chopped celery
½ small lemon, sliced
1 teaspoon dill weed
2 tablespoons water
1 tablespoon flour
Juice of ½ lemon
Pepper to taste
1 teaspoon dill weed.

Cut veal into 1-inch cubes. Place veal, onions, peppercorns, cloves, Lite Salt, carrots, celery, lemon slices and 1 teaspoon dill weed in a large cooking pot. Add enough water to cover the meat. Heat to boiling; reduce heat and cover pan. Simmer until meat is tender —about 1 hour.

Remove meat to serving dish. Keep warm. Strain cooking liquid into a saucepan. Reserve the cooked vegetables and lemon slices. Mix 2 tablespoons water and flour until smooth. Stir into cooking liquid. Heat to boiling, stirring constantly until slightly thickened. Put vegetables and lemon in a blender container, blend into a puree, add to the sauce, mix. Add lemon juice and pepper. Stir and heat through.

Pour sauce over meat. Sprinkle with dill weed. Serve with rice, steamed potatoes or pasta.

Makes 8 servings (about 8 cups).

Elegant Entrées

BEEF STROGANOFF

A delicious low-fat version without the traditional sour cream.

    1 pound trimmed round steak
    2 tablespoons flour
    1 teaspoon paprika
    ½ onion, chopped
    1 clove garlic, crushed
    1 tablespoon oil
    1 can (4 ounces) mushrooms, undrained
    1 cup plain low-fat yogurt
    1 cube beef bouillon

Slice beef in thin, diagonal strips (may be easier to do if partially frozen). Mix flour and paprika, and shake beef strips in it to coat. Brown beef, onion and garlic in oil over high heat until brown. Stir in mushrooms, yogurt and bouillon cube. Heat to boiling, stirring constantly. Reduce heat, cover and simmer for 12–15 minutes. Serve over eggless noodles or macaroni ribbons.

Makes 4 servings (about 4 cups).

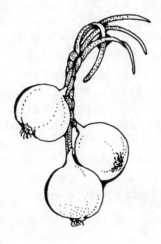

FLANK STEAK TERIYAKI

The sweet and sour sauce is delicious over Bulgur Pilaf. A good way to serve a grain and small amount of meat.

    1 tablespoon oil
    ¼ cup lower-sodium soy sauce
    ¼ cup honey
    2 tablespoons vinegar
    1½ teaspoons ground ginger
    2 tablespoons finely chopped green onion
    2 cloves garlic, minced
    1½ pounds flank steak

Combine ingredients and pour over flank steak. Marinate 4 hours or more, turning occasionally.

Grill over charcoal or broil on each side, turning once. Baste occasionally. Be careful not to overcook. Slice in thin slices, cutting on the diagonal across grain from top to bottom.

Makes 6 servings.

MOO SHOO PORK

For your Oriental dinner—this dish is usually accompanied by thin pancackes called Peking Doilies.* Hoisin sauce* is spread on the pancakes, then the Moo Shoo Pork mixture is placed on top. The pancake is then rolled up to enclose the filling.

    1 cup bean sprouts
    ⅓ cup lily buds*
    ⅓ cup black fungus (cloud ears*)
    1 tablespoon lower-sodium soy sauce
    1 teaspoon sugar
    4 ounces pork chop, well-trimmed and
       cut in match-sized pieces
    2 green onions

4 egg whites
¼ cup egg substitute (commercial *or*
  Homemade Egg Substitute, page 241)
1 tablespoon oil, divided
2 slices fresh ginger, peeled and minced

Blanch bean sprouts in boiling water for 10 seconds. In separate bowls, soak lily buds and black fungus in boiling water until soft, about 30 minutes. Combine soy sauce and sugar, add to shredded pork and toss. Shred white part of green onions and cut green part into 2-inch sections. Lightly beat egg whites and egg substitute together. Shred black fungus, discarding thicker part. Cut ends off lily buds and cut each in half.

In a large wok or skillet, heat 1 teaspoon of the oil. Add the beaten eggs and scramble quickly. Remove eggs while still moist and cut into slivers.

Heat the remaining 2 teaspoons oil. Add minced ginger and stir-fry. Add pork and stir-fry with ginger until pork loses its pinkness. To the pork, add bean sprouts, lily buds, black fungus and green onions. Stir-fry 1 minute, then cook covered, 1–2 minutes longer over medium heat.

Return scrambled eggs to pan and stir in to reheat. Serve at once.

Makes 4–6 servings (about 2½ cups).

* Available in Chinese grocery stores.

STUFFED FLANK STEAK FLORENTINE

Nice to serve for a special occasion with Mushroom Barley Pilaf and a salad.

2 pounds flank steak
3 egg whites, slightly beaten *or* ½ cup egg
  substitute (commercial *or* Homemade
  Egg Substitute, page 241)
2 packages (10 ounces each) frozen
  chopped spinach, cooked and drained
1 cup grated low-fat cheese
1 teaspoon sage
Dash pepper
1½ cups bread crumbs
3 tablespoons flour
1 tablespoon oil
2 cans (8 ounces each) unsalted tomato
  sauce
1 cup dry red wine
1 cup chopped onion
2 cloves garlic, minced

Preheat oven to 350°. Pound steak with meat mallet to ¼-inch thickness; set aside. Combine egg whites *or* egg substitute, spinach, cheese, sage and pepper; stir in bread crumbs. Spread mixture over steak. Starting from narrow side, roll up jelly-roll fashion; tie with string. Coat lightly with flour. In large skillet, heat oil and carefully brown steak rolls on all sides. Place in 9-by-13-inch baking dish.

Combine tomato sauce, wine, onion and garlic. Pour over meat. Cover with foil and bake for 1–1½ hours or until meat is tender. To serve meat, remove string and slice. Spoon sauce over steak rolls.

Makes 8 to 10 servings.

VEAL ROLL-UPS

Small cutlets with bread stuffing and a delicious mustard sauce.

- 2 cups bread stuffing cubes
- ½ cup water
- 8 boneless veal cutlets (about 2 pounds)
- 8 teaspoons Dijon mustard
- 3 tablespoons flour
- ½ cup egg substitute (commercial *or* Homemade Egg Substitute, page 241)
- 1 cup Italian bread crumbs
- 1 tablespoon oil
- 3 tablespoons snipped parsley

Prepare Mustard Sauce (see below). Mix bread stuffing cubes with water and stir with a fork. Pound meat until ¼ inch thick. Spread 1 teaspoon Mustard Sauce on each cutlet, then top with about 3 tablespoons bread stuffing. Roll up and secure with a wooden pick.

Coat rolls with flour, then dip into egg substitute and roll in bread crumbs. Heat oil in nonstick fry pan and brown—about 4 minutes. Transfer to lightly oiled baking dish. Pour half the mustard sauce over the top of the roll-ups; cover and bake in 325° oven until tender (about 30 minutes). Sprinkle parsley on rolls and serve with remaining Mustard Sauce.

MUSTARD SAUCE
- ¼ cup Dijon mustard
- 2 tablespoons sugar
- 1 tablespoon oil
- 2 tablespoons white wine
- 1 tablespoon dill weed

In a bowl, stir mustard and sugar with a wire whisk. Gradually add oil, wine and stir in the dill weed.

Makes about ½ cup sauce. Serves 8.

Casual Meals

BEEF-MUSHROOM SPAGHETTI SAUCE (with TVP)

Textured Vegetable Protein (TVP) is very low in fat and inexpensive! We recommend combining it with lean ground beef, such as in this spaghetti sauce, when using it for the first time.

- ½ cup TVP reconstituted with 1 cup water
- ½ cup minced onion
- 2 ounces ground beef (10 percent fat)
- ½ cup sliced fresh mushrooms *or* 1 can (4 ounces) mushrooms, drained
- 2 cloves garlic, minced
- 1 can (16 ounces) unsalted tomatoes
- 1 can (6 ounces) unsalted tomato paste
- 1 teaspoon parsley flakes
- 1 bay leaf
- ¾ teaspoon basil leaves
- ½–1 teaspoon oregano leaves
- ⅛ teaspoon pepper
- ¼ cup chopped green pepper (optional)
- ¼ cup grated Parmesan cheese for topping

Reconstitute TVP with water. Sauté onions and ground beef together; stir until browned. Mix in reconstituted TVP, mushrooms, garlic, tomatoes, tomato paste, parsley, bay leaf, basil, oregano and pepper. Simmer gently for 30 minutes. Add green peppers, if desired, the last 10 minutes of cooking. Serve over cooked spaghetti. Sprinkle with Parmesan cheese.

Makes about 4 cups of sauce.

TACO SALAD

Summer is here!

   2 cups Baked Corn Chips, page 220
   1 cup Thousand Island Salad Dressing,
      page 372, *or* commercial low-fat
      dressing
   ½ pound ground beef (10 percent fat)
   1 can (16 ounces) kidney beans,
      drained *
   1 teaspoon chili powder
   1 large head lettuce, chopped
   4 tomatoes, chopped
   ½ avocado, sliced
   ⅓ cup grated low-fat cheese
   2 tablespoons hot taco sauce

Prepare Baked Corn Chips and Thousand Island Salad Dressing according to directions.

Brown ground beef in a nonstick fry pan. Drain off fat. Add beans and chili powder and simmer 5 minutes. Chop vegetables and put in salad bowl.

Before serving, toss vegetables and grated cheese with bean/beef mixture and put in large salad bowl. Arrange Corn Chips around edge. Combine salad dressing and taco sauce. Serve in a pitcher along with salad.

Makes 6 to 8 servings (about 16 cups).

* Use low-sodium beans if available.

VEGETABLE-BEEF SOUP

An old standby made with lots of vegetables and enough meat for a good flavor. Serve with Old-Style Wheat Biscuits and Rhubarb Buckle.

   1 teaspoon oil
   ½ pound beef stew meat, well trimmed
   1 clove garlic, minced
   1 large onion, chopped
   2 carrots, julienned
   3 medium potatoes, peeled and chopped
   2 cans (16 ounces each) unsalted
      tomatoes
   5 cups water
   1½ teaspoons Lite Salt or less
   ⅛ teaspoon pepper
   ½ teaspoon basil leaves

Heat oil in fry pan. Add meat, garlic and onions. Stir rapidly until brown. Add carrots, potatoes, tomatoes, water, Lite Salt, pepper and basil. Bring to boil. Reduce heat. Cover and simmer at least 2 hours. Add water as needed to keep volume unchanged.

Makes 12 cups.

DESSERTS

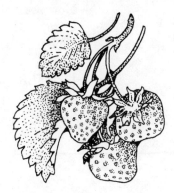

This section contains several ideas for a nice meal finale. An excellent choice is fruit or a fruit compote combination. Here we offer a wide variety of our favorite suggestions. Certainly a baked item is not a necessary part of every sack lunch or evening meal, but for an occasional treat these have been modified to be lower in fat, cholesterol, sugar and salt. Fiber has been increased by replacing part of the white flour with whole wheat flour. You will note serving sizes are often small—another example of low-fat eating.

CAKES
Angel Quickie
Apple Loaf Cake
Baba au Rhum
Baked Doughnut Holes
Chewy Wheat Germ Brownies
Chocolate Zucchini Cake

Cocoa Cake
Creme de Menthe Cheesecake
Depression Cake
Hot Fudge Pudding Cake
Party Carrot Cake
Pinto Fiesta Cake
Poppy Seed Cake
Ricotta Cheesecake

FRUIT DESSERTS
All Season Shortcake
Apple Crisp
Apricot Bavarian
Baked Apples
Bananas en Papillote
Fresh Fruit Crepes
Fruit Salad Alaska
Peach Cardinal
Pears in Wine
Rhubarb Buckle

FROZEN DESSERTS
Blueberry Ice
Frozen Fruit Yogurts
Strawberry Ice

PUDDINGS
Chocolate Pudding
Pumpkin Bread Pudding
Vanilla Pudding

PIES
Pumpkin Pie
Strawberry Yogurt Pie

COOKIES AND BARS
Apricot Meringue Bars
Carob Cookies
Crispy Spice Cookies
Forgotten Kisses
Gingies
Lebkuchen
Molasses Orange Bars
Northwest Harvest Bars
Oatmeal Cookies
Walnut Squares

DESSERT SPECIALTIES
Crepes
Graham Cracker Crust

Cakes

ANGEL QUICKIE

Tastes and looks wonderful! No need for a frosting. Leftover slices are very good toasted under the broiler and topped with fruit.

   1 package angel food cake mix
   ⅓ cup cocoa
   2 teaspoons powdered instant coffee
   (instant espresso is delicious)

Preheat oven to 350°. Follow directions on angel food mix package, stirring cocoa and coffee powder into dry mix. Beat 1½ minutes, scraping bowl often. Bake 40–50 minutes in *unoiled* tube pan. Invert and cool thoroughly.

   Makes 12 servings.

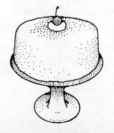

APPLE LOAF CAKE

   ½ cup apple juice *or* water
   ½ cup oil
   2 cups sugar
   3 egg whites *or* ½ cup egg substitute
   (commercial *or* Homemade Egg
   Substitute, page 241)
   1 teaspoon vanilla
   3 cups chopped unpeeled apples
   ¼ cup chopped nuts
   2 cups white flour
   1 cup whole wheat flour
   ¾ teaspoon nutmeg
   ¾ teaspoon cinnamon
   1½ teaspoons baking soda

Preheat oven to 325°. Mix ingredients in order given. Lightly oil a 10-inch tube or bundt pan and bake for 1 hour. Let cool before removing from pan.

   Makes 24 servings.

BABA AU RHUM (Savarin)

A rum-flavored yeast cake with red berry sauce served over it.

2 packages active dry yeast
1 cup skim milk, lukewarm
4 cups white flour
6 egg whites
2 teaspoons sugar
½ teaspoon Lite Salt
5 tablespoons margarine, melted

Dissolve yeast in lukewarm milk. In a large bowl, mix flour, egg whites and dissolved yeast. The dough should be smooth. Cover and let rise in a warm place for at least 1 hour and until the dough has doubled in volume.

Add sugar, Lite Salt and melted margarine to the dough. Mix well. It will be a soft, sticky dough this time. Oil a 12 cup mold (a ring mold works well) or a bundt cake pan. Put the dough in the pan to fill about halfway to the top. Let rise again, in the mold, from 1–2 hours.

Bake in a 375° oven. If the top becomes too brown cover for a while with foil. Bake 30 minutes or until "baba" pulls away from sides of pan.

Unmold while still warm. After cooling, put back in the mold to soak up the Rum Syrup.

RUM SYRUP
2 cups sugar
2 cups water
1 cup rum

Dissolve sugar in water. Bring to a boil and simmer for about 5 minutes, then add rum. Pour over the cooked and cooled baba, a tablespoon at a time, until all syrup is absorbed.

Unmold and serve with Strawberry or Raspberry Sauce, page 377, or any sauce of your choice to spoon over the top of each serving.

Makes 24 servings.

BAKED DOUGHNUT HOLES

Everyone loves these lower-fat little cakes. The fresher they are the better!

2 tablespoons oil
½ cup sugar
2 egg whites *or* ¼ cup egg substitute (commercial *or* Homemade Egg Substitute, page 241)
1 teaspoon vanilla
⅔ cup skim milk
2 cups white flour
1 tablespoon baking powder
½ teaspoon nutmeg

TOPPING
1½ tablespoons margarine
½ cup sugar
2 teaspoons cinnamon

Preheat oven to 400°. Cream oil, ½ cup sugar and egg whites *or* egg substitute. Add vanilla and skim milk; stir well. Sift dry ingredients and add gradually to the creamed mixture. Lightly oil *small* muffin tins and fill ⅔ full with batter. Bake 15–18 minutes.

While doughnuts are baking, prepare topping. Melt margarine and place in a small bowl. Mix sugar and cinnamon together in another small bowl. Brush warm doughnuts lightly with the melted margarine and then roll in the cinnamon-sugar mixture.

Makes 36 doughnuts.

CHEWY WHEAT GERM BROWNIES

2 tablespoons oil
1 tablespoon molasses
⅔ cup sugar
½ cup egg substitute (commercial or Homemade Egg Substitute, page 241)
2 teaspoons vanilla
1 cup wheat germ
½ cup powdered nonfat milk
½ teaspoon baking powder
¼ cup chopped walnuts

Preheat oven to 350°. Combine first 5 ingredients and stir well. Mix dry ingredients together in a separate bowl. Add walnuts to dry ingredients.

Combine the wet and dry ingredients, stirring only enough to blend. Spread in an 8-by-8-inch pan that has been completely lined with wax paper. Bake for 30 minutes. Turn out of pan and remove wax paper immediately. Cut into bars while hot.

Makes 16 small bars.

CHOCOLATE ZUCCHINI CAKE

A very nice cake which does not need to be frosted.

1 teaspoon vanilla
½ cup oil
1½ cups sugar
4 egg whites
½ cup skim milk
1 teaspoon baking soda
1¼ cups white flour
1¼ cups whole wheat flour
¼ cup cocoa powder
½ teaspoon cinnamon
½ teaspoon nutmeg
¼ teaspoon Lite Salt or less
2 cups grated zucchini

Preheat oven to 350°. Combine vanilla, oil, sugar, egg whites, and skim milk. Sift together baking soda, flours, cocoa, cinnamon, nutmeg and Lite Salt. Add dry ingredients alternately with zucchini to the first mixture.

Bake for 60–65 minutes in a lightly oiled bundt pan, or about 45 minutes in a 9-by-13-inch pan.

Makes 24 servings (about 2 by 2 inches).

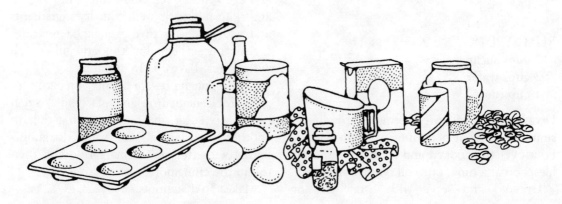

COCOA CAKE

Very versatile—can be made into cupcakes or into a cake. Serve unfrosted or top with berries.

1½ cups flour
1 cup sugar
1 teaspoon baking soda
3 tablespoons cocoa powder
3 tablespoons oil
1 teaspoon vanilla
1 tablespoon vinegar
1 cup cold water

Preheat oven to 350°. Sift dry ingredients together. Pour the liquid ingredients over the dry ingredients and stir until smooth. If making cupcakes, turn into 12 paper-lined muffin tins and bake for 25–30 minutes. For a cake, bake in ungreased 9-inch square pan for 35 minutes. Cool.

Makes 9 servings of cake or 12 cupcakes.

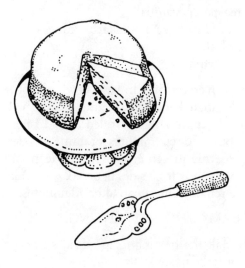

CREME DE MENTHE CHEESECAKE

A beautiful treat!

1 cup chocolate cookie crumbs (use Nabisco's "Famous Wafers"); reserve 2 tablespoons for topping
1 teaspoon sugar
2 tablespoons melted margarine
2½ cups part-skim ricotta cheese
⅔ cup plain low-fat yogurt
4 egg whites
¾ cup sugar
1 tablespoon cornstarch
⅓ cup creme de menthe

Preheat oven to 350°. To prepare crumbs, grind cookies in a blender (save 2 tablespoons for topping). Combine remaining chocolate crumbs, 1 teaspoon sugar and melted margarine in a small mixing bowl. Press firmly into the bottom of a 10-inch springform pan. Bake for 10 minutes; cool.

Blend approximately a third of the ricotta cheese, all the yogurt and egg whites in a covered blender until very smooth. *Note:* It is very important to blend this mixture until very smooth to obtain the desired texture. Add small amounts of the remaining ricotta cheese and blend until smooth. Gradually blend in ¾ cup sugar and cornstarch. Beat well. Blend in crème de menthe.

Pour over baked crust and bake for 1 hour and 10 minutes or until the cake feels firm when lightly touched near the center. Turn off oven heat and let the cake cool for 2 hours in the oven with the door ajar. *Note:* The cake will fall to approximately half its height. Chill. Release sides of pan. Sprinkle 2 tablespoons remaining chocolate crumbs over top.

Makes 12 servings.

DEPRESSION CAKE

From the days when sugar and eggs were scarce—now, it means healthful food.

- 1 cup raisins
- 2 cups water
- 2 tablespoons oil
- 1 cup brown sugar
- 1 cup white flour
- 1 cup whole wheat flour
- 1½ teaspoons baking soda
- 1 teaspoon cinnamon
- 1 teaspoon nutmeg

Preheat oven to 325°. Cook raisins in water. Simmer until 1 cup liquid remains. Set aside to cool. Cream sugar and oil. Add raisins and liquid. Beat with a spoon. Add flours, baking soda, spices and beat well. Bake in a lightly oiled 9-inch-square pan for 30–40 minutes.

Makes 9 servings.

HOT FUDGE PUDDING CAKE

A delicious treat!

- 1 cup flour
- 2 teaspoons baking powder
- ¾ cup sugar
- 2 tablespoons cocoa
- ½ cup skim milk
- 1 tablespoon oil
- ¼ cup chopped walnuts

TOPPING
- ¼ cup cocoa
- 1 cup brown sugar
- 1¾ cups *hot* water

Preheat oven to 350°. Sift together first 4 ingredients. Stir in skim milk and oil and then walnuts. Spread in a 9-inch-square unoiled pan. Prepare topping. Combine cocoa and brown sugar and sprinkle over batter. Pour the hot water over entire batter and topping. Bake for 45 minutes. During baking the cake mixture rises to the top and the chocolate sauce settles to the bottom. Invert square of pudding on dessert plates. Dip sauce from pan over each. Or, the entire pudding can be inverted in a deep serving platter.

Makes 12 servings (about 2¼ by 3 inches).

PARTY CARROT CAKE

- 2 cups sugar
- ½ cup oil
- 1½ cups whole wheat flour
- 1½ cups white flour
- 2½ teaspoons baking soda
- 2½ teaspoons cinnamon
- ½ teaspoon Lite Salt or less
- 2 cups shredded carrots
- 2 teaspoons vanilla
- 1 can (11 ounces) mandarin oranges, undrained
- 5 egg whites

Preheat oven to 350°. In large bowl, combine all cake ingredients. Beat 2 minutes at high speed. Pour into lightly oiled 9-by-13-inch pan. Bake 50–60 minutes or until wooden pick inserted in center comes out clean and cake pulls away from sides of pan. Cool. Cake can be removed from pan after 30 minutes.

"CREAM" CHEESE FROSTING

Make half the frosting recipe if sides of cake are not to be frosted.

- ½ package (4 ounces) light cream cheese or Neufchâtel, softened

1 teaspoon vanilla
2 cups powdered sugar

Blend ingredients in medium bowl; beat until smooth. Adjust powdered sugar as desired for proper firmness. Spread over cake. Store frosted cake in refrigerator.

Makes 24 servings (about 2 by 2 inches).

PINTO FIESTA CAKE

An unusual use of legumes, to say the least!

1 cup sugar
¼ cup margarine
2 egg whites, lightly beaten
2 cups cooked pinto beans, mashed, *or* refried beans *
1 cup flour
1 teaspoon baking soda
1 teaspoon cinnamon
½ teaspoon cloves
½ teaspoon allspice
2 cups diced raw apples
1 cup raisins
¼ cup chopped walnuts
2 teaspoons vanilla

Preheat oven to 375°. Cream sugar and margarine, add beaten egg whites. Add mashed beans. Mix well. Sift all dry ingredients (including spices) together and add to sugar mixture. Add apples, raisins, chopped walnuts and vanilla. Pour into lightly oiled 10-inch tube or bundt cake pan and bake for 45 minutes.

Makes 16 servings.

* Use low-sodium beans if available.

POPPY SEED CAKE

2 ounces poppy seeds
1 cup skim milk
½ cup egg substitute (commercial *or* Homemade Egg Substitute, page 241) *or* 3 egg whites
⅓ cup oil
1 cup sugar
1 teaspoon almond extract
Grated rind of 1 lemon
2 cups whole wheat flour
¼ cup powdered nonfat milk
½ teaspoon cinnamon
¼ teaspoon nutmeg
2½ teaspoons baking powder

Soak poppy seeds in skim milk for 1 hour. Preheat oven to 350°. Add egg whites, oil, sugar, almond extract and lemon rind to poppy seeds. Mix well, and combine with remaining ingredients, stirring only to just moisten the batter. Pour in lightly oiled 9-by-5-inch loaf pan. Bake 45–60 minutes. Prepare glaze and spread over warm cake.

GLAZE
2 tablespoons powdered sugar (approximate)
½ teaspoon vanilla, rum *or* brandy extract *or* lemon juice
1 tablespoon cornstarch
1–2 tablespoons hot water (depends on desired thickness)

Blend ingredients until glaze is smooth.

Makes 16 servings (½ inch each).

RICOTTA CHEESECAKE

Made with ricotta cheese and egg whites, this cheesecake tastes light and delicious.

1 cup graham cracker crumbs
2 tablespoons sugar
¼ teaspoon cinnamon
2 tablespoons melted margarine
2½ cups part-skim ricotta cheese
1 cup plain low-fat yogurt
4 egg whites
1 cup sugar
1 tablespoon cornstarch
1 teaspoon vanilla
3 tablespoons freshly squeezed lemon
  juice
Yogurt Dessert Sauce, page 377 (optional
  for topping)

Preheat oven to 350°. In a small bowl combine the cracker crumbs, sugar, cinnamon and margarine. Press firmly into the bottom of a 10-inch springform pan. Bake for 10 minutes. Cool.

Blend approximately a third of the ricotta cheese and all the yogurt and egg whites in a covered blender until very smooth. *Note:* It is very important to blend this mixture until very smooth to obtain the desired texture. Add small amounts of the remaining ricotta cheese and blend until smooth. Gradually blend in sugar and cornstarch. Beat well. Blend in vanilla and lemon juice.

Pour over crust in prepared pan and bake for 1 hour and 10 minutes or until the cake feels firm when lightly touched near the center. Turn off oven heat and let the cake cool for 2 hours in the oven with the door ajar. *Note:* The cake will fall to approximately half its height. Chill. Release sides of pan and place on serving dish.

If a topping is desired, Yogurt Dessert Sauce or a fruit sauce works well.

Makes 12 servings.

Fruit Desserts

ALL SEASON SHORTCAKE

Serve this easy shortcake all year long with berries, nectarines or peaches and vanilla yogurt.

3 egg whites
¾ cup sugar
1 teaspoon grated orange peel
½ teaspoon vanilla
½ cup skim milk
1 tablespoon margarine
1 cup flour
1 teaspoon baking powder
¼ teaspoon Lite Salt or less
¼ teaspoon ground nutmeg

6 cups fresh fruit, sliced as for shortcake
½ cup sugar
3 cups low-fat vanilla yogurt *or* Dream
  Whip prepared with skim milk

Cut a piece of waxed paper to fit the bottom of a 9-inch square baking pan. Lightly oil pan sides and paper.

Preheat oven to 350°. With a mixer, beat together the egg whites, sugar, orange peel and vanilla until very light and fluffy. In a small saucepan, heat the milk and margarine until hot, then stir into the egg mixture. In a bowl, stir together the flour, baking powder, Lite Salt and nutmeg. Add to the batter and stir to blend well. Pour batter into prepared pan.

Bake cake for 15 minutes, until center springs back when touched. Cool in pan for 5 minutes, then run a knife around sides to loosen. Turn out onto rack, peel off paper and cool completely.

Prepare fruit and mix with sugar. Chill until serving time.

When ready to serve, slice shortcake in half horizontally and place ½ on serving platter. Layer with 1½ cups yogurt or Dream Whip and 3 cups prepared fruit. Top with remaining cake half, 1½ cups yogurt or Dream Whip and 3 cups fresh fruit. Cut in squares to serve.

Makes 9 servings.

APPLE CRISP

Crispy! Crunchy! For a larger crowd you can double the recipe and use a 9-by-13-inch baking dish.

> 4 cups sliced peeled tart apples (about 4 medium)
> ⅓ cup brown sugar
> ¼ cup flour
> ¼ cup oatmeal
> ½ teaspoon cinnamon
> ¼ teaspoon nutmeg
> 2 tablespoons margarine, softened
> Vanilla yogurt *or* Yogurt Dessert Sauce, page 377 (optional for topping)

Preheat oven to 375°. Lightly oil an 8-inch square baking pan. Place apple slices in pan. Mix remaining ingredients thoroughly. Sprinkle over apples.

Bake 30 minutes or until apples are tender and topping is golden brown. Serve warm and, if desired, with vanilla yogurt or Yogurt Dessert Sauce.

Makes 4–6 servings.

APRICOT BAVARIAN

Unusual and very attractive.

> ½ cup dried apricots
> ½ cup frozen orange juice concentrate

> 1 envelope plus 1 teaspoon unflavored gelatin
> ¼ cup cold water
> 2 tablespoons freshly squeezed lemon juice
> ¾ cup plus 2 tablespoons granulated sugar
> 3 cups plain low-fat yogurt, divided in half
> 3 egg whites
> 3 oranges, thinly sliced

Cook apricots in the orange juice concentrate until tender. Sprinkle gelatin over cold water in a heatproof cup and let stand 5 minutes or longer. Place container in small saucepan with hot water and set over moderate heat until gelatin is dissolved, about 5 minutes. Stir occasionally. Put apricot-orange juice mixture, ¾ cup sugar, dissolved gelatin, lemon juice and 1½ cups yogurt in a blender. Mix well. Beat egg whites until frothy. While beating, gradually add 2 tablespoons sugar and beat until peaks form. Gently fold egg whites into apricot/yogurt mixture. Do not overmix. Gently transfer the apricot mixture to a lightly oiled 8-inch ring mold. Cover with plastic and refrigerate at least 4 hours.

To serve, run a small sharp knife around edge of mold to loosen. Invert large serving platter over mold, then, invert the two together. Carefully lift off mold. (*Note:* If you lightly oil the platter first, you can readjust the position of the unmolded dessert in case you were off center.) Arrange overlapping slices of orange around the outside of the dessert. Put remaining 1½ cups yogurt into a small bowl and place in center of dessert. Spoon 2–3 tablespoons of yogurt beside each serving of Bavarian.

Makes 8 to 12 servings.

BAKED APPLES

Use tart baking apples for this classic dessert. The aroma from the cinnamon and apples is terrific!

4 apples
Water
3 tablespoons brown sugar
4 teaspoons raisins
Dash cinnamon or nutmeg
Yogurt Dessert Sauce, page 377
  (optional)

Preheat oven to 350°. Wash and core apples. Peel upper ¼ of the apple to prevent the skin from splitting. Place apple upright in baking dish filled about ¼-inch deep with water. Combine brown sugar, raisins and cinnamon. Fill the center core of the apple with the mixture. Bake 30–45 minutes or until tender. Serve hot or cold with Yogurt Dessert Sauce if desired.

Makes 4 servings.

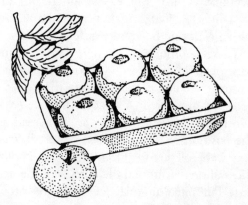

BANANAS EN PAPILLOTE
(Baked Bananas)

½ cup water
2 tablespoons sugar
½ cup mashed fresh fruit (apricots,
  berries, peaches, etc.)
½ teaspoon vanilla
4 small bananas, peeled
Fresh mint leaves, for garnish

Preheat oven to 425°. Heat water in a saucepan, add sugar and stir to dissolve. Remove from the heat, add the mashed fruit and the vanilla. Mix well.

Fold 4 sheets of foil (12 by 8 inches) in half lengthwise. At the end of the fold turn up and pinch the corners to make a "boat" to hold the bananas and the sauce. Put a whole banana in each "boat." Pour about 3 tablespoons of fruit sauce over the banana. Close the foil by folding over the edges and pinching them together tightly.

Place on a baking sheet. Bake for 15–20 minutes. Serve on heated plates after having opened the foil and decorated the bananas with mint leaves.

Serve with plain yogurt and more fruit sauce, if needed.

Makes 4 servings.

FRESH FRUIT CREPES

Fill prepared crepes with sweetened fruit at the last minute for a lovely finishing touch to your meal.

2 cups strawberries, raspberries,
  blueberries, sliced bananas, peaches *or*
  sliced papaya
1 cup plain low-fat yogurt

2 tablespoons sugar
1 tablespoon brandy (optional)

Prepare Crepes, page 368.

Mix fruit with yogurt, sugar and brandy, if desired. At serving time spoon 2 tablespoons filling over flat crepes; roll. Dust with powdered sugar and serve.

Makes filling for 16 crepes (about 3 cups).

FRUIT SALAD ALASKA

Fruit salad with a baked meringue on top.

  3 tablespoons orange marmalade
  1 tablespoon Cointreau or Grand
    Marnier liqueur
  1 orange, peeled and diced
  1 can (16 ounces) pineapple chunks
    packed in own juice (drained) *or* 1 cup
    fresh pineapple cubes
  12–16 fresh strawberries
  1 large fresh peach, peeled and diced
  3 egg whites
  ⅛ teaspoon cream of tartar
  1–2 tablespoons sugar
  ½ teaspoon vanilla

Preheat oven to 450°. In a saucepan, mix the marmalade and liqueur. Bring to a boil. Let cool. Prepare the fruit. Drain well. Pour the mixed fruit into 4 individual soufflé-type baking dishes. Pour marmalade sauce over fruit. Beat the egg whites until stiff. Add the cream of tartar, beat, add the sugar, and beat until stiff. Fold in the vanilla. Spread the egg white mixture on top of the fruit salad, heaping it thick and spreading it to the edge of the dishes. Bake for 5 minutes or until the meringue is lightly browned.

Makes 4 servings.

PEACH CARDINAL

Fresh peaches, poached and served with a raspberry sauce.

  4 cups water
  1 cup sugar
  1 tablespoon vanilla
  1 tablespoon freshly squeezed lemon juice
  6 ripe fresh peaches, 2½-inch diameter
  3 cups fresh or frozen raspberries
  3 tablespoons sugar
  Mint leaves, for decoration (optional)

Simmer water, sugar, vanilla and lemon juice in a large saucepan. Stir until sugar has dissolved. Add unpeeled peaches to simmering syrup. Keep just below simmering point for 8 minutes, or until peaches are soft when carefully tested with a sharp knife. Remove pan from heat. Let peaches cool in syrup 20 minutes. Drain peaches. Peel while warm and arrange in serving dish or individual cups.

Put raspberries and sugar in blender and whirl until raspberries are well mashed. Pour raspberry puree over peaches. Keep chilled until serving time. Decorate with mint leaves, if desired.

Makes 6 servings.

PEARS IN WINE

  6 medium-size firm ripe pears
  2 cups cold water
  3 tablespoons freshly squeezed lemon
    juice, divided
  2 cups red wine
  ½ teaspoon cinnamon
  ½ cup sugar
  ¼ cup red currant jelly
  ¼ cup slivered almonds, to decorate

Peel pears. They may be left whole, or cut in halves. If served whole, cut a small slice off the bottoms so that the pears will stand up easily. Carefully remove the core from the bottoms. If served in halves, cut the cores out. Drop quickly in water and 1 tablespoon of lemon juice to prevent discoloration. Bring wine, cinnamon, and rest of the lemon juice and sugar to boil in a saucepan. Drain pears and drop in boiling syrup. Reduce to simmer for 10 minutes or until pears are soft when pierced with a knife. Do not overcook. Remove pan from heat. Let cool in syrup for 20 minutes. Drain, reserving the syrup. Set pears in a serving dish or in individual cups. Continue boiling syrup until it measures ½ cup. Add red currant jelly and simmer briefly. Pour sauce over pears. Chill well and decorate with almonds.

Makes 6 servings.

RHUBARB BUCKLE

A true family favorite! Any fresh fruit can be used.

5 cups rhubarb, cut into 1-inch pieces
½ cup sugar
½ cup water

1 cup flour
½ cup sugar
1 teaspoon baking powder
3 egg whites

Preheat oven to 350°. Put rhubarb pieces into 10-inch baking dish. Sprinkle with ½ cup sugar and mix until fruit is coated. Add water. In small bowl, mix flour, ½ cup sugar, baking powder and egg whites. Drop by spoonfuls over fruit. Bake 45–55 minutes until fruit is tender and the dough is lightly browned.

Makes 8 servings.

Frozen Desserts

BLUEBERRY ICE

No handcranking required to make this frozen dessert!

1 pint blueberries *or* huckleberries
½ cup cold water
1 cup sugar, divided
1 cup boiling water
½ cup freshly squeezed lemon juice
1 egg white

Place berries in blender or food processor with cold water and ¼ cup sugar. Blend until mixture is a puree, and pour into a 1½-quart stainless-steel bowl.

Combine remaining sugar, boiling water and lemon juice and stir until sugar is dissolved. Add to blueberry mixture and mix thoroughly. Beat egg white until stiff, but not dry, and fold into blueberry mixture.

Place in coldest part of freezer. When ice begins to freeze around the edges, stir toward center, checking every half hour and repeating until mixture is slushy.

Beat with a rotary beater and return to freezer. Repeat at least once more until ice is quite solid. Can be served immediately, but tastes better if made a day ahead, covered, and frozen until serving time.

Makes 8 servings (½ cup each).

FROZEN FRUIT YOGURTS

Get out your ice-cream freezer! This is a basic mixture with several choices of sweetened fruits to add to it. (Suggestions for uncooked or cooked fruits are below.)

3 egg whites
¼ teaspoon cream of tartar
2 quarts plain low-fat yogurt

Prepare the sweetened fruit mixture of your choice; see below.

Beat egg whites with cream of tartar until stiff. Add yogurt and prepared fruit mixture. Transfer to a gallon or larger ice-cream freezer and assemble and freeze according to manufacturer's directions. Use about 4 parts ice to 1 part rock salt. When yogurt is done, remove dasher and pack with more ice or transfer to your freezer to allow further hardening.

UNCOOKED FRUIT MIXTURES
General Rule: Use any fruit (or flavoring) that tastes good mixed with yogurt. Sweeten the fruit/yogurt mixture to taste, keeping in mind that the mixture will not taste as sweet after it is frozen, so make it a little "too sweet" beforehand. Remember that there is quite a variation in the sweetness of individual fruits, so the amount of added sugar will vary according to your taste buds.

—**Lemon:** Use juice of 6 lemons, grated rind of 2–3 lemons, and 2½–3 cups sugar.
—**Lime:** Use juice of 10–12 limes, grated rind of 4–5 limes, and 2½–3 cups sugar.
—**Orange:** Use juice of 4–5 oranges, grated rind of 3–4 oranges, and 1½–2 cups of sugar.
—**Strawberry, blackberry, raspberry:** Use 4 cups lightly packed fresh (or unsweetened frozen, defrosted) berries. Mash berries,

then add 2 cups sugar and 4 teaspoons *each* lemon juice and vanilla.
—**Banana-honey:** Measure 4 cups thinly sliced ripe bananas, then coarsely mash them. Add 1¼ cups sugar, ¾ cup honey, 3 tablespoons lemon juice and 2 tablespoons vanilla.
—**Pear:** Puree in blender 4 cups sliced pears, 1½–2 cups sugar, 2 teaspoons lemon juice and ½ teaspoon nutmeg.
—**Cantaloupe:** Puree in blender 3 cups sliced cantaloupe and 1–1½ cups sugar.
—**Pumpkin:** Mix 3½ cups (1 large can) cooked pumpkin with 2–2½ cups sugar (brown, white or a combination), 2 teaspoons cinnamon, 1 teaspoon allspice and ½ teaspoon nutmeg. Mixture can be warmed slightly to hasten mixing.

COOKED FRUIT MIXTURES
General Rule: Combine the fruit and sugar or honey in a 3-quart pan. Bring to a boil, stirring over high heat. Reduce heat to medium and cook, stirring constantly, until fruit softens and partially disintegrates (it takes 1 to 4 minutes, depending on the ripeness of the fruit); break up any large pieces with a fork. Remove from heat and stir in the fruit juices, spices and flavorings listed under each flavor version.

—**Apricot-orange:** Use 4 cups thinly sliced unpeeled ripe apricots. 2 cups sugar, 2 tablespoons lemon juice, ½ cup orange juice, 1 teaspoon grated orange peel and 4 teaspoons vanilla.
—**Blueberry:** Use 4 cups whole fresh (or unsweetened frozen, defrosted) blueberries, 1¾ cups sugar, 2 tablespoons lemon juice and 1 tablespoon vanilla.

—*Peach:* Use 4 cups sliced peeled peaches, 2 cups firmly packed brown sugar, 3 tablespoons lemon juice, 2 tablespoons vanilla, ¾ teaspoon ground nutmeg and ¾ teaspoon ground cinnamon.

Makes 1 gallon or 16 servings.

STRAWBERRY ICE (Sorbet)

¾ cup sugar
1 cup hot water
2 tablespoons freshly squeezed lemon juice
1 tablespoon orange juice
1 pint strawberries, hulled

Dissolve sugar in hot water and cool. Add juices. Put strawberries and sugar syrup into the blender and whirl until it is smooth. Place in a freezer-proof dish, and freeze until firmish, then whirl in blender again. Freeze until hard.

Makes 3 cups.

Puddings

CHOCOLATE PUDDING

3 tablespoons cornstarch
1½ tablespoons cocoa
2 cups skim milk
½ cup sugar
1 teaspoon vanilla

Combine cornstarch and cocoa. Add milk slowly and stir until blended. Cook over medium heat, stirring continuously, until smooth and thick.

Remove from heat and stir in sugar and vanilla. Be sure the sugar is completely dissolved in the hot pudding. Pour into dessert dishes and chill.

Makes 6 servings (about 3 cups).

PUMPKIN BREAD PUDDING

For bread pudding lovers! Serve warm or cold with Yogurt Dessert Sauce

8 slices whole wheat bread
1 cup egg substitute (commercial or Homemade Egg Substitute, page 241)
2¼ cups skim milk
1 can (16 ounces) pumpkin
1 cup brown sugar
1½ teaspoons cinnamon
1½ teaspoons pumpkin pie spice
½ teaspoon nutmeg
1 teaspoon vanilla
¾ cup raisins

Preheat oven to 375°. Crumble bread by hand or in a blender or food processor to make bread crumbs. Combine egg substitute, skim milk, pumpkin, brown sugar, cinnamon, spices and vanilla; add raisins and combine with bread crumbs in a lightly oiled 2-quart casserole dish.

Set 2-quart casserole dish in larger baking dish filled partially with hot water. Bake 1 hour or until knife inserted in center comes out clean.

Makes 12 servings (about 6 cups).

VANILLA PUDDING

Nice to serve over sliced fruit or also makes a marvelous summer dessert. (Prepare a Graham Cracker Crust, fill it with berries or other fruit; pour pudding over and chill.)

2 cups skim milk
2 tablespoons cornstarch

¼ cup (or less) brown sugar
1–2 teaspoons vanilla

Gently heat 1½ cups milk in a heavy saucepan. Combine cornstarch with the reserved milk. Add this to the heated milk. Stir in remaining ingredients and cook over low heat until thick, stirring often. Reduce heat and cook gently about 8 minutes more, stirring constantly.

Serve warm or pour into bowl and chill.
Makes 4 servings (about 2 cups).

Pies

PUMPKIN PIE

A harvest special!

1 9-inch Graham Cracker Crust, page 368

2 cups canned or cooked pumpkin
1½ cups evaporated skim milk
¼ cup brown sugar
½ cup white sugar
1 teaspoon cinnamon
½ teaspoon ground ginger
¼ teaspoon nutmeg _or_ allspice
⅛ teaspoon ground cloves
3 egg whites

Yogurt Dessert Sauce, page 377

Earlier in the day, prepare Graham Cracker Crust. Bake 10 minutes and cool.

To prepare filling, preheat oven to 350° and mix all the ingredients until well blended. Pour mixture into cooled pie shell. Bake 1 hour or until an inserted knife comes out clean.

Serve with Yogurt Dessert Sauce.
Makes 8 servings.

STRAWBERRY YOGURT PIE

1 9-inch Graham Cracker Crust, page 368

1½ cups plain low-fat yogurt
1½ cups low-fat cottage cheese, drained
4 tablespoons honey
1 teaspoon vanilla
¼ teaspoon freshly squeezed lemon juice
1 envelope unflavored gelatin
3 cups sliced fresh strawberries

Earlier in the day, prepare Graham Cracker Crust. Bake 10 minutes and cool.

To prepare filling, combine yogurt, cottage cheese, honey, vanilla and lemon juice in blender. While blender is running, dissolve gelatin by first sprinkling over 1 tablespoon cold water, then stirring in 3 tablespoons boiling water. Add dissolved gelatin to blender and blend well. Spread sliced strawberries in bottom of pie shell and pour yogurt mixture over them. Chill several hours.

Makes 8 to 12 servings.

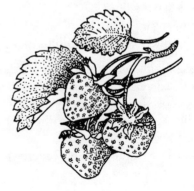

Cookies and Bars

APRICOT MERINGUE BARS

A very dainty and sweet cookie.

2½ cups flour
½ teaspoon baking soda
½ cup margarine
2 egg whites
¼ cup sugar
½ teaspoon vanilla
1 cup apricot jam

Preheat oven to 375°. Sift flour and baking soda. Cream margarine, egg whites, sugar and vanilla. Combine flour mixture and creamed mixture. Press out onto an unoiled baking sheet, about ¼ inch thick. Spread the apricot jam evenly on the dough. Bake for 15 minutes or until very lightly browned. Remove bars from oven and turn oven down to 300°.

MERINGUE TOPPING
2 egg whites
2 tablespoons flour
½ cup sugar
½ cup finely chopped walnuts

Beat egg whites until stiff. Stir in the flour and sugar. Spread meringue topping over the slightly cooked jam and the bars and sprinkle with the walnuts. Return to the 300° oven and bake for 15 minutes more.
Makes 42 bars (about 2 by 2 inches).

CAROB COOKIES

By substituting carob powder for cocoa, this cookie is very low-fat.

1½ cups white flour
1½ cups whole wheat flour
½ cup carob powder
1 tablespoon powdered instant coffee (decaffeinated works well)
½ teaspoon baking soda
1½ teaspoons baking powder
1 cup sugar
5 egg whites
¾ cup oil
1 teaspoon vanilla
¼ cup chopped nuts

Mix dry ingredients together. Beat egg whites slightly and add oil and vanilla; add to dry ingredients. Add chopped nuts and form into small balls. Bake for 15 minutes.
Makes 48 cookies.

CRISPY SPICE COOKIES

3 cups flour
2 teaspoons ground ginger
1½ teaspoons cinnamon
1 teaspoon ground cloves
¾ cup margarine
½ cup sugar
½ cup dark corn syrup

Preheat oven to 350°. Sift first 4 ingredients. Cream margarine and sugar; stir in corn syrup. Mix in flour. Roll out ⅛-inch thick on floured surface. Cut into shapes. Place on baking sheet. Bake about 10 minutes. Decorate, if desired.
Makes 54 cookies (2 inches each).

FORGOTTEN KISSES

Pretty "party" cookies. This recipe makes half the batch with coffee flavoring added and the other half with lemon and nuts.

- 2 egg whites
- ⅛ teaspoon Lite Salt or less
- ½ teaspoon cream of tartar
- ¾ cup sugar
- ½ teaspoon vanilla
- ½ teaspoon powdered instant coffee
- Dash nutmeg
- ¼ cup finely chopped walnuts
- ¼ teaspoon grated lemon peel

Preheat oven to 350°. Beat egg whites until fluffy. Add Lite Salt and cream of tartar and beat. Add sugar slowly, beating all the time. Continue beating until glossy and mixture stands in stiff peaks. Add vanilla. Place half the mixture in small bowl and fold in coffee powder and nutmeg. Fold nuts and lemon peel into remaining mixture. Drop by tablespoons onto unoiled baking sheet. Put in 350° oven. Turn *off* oven heat immediately. Leave cookies until cool (at least 2 hours). Do not open oven door. Remove onto racks.

Makes 36 small kisses.

GINGIES

- ⅓ cup margarine
- 1 cup brown sugar
- 1½ cups dark molasses
- ½ cup cold water
- 3 cups whole wheat flour
- 3 cups white flour
- 1 teaspoon allspice
- 1 teaspoon ground ginger
- 1 teaspoon ground cloves
- 1 teaspoon cinnamon
- 2 teaspoons baking soda
- 1 tablespoon cold water

Mix the margarine, brown sugar and molasses together thoroughly. Stir in ½ cup cold water. Sift the flours and spices together and add to above mixture. Dissolve the baking soda in 1 tablespoon cold water and add to dough. Mix well, cover bowl and chill dough.

When ready to bake, preheat oven to 350°. Roll out cookie dough thick (½ inch). Cut with 2½-inch round cutter. Place far apart on lightly oiled baking sheet. Bake until no imprint remains when touched lightly with finger, about 15–18 minutes.

Makes 45 large, puffy cookies.

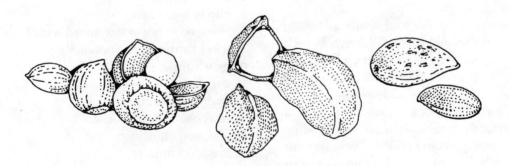

LEBKUCHEN

Make these cookies a week before eating. An old German favorite.

2¾ cups flour
1 teaspoon cinnamon
1 teaspoon ground cloves
1 teaspoon allspice
1 teaspoon nutmeg
½ teaspoon baking soda
½ cup honey
½ cup molasses
¾ cup brown sugar
2 egg whites
1 tablespoon freshly squeezed lemon juice
1 teaspoon freshly grated lemon rind
⅓ cup finely chopped nuts
⅓ cup candied fruit peel

GLAZE
½ cup powdered sugar
2 tablespoons cornstarch
1–3 tablespoons hot water
½ teaspoon vanilla *or* brandy

Sift flour with spices and baking soda; set aside. Heat the honey, molasses and brown sugar to a boil; cool to lukewarm. Stir in egg whites and juice, and grate the lemon rind into the mixture. Stir in flour in several additions, then work in nuts and peel. Cover and chill *overnight.*

Preheat oven to 400° and lightly oil baking sheets. On a floured board roll dough ¼-inch thick in small batches (keep rest chilled), and cut into rectangles 1½ by 2½ inches. Place 1 inch apart and bake 10–12 minutes.

Mix ingredients for glaze together (make a thick, smooth paste), and brush cookies while still hot (using a pastry brush). Decorate with more candied fruit if desired. Store cookies in airtight tins to age at least a week before eating.

Makes about 60 cookies.

MOLASSES ORANGE BARS

1 can (6 ounces) frozen orange juice
  concentrate, thawed
½ cup oatmeal
1 cup raisins
½ cup margarine
½ cup sugar
½ cup molasses
2 egg whites
2 cups flour
1½ teaspoons baking soda
1 teaspoon ground ginger
1 teaspoon cinnamon

Preheat oven to 325°. Combine orange juice, oatmeal and raisins and set aside. Cream margarine, sugar and molasses until fluffy. Blend in egg whites. Mix together flour, baking soda and spices and add to molasses mixture. Add raisin mixture and mix well. Pour into lightly oiled 9-by-13-inch baking pan. Bake 45 minutes. Cool, then cut into bars.

Makes 28 bars (about 2 by 2 inches).

NORTHWEST HARVEST BARS

A delicious low-fat bar.

¼ cup margarine
⅔ cup brown sugar
2 tablespoons hot water mixed with 1
  packet Butter Buds (optional)
4 egg whites
¾ cup flour
½ teaspoon baking powder
½ teaspoon Lite Salt or less
½ teaspoon cinnamon
½ teaspoon nutmeg
½ teaspoon ground ginger
¼ teaspoon baking soda

⅔ cup canned pumpkin
½ cup raisins
½ teaspoon vanilla

Preheat oven to 350°. Spray a 9-inch square baking pan with nonstick coating. In large saucepan, melt margarine over low heat. Remove from heat and stir in brown sugar, water and Butter Buds, if used; beat in egg whites. Add dry ingredients and mix until well blended. Stir in pumpkin, raisins and vanilla. Pour into prepared pan and bake 25–30 minutes. Cool and cut into bars.

Makes 16 bars (about 2¼ by 2¼ inches).

OATMEAL COOKIES

These are cholesterol free but not low in fat so should be eaten only occasionally.

1 cup shortening
1 cup brown sugar
1 cup granulated sugar
3 egg whites
1 teaspoon vanilla
1½ cups flour
1 teaspoon baking soda
3 cups oatmeal
1 cup raisins

Thoroughly cream shortening and sugars. Add egg whites and vanilla. Beat well. Sift together flour and soda; add to creamed mixture. Stir in oatmeal and raisins. Mix well. Form dough in rolls 1–1½ inches in diameter. Wrap in foil or plastic. Chill thoroughly.

Preheat oven to 350°. With sharp knife, slice cookies about ¼ inch thick. Bake on ungreased baking sheet for 10 minutes or until lightly browned.

Makes about 60 cookies.

WALNUT SQUARES

Sweet and nutty, these bars make good tea cookies.

1 cup finely ground whole wheat bread crumbs
¾ cup brown sugar
4 egg whites
½ teaspoon cream of tartar
1 teaspoon vanilla
½ cup chopped walnuts

Preheat oven to 350°. Mix together bread crumbs and sugar. In a separate bowl, beat egg whites with cream of tartar until stiff.

Gently fold the vanilla, crumb mixture and walnuts (in order listed) into the egg whites. Bake in an unoiled 8-by-8-inch square pan for 20 minutes, then reduce heat to 300° and bake an additional 10 minutes. Cut into small squares.

Makes about 30 (1½ inch) squares.

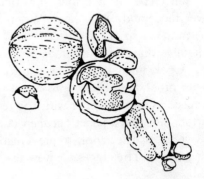

Dessert Specialties

CREPES

The following basic recipe is a low-fat, low-cholesterol version of the original one which called for whole eggs, whole milk and butter.

1 cup cold water
1 cup cold skim milk
6 egg whites
½ teaspoon Lite Salt or less
2 cups sifted flour
2 tablespoons oil

Put liquids, egg whites and salt into blender jar; add flour, then oil. Blend at top speed, scraping any flour adhering to the sides of the jar. Cover, refrigerate 2 hours. This is an important step—it allows the flour particles to expand in the liquid and ensures a tender, thin crepe. The batter should be a very light creamy texture—just thick enough to coat a wooden spoon.

For each crepe, heat 6-inch nonstick fry pan over moderately high heat. When hot, pour a scant ¼ cup of the batter into skillet; immediately rotate pan until batter covers bottom. Cook until light brown; turn and brown on other side. Slide onto warm plate and proceed in same manner with the rest of the batter. Put waxed paper between crepes. Keep covered, as they cool, to prevent them from drying out. The crepes are now ready to be filled.

Makes 20 crepes, 6 inches each.

SERVING, STORING, FREEZING OF CREPES

These versatile crepes can be:
—Filled, folded or rolled and served immediately. Several recipes for fillings are on pages 240, 301, 310, 326 and 358.
—Prepared ahead of time, piled up with layers of waxed paper between each one, wrapped in foil, refrigerated and reheated when ready to be filled and served.
—Prepared in advance, frozen and reheated at the last minute. Wrap in heavy foil to freeze. They will keep for weeks.

CREPES—1001 WAYS TO SERVE AND ENJOY THEM!

Crepes are thin relatives of the American pancake. They are easy to make, fun and can be eaten in a variety of ways.
—Festive and delicate desserts can be made using crepes, filling them with jams, jellies, puddings, or fresh or stewed fruit.
—Try a crepe cake! Layers of crepes are piled upon each other, each one spread with a low-fat filling and served cut in pie-shaped wedges. Appetizers, main dishes and desserts can be made that way.
—They can be served as a simple breakfast dish very much like pancakes.
—They become a nourishing main course dish when filled with a myriad of poultry, seafood, meat or vegetable fillings—rolled into cylinders or folded and served with or without a sauce. They afford a marvelous opportunity for using leftovers in an elegant disguise.

GRAHAM CRACKER CRUST

1½ cups graham cracker crumbs
2 tablespoons honey
1 tablespoon oil

Preheat oven to 350°. Blend graham cracker crumbs, honey and oil and mix well. Pat into 9-inch pie pan. Bake for 10 minutes. Allow shell to cool before filling.

Makes 1 9-inch crust.

BEVERAGES

Cranberry Wassail
Egg Nog
Fruited Punch
Mulled Cider
Orange Frosty
Quick Hot Spiced Cider
Strawberry-Banana Smoothie

CRANBERRY WASSAIL

A holiday nonalcoholic favorite.

2½ cups boiling water
2 tablespoons tea leaves *or* 6 tea bags
¼ teaspoon allspice
¼ teaspoon cinnamon
¼ teaspoon nutmeg
¾ cup sugar
2 cups cranberry juice cocktail
1½ cups water
½ cup orange juice
⅓ cup freshly squeezed lemon juice

Pour boiling water over tea and spices. Cover and let steep 5 minutes. Strain. Add sugar and stir to dissolve. Add remaining ingredients and heat just to boiling. Serve hot.

Makes 7½ cups.

EGG NOG

½ cup egg substitute (commercial *or* Homemade Egg Substitute, page 241)
2–4 tablespoons sugar
1 can (13 ounces) evaporated skim milk
¾ cup skim milk
1 teaspoon vanilla
1 teaspoon rum flavoring *or* use 3 ounces of rum *or* dry sherry
Nutmeg

Whip egg substitute and sugar together and combine with the two kinds of milk, vanilla and rum flavoring *or* rum *or* dry sherry. Mix well. Chill. Top with nutmeg. The flavor is enhanced by chilling overnight.

Makes 3 cups.

FRUITED PUNCH

A very popular punch—we serve it with Mexican foods, but it's great for all parties!

1 can (12 ounces) lemonade concentrate
4½ cans water
2 cups grape juice
2 oranges, thinly sliced
1 lemon, thinly sliced
½ of 20-ounce can sliced peaches and juice (cut slices in half)
½ of 20-ounce can chunk pineapple and juice

Mix lemonade, water and grape juice. Add remaining ingredients. Serve chilled.
Makes 11 cups.

ORANGE FROSTY

1 can (6 ounces) orange juice concentrate
1 cup skim milk
½ cup water
½ cup sugar
1 tablespoon vanilla

Blend; add 1 tray crushed ice and blend again.
Makes 5 cups.

QUICK HOT SPICED CIDER

Put the amount of cider you want to serve into a kettle. Sprinkle top with ground cinnamon and cloves. Stir and taste. Heat to just below boiling. Serve warm.

Or, if you have more time . . .

MULLED CIDER

Put from 1–3 quarts of cider into a kettle. Push whole cloves into an orange and add to cider. Add 1 long or 2 shorter pieces of stick cinnamon. Heat to just below boiling. Reduce heat to simmer for 30 minutes or until cider tastes spicy. Serve warm.
Makes 4–12 cups.

STRAWBERRY-BANANA SMOOTHIE

1 cup buttermilk
½ ripe banana
2 tablespoons frozen or fresh strawberries (sweetened)
1 tablespoon orange juice concentrate

Combine all ingredients in an electric blender; mix for a few seconds or until mixture is uniform in color and consistency.
Makes 2 cups.

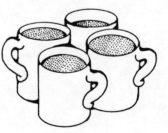

SAUCES, GRAVIES AND SALAD DRESSINGS

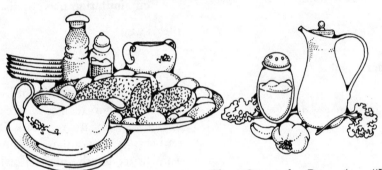

FOR SALADS

Red French Salad Dressing
Russian Salad Dressing
Tangy Salad Dressing
Thousand Island Salad Dressing
Vinaigrette Salad Dressing with Greens
Western Salad Dressing Mix
Yogurt-Chive Dressing (see "Chicken, Turkey and Rabbit" section)

FOR MEAT, FISH OR POULTRY

Dilly Sauce
Oriental Sauce for Fish
Tartar Sauce
Turkey Gravy

FOR PASTA OR VEGETABLES

Basic White Sauce
Beef-Mushroom Spaghetti Sauce (see "Beef, Veal and Pork" section)

Clam Sauce for Pasta (see "Fish and Shellfish" section)
Light Mushroom Sauce for Pasta
Marinara Sauce
Mock Hollandaise Sauce
Mock Sour Cream (see "Appetizers and Hors D'Oeuvres" section)
Tomato-Mushroom Spaghetti Sauce
Turkey-Mushroom Spaghetti Sauce (see "Chicken, Turkey and Rabbit" section)

FOR FALAFEL (see "Soups and Sandwiches" section)

Tahini Dressing
Yogurt Dressing

FOR DESSERTS, PANCAKES OR WAFFLES

Glorious Blueberries
Strawberry or Raspberry Sauce
Yogurt Dessert Sauce

For Salads

RED FRENCH SALAD DRESSING

The secret is to have this prepared and ready to use.

> **1 cup low-sodium ketchup**
> **½ cup sugar**
> **⅓ cup oil**
> **½ cup vinegar**
> **Onion powder**
> **Pepper**

Combine all ingredients and mix well.
Makes about 2⅓ cups.

RUSSIAN SALAD DRESSING

A delicious low-salt and low-fat version.

> **1 can (10½ ounces) low-sodium tomato soup**
> **¼ cup oil**
> **Peel of ½ lemon, grated**
> **2 tablespoons freshly squeezed lemon juice**
> **2 tablespoons chopped green onion**
> **1 teaspoon prepared horseradish**
> **Dash ground cinnamon (optional)**
> **1 clove garlic, crushed (optional)**

Blend tomato soup. Combine all ingredients in jar with lid. Chill. Shake well before serving.
Makes about 1¾ cups.

TANGY SALAD DRESSING

We've found this combination to be creamy enough in taste for mayonnaise lovers, yet low enough in fat to be a real improvement over commercial "imitation" salad dressings which still contain considerable fat.

> **1 cup low-fat yogurt**
> **¼ cup imitation mayonnaise**

Blend well.
Makes 1¼ cups.

NOTE: This makes an excellent homemade creamy salad dressing. Use it for coleslaw, potato salad or in recipes where large amounts of mayonnaise are required. It is somewhat tarter than mayonnaise alone, so you may want to reduce the vinegar or lemon juice in your tried-and-true recipes.

THOUSAND ISLAND SALAD DRESSING

A low-fat version of an all-time favorite.

> **½ cup low-fat cottage cheese**
> **2 tablespoons plain low-fat yogurt**
> **2 tablespoons imitation mayonnaise**
> **2 tablespoons low-sodium ketchup**
> **Dash cayenne pepper**
> **1 tablespoon skim milk (or more for desired thickness)**

Combine ingredients and blend thoroughly.
Add:

> **1 tablespoon chopped dill pickles**
> **1 tablespoon finely chopped onion**

Makes 1 cup.

VINAIGRETTE SALAD DRESSING WITH GREENS

A quick dressing made directly in the salad bowl. When you toss the salad this way, not much dressing is required. A simple salad of romaine becomes very elegant.

1 clove garlic, peeled
1 tablespoon olive oil
1 tablespoon garlic-flavored wine vinegar
1 teaspoon Dijon mustard
6 cups torn lettuce, preferably romaine
Pepper

Rub a large salad bowl with the whole garlic clove, then mince it. Add minced garlic, oil, vinegar and mustard and stir well to combine. Cover bowl until ready to serve. Remove cover and add lettuce. Mix until all pieces are very well coated. Grate fresh pepper over the salad.

Makes 6 cups of salad.

OPTION

For special treats, add up to 1 teaspoon Parmesan cheese before tossing.

WESTERN SALAD DRESSING MIX

Homemade Ranch Salad Dressing—much lower in salt than the commercial versions.

¾ teaspoon Lite Salt or less
2 teaspoons dried parsley flakes
1 teaspoon garlic powder
1 teaspoon pepper
½ teaspoon onion powder

Put all ingredients in a small jar and shake well to mix. Store in airtight container. Shake before measuring out to use.

Makes 5 teaspoons.

DRESSING
1 teaspoon Western Dressing Mix
¼ cup imitation mayonnaise
¾ cup plain low-fat yogurt
1 cup buttermilk

In bowl stir together all ingredients. Store in an airtight container in the refrigerator. (Flavor is best when stored 24 hours before using.)

Makes 2 cups.

For Meat, Fish or Poultry

DILLY SAUCE

Wonderful to serve with Salmon Mousse or Fish Almondine.

2 tablespoons imitation mayonnaise
1 cup plain low-fat yogurt
¾ teaspoon tarragon leaves
1½ teaspoons dill weed

Put mayonnaise and yogurt in a mixing bowl. Mix thoroughly with a wire whisk. Add the other ingredients and mix well. Pour into a container with a tight-fitting lid and refrigerate a few hours before serving.

Makes about 1 cup.

ORIENTAL SAUCE FOR FISH

Quick and easy!

  ½ cup orange juice
  1 tablespoon lower-sodium soy sauce
  2 tablespoons low-sodium ketchup
  ½ bunch parsley, chopped
  ⅓ cup freshly squeezed lemon juice
  ½ teaspoon oregano leaves
  ½ teaspoon pepper
  Pinch garlic powder

Combine ingredients. Pour over fish. Cover and bake for 20–30 minutes at 350° until fish flakes easily with a fork.

Makes enough marinade for 2 pounds of fish fillets (about 1 cup).

TARTAR SAUCE

Especially nice served with Skinny Sole.

  1 cup low-fat cottage cheese
  2 tablespoons buttermilk
  3 tablespoons chopped onion
  3 tablespoons chopped parsley
  3 tablespoons chopped sweet pickle *or* drained sweet pickle relish

Combine cottage cheese and buttermilk in blender until smooth. Add this mixture to chopped vegetables in bowl and mix.

Makes 1¾ cups.

TURKEY GRAVY

You can get your turkey gravy base all made ahead of time, which will save you that much fussing at the last minute. This is a white wine turkey stock thickened at the end with cornstarch. When the turkey is done and the roaster degreased, blend the gravy base into the roasting juices.

  Turkey neck and gizzard
  2 tablespoons oil
  1 cup chopped onion
  1 cup chopped carrots
  1 cup dry white wine *or* ⅔ cup dry white vermouth
  2 cups chicken broth
  Water as needed
  ½ teaspoon Lite Salt or less
  1 bay leaf
  ½ teaspoon thyme leaves *or* sage
  3 tablespoons cornstarch blended with ¼ cup port or cold chicken broth

Early in the day: Chop neck into 2-inch pieces and quarter the gizzard. Dry on paper towels. Heat oil in a heavy 3-quart saucepan, stir in the neck and gizzard and brown rapidly on all sides. Remove them and stir the vegetables into the pan. Cover and cook slowly 5–8 minutes, or until tender. Uncover, raise heat and brown lightly for several minutes. Return neck and gizzard to pan, add the wine, broth and enough water to cover ingredients by an inch. Add Lite Salt and herbs and simmer partially covered for 2½–3 hours. Strain and return stock to pan. There should be about 3 cups. Beat in cornstarch mixture and simmer 2–3 minutes. Liquid will be lightly thickened. When cool, cover and refrigerate until turkey is done.

Finishing the sauce or gravy: When the turkey is roasted, skim all fat out of roasting pan and discard. Pour remaining drippings into saucepan with thickened turkey stock and stir over moderately high heat for several minutes. Pour into a warm gravy bowl.

Makes about 4 cups.

For Pasta or Vegetables

BASIC WHITE SAUCE

A white sauce can be prepared low-fat. Serve over vegetables for "creamed" or "scalloped" dishes or as a base for "creamed" soups.

2 tablespoons margarine
2 tablespoons flour
¼ teaspoon Lite Salt or less
¼ teaspoon pepper
2 cups skim milk

Melt margarine in small saucepan over low heat. Add flour, Lite Salt and pepper, stirring until mixture is smooth and bubbly. Remove from heat. Add skim milk. Heat to boiling, stirring constantly. The consistency should be like heavy cream.

Makes 2¼ cups.

OTHER USES
This typical white sauce can be used in many ways. A number of spices or ingredients can be added to it to create interesting and varied dishes. Add:

—½ teaspoon curry powder as an accompaniment for chicken, rice or shrimp.
—½ teaspoon dill weed as an accompaniment for fish.

—½ teaspoon nutmeg for vegetable dishes.
—Chopped or minced clams or mushrooms as toppings for pasta.

LIGHT MUSHROOM SAUCE FOR PASTA

For mushroom lovers who enjoy a thin, light sauce over fresh cooked pasta! Very attractive when served over fresh spinach pasta.

1 pound small mushrooms
1 tablespoon margarine
1 clove garlic, minced
2 tablespoons flour
2 cups skim milk
¼ cup chopped parsley
½ teaspoon Lite Salt or less
¼ teaspoon pepper
1 tablespoon freshly squeezed lemon juice
¼ cup freshly grated Parmesan cheese
Fresh pasta for 4

Wash and dry mushrooms thoroughly and slice thin. Melt margarine in a large skillet. Sauté garlic. Add sliced mushrooms and sauté over high heat until mushrooms are brown and liquid is mostly evaporated. Stir in flour and cook for a few minutes, then add milk, parsley, Lite Salt and pepper. Stir and cook for 5 minutes or until it begins to thicken. Add lemon juice.

Fill a large saucepan ⅔ full with water. Bring to a boil. Add pasta. Bring water back to a boil and cook uncovered until pasta is tender, but firm to bite. Drain pasta and mix with sauce. Sprinkle with ¼ cup Parmesan cheese. Serve immediately.

Makes 4 cups sauce (enough for 8 cups pasta).

MARINARA SAUCE (tomato sauce)

Wonderful over fresh pasta or whenever you need a nicely flavored tomato sauce. Double the recipe and keep some in the freezer.

1 clove garlic, minced
1 tablespoon olive oil
2 cans (16 ounces each) unsalted tomatoes
2 cans (8 ounces each) unsalted tomato sauce
1 teaspoon oregano leaves
1 tablespoon chopped or dried parsley

Sauté garlic in olive oil. Add tomatoes and tomato sauce slowly. Stir in oregano and parsley. Bring to a boil and simmer covered for 20 minutes to 2 hours. (The longer the better!) Break up the tomatoes with a potato masher and stir sauce occasionally.

This sauce has great versatility. Use it as a pizza sauce and in any other dishes calling for tomato sauce. For Mexican flavors, add ground cumin (½–1 teaspoon) and hot sauce.

Makes about 4 cups.

MOCK HOLLANDAISE SAUCE

Serve this sauce over Breakfast Volcanos for a special meal.

1 tablespoon cornstarch
1 cup chicken broth
4 teaspoons freshly squeezed lemon juice
2 tablespoons margarine
¼ cup grated low-fat cheese

Mix cornstarch with a little broth to a smooth paste. Add the remaining broth, lemon juice and margarine. Heat slowly to boiling, stir-ring constantly. Cook 3 minutes longer, stir-ring occasionally; add cheese and stir until melted.

Makes about 1 cup.

TOMATO-MUSHROOM SPAGHETTI SAUCE

A meatless spaghetti sauce which is very tasty.

1 cup sliced fresh mushrooms
½ cup minced onions
2 cloves garlic, minced
1 can (16 ounces) unsalted tomatoes
1 can (6 ounces) unsalted tomato paste
½ cup water
1 tablespoon chopped parsley
1 bay leaf
1 teaspoon basil leaves
2 teaspoons oregano leaves
⅛ teaspoon pepper
¼ cup chopped green pepper (optional)
¼ cup grated Parmesan cheese, for topping

Mix mushrooms, onions, garlic, tomatoes, tomato paste, water, parsley, bay leaf, basil, oregano and pepper. Simmer gently 1–2 hours, adding green peppers, if desired, the last 10 minutes of cooking. Serve over cooked spaghetti. Sprinkle with Parmesan cheese.

Makes 4 cups of sauce.

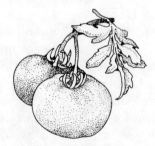

For Desserts, Pancakes or Waffles

GLORIOUS BLUEBERRIES

A beautiful dessert sauce to serve with fresh fruit.

2 cups blueberries
2 tablespoons water
3 tablespoons cornstarch
¼ cup sugar
1 cup plain low-fat yogurt

Wash berries and place in saucepan with water. Bring to a boil, stirring frequently, until soft. Put in blender with cornstarch and sugar and mix until smooth.

Return mixture to saucepan and cook over low heat until thickened, stirring often. Cool. Fold in yogurt. Serve cold in a small bowl surrounded with pieces of fresh fruit. Wooden picks may be served to spear the fruit so it can be dipped into the sauce.

Makes 10–12 servings (about 3 cups).

STRAWBERRY OR RASPBERRY SAUCE

Can be used as a topping for Baba au Rhum, frozen desserts, fruit desserts, pancakes, waffles etc.

1 quart of strawberries or raspberries
⅓ cup (or less) sugar according to taste
Juice of 1 lemon *or* 2 tablespoons sherry

Stem, wash and drain berries. Put berries in an electric blender and puree until smooth (or push berries through a food mill). Add sugar, lemon juice *or* sherry and mix all together.

Makes 4 cups.

YOGURT DESSERT SAUCE

This light sauce can be used with Pumpkin Bread Pudding, Baked Apples, Apple Crisp or any other fruit dessert. Wonderful over fresh strawberries!

2 cups plain low-fat yogurt
1 teaspoon vanilla extract
¼ cup sugar

Combine all ingredients and stir well.

Makes enough topping for 8 servings (about 2 cups).

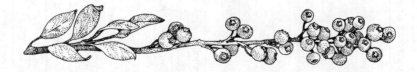

NUTRIENT ANALYSIS OF RECIPES

Recipes	Amount	Calories	Protein (gm)	Carbohydrate (gm)	Total Fat (gm)	CSI* (units)	Dietary Fiber (gm)	Sodium (mg)	Potassium (mg)	Calcium (mg)	Iron (mg)
Appetizers and Hors D'oeuvres											
Antipasto	½ cup	27	1.3	3.9	1.1	0.1	1.5	74	185	23	0.6
Baked Corn Chips	1 cup	114	3.4	20.3	2.7	0.3	1.6	97	83	67	0.9
Bean Dip	¼ cup	59	3.2	9.8	1.0	0.3	5.7	243	242	22	1.0
Broccoli Canapés	¼ cup	18	0.9	1.7	1.1	0.1	1.0	107	112	27	0.3
Chowchow	¼ cup	49	1.0	5.8	2.7	0.4	0.5	74	425	16	0.6
Cream Puff Shells	1 shell	48	2.0	4.2	2.6	0.5	0.1	64	48	15	0.2
Dill Dip	¼ cup	66	5.5	3.7	3.3	1.1	0.0	311	55	37	0.2
Eggplant Delight	¼ cup	35	0.5	2.4	2.8	0.4	0.8	1	79	6	0.3
Great Little Snackers	2 crackers	64	2.1	9.4	2.1	0.6	1.0	101	60	18	0.6
Herbed Tofu Dip	¼ cup	47	4.4	3.0	2.4	0.3	0.3	93	154	83	1.4
Hummous	¼ cup	106	5.6	15.7	2.8	0.4	2.7	125	191	34	2.0
Marinated Mushrooms	1/10 recipe	39	1.0	2.9	2.8	0.4	0.7	25	162	5	0.5
Mock Sour Cream	¼ cup	54	8.0	2.5	1.2	0.9	0.0	238	68	48	0.1
Mushroom Nut Pâté	2 Tbsp.	31	1.3	2.0	2.3	0.2	0.7	5	144	9	0.4
Pita Chips	½ cup	67	2.5	13.0	0.4	0.1	0.0	135	29	19	0.6
Popeye's Spinach Dip	¼ cup	37	2.0	4.6	1.4	0.5	0.6	108	107	51	0.4
St. Helens Appetizer	1/12 recipe	143	6.3	23.0	3.4	0.9	5.5	258	304	96	1.4
Spicy Stuffed Mushrooms	3 mushrooms	35	1.7	4.8	1.2	0.2	0.8	65	207	11	0.7
Steamed Buns	1 bun	73	1.7	9.6	3.1	0.9	0.5	179	85	58	0.5
Beef, Veal and Pork											
Bayou Red Beans	1 cup	202	15.1	30.9	3.6	1.5	7.0	620	702	80	4.1
Bean Hot Dish	1 cup	231	16.0	38.1	3.4	1.8	6.8	441	719	73	4.4
Beef and Bean Ragout	1 cup	101	8.7	12.2	2.5	1.3	3.6	39	445	26	2.0
Beef Barley Skillet†	1 cup	369	17.6	66.7	3.6	2.8	6.9	236	484	29	3.3

Source: Computer analysis done using the National Heart, Lung and Blood Institute Nutrition Data Base. Nutrition Coordinating Center, Minneapolis, Minnesota.
* Cholesterol-Saturated Fat Index.
† Calculation includes rice or other grain, potatoes, pasta or bread.

Recipes	Amount	Calories	Protein (gm)	Carbohydrate (gm)	Total Fat (gm)	CSI* (units)	Dietary Fiber (gm)	Sodium (mg)	Potassium (mg)	Calcium (mg)	Iron (mg)
Beef-Mushroom Spaghetti Sauce	1 cup	150	14.2	19.0	2.9	2.0	2.8	173	1053	133	4.0
Beef Stroganoff	1 cup	242	29.2	8.8	9.7	6.2	0.7	442	466	85	3.4
Beef-Tomato Chow Yuk	¼ recipe	211	15.6	23.5	6.5	3.0	2.1	242	574	30	2.5
Flank Steak Teriyaki	⅙ recipe	226	26.0	13.7	7.4	5.2	0.1	477	365	15	3.4
Moo Shoo Pork—Filling	½ cup	99	9.8	3.5	5.1	1.9	0.9	206	169	19	1.1
Pepper Steak	¼ recipe	217	27.0	8.8	7.1	5.4	1.0	538	488	22	3.8
Pizza Rice Casserole	1 cup	137	13.0	14.1	3.3	2.8	1.5	194	247	82	1.3
Stay-Abed Stew	1 cup	121	10.2	16.3	1.9	1.6	2.7	215	477	28	2.0
Stuffed Flank Steak Florentine	⅛ recipe	281	33.3	14.5	10.2	7.5	2.3	221	599	166	4.4
Taco Salad	1 cup	126	8.7	14.9	4.1	1.8	2.9	197	359	70	1.8
Tamale Pie	1 cup	205	13.5	31.0	4.3	2.7	5.7	367	499	88	3.0
Veal Roll-Ups	1 roll	344	34.0	22.2	12.3	9.1	0.6	460	504	64	5.2
Veal Stew with Dill	1 cup	182	27.8	4.0	5.4	6.3	1.1	120	544	27	3.8
Vegetable-Beef Soup	1 cup	80	5.9	10.9	1.7	1.1	2.0	130	527	18	1.2
Beverages											
Cranberry Wassail	½ cup	66	0.1	16.5	0.1	0.0	0.1	3	40	3	0.1
Egg Nog	½ cup	100	8.3	16.3	0.2	0.2	0.0	134	294	240	0.6
Fruited Punch	½ cup	63	0.4	15.7	0.1	0.0	1.2	1	91	11	0.1
Mulled Cider	½ cup	61	0.2	14.9	0.2	0.0	0.4	4	152	13	0.4
Orange Frosty	1 cup	168	2.7	39.3	0.2	0.1	0.6	27	368	74	0.2
Quick Hot Spiced Cider	½ cup	61	0.2	14.9	0.2	0.0	0.4	4	152	13	0.4
Strawberry-Banana Smoothie	1 cup	102	4.6	19.4	1.2	1.0	0.9	130	359	148	0.3
Breads and Muffins											
A Barrel of Muffins	1 muffin	105	3.0	16.4	4.0	0.7	2.3	166	127	27	1.6
Apricot Nut Bread	½" slice	162	2.8	28.4	4.1	0.6	0.8	135	90	79	0.7

* Cholesterol-Saturated Fat Index.
† Calculation includes rice or other grain, potatoes, pasta or bread.

Recipes	Amount	Calories	Protein (gm)	Carbohydrate (gm)	Total Fat (gm)	CSI* (units)	Dietary Fiber (gm)	Sodium (mg)	Potassium (mg)	Calcium (mg)	Iron (mg)
Baking Mix	1 cup	491	13.5	72.9	16.9	4.2	7.1	738	674	376	2.9
Blueberry Bran Muffins	1 muffin	146	5.3	34.6	0.5	0.1	4.7	354	288	137	3.0
Caraway Dinner Rolls	1 roll	108	5.9	19.6	0.7	0.3	1.7	111	106	20	0.8
Carrot and Bran Muffins	1 muffin	133	3.6	21.4	5.1	0.7	4.0	102	329	68	2.1
Cereal Bran Muffins	1 muffin	116	4.4	19.5	3.9	0.6	3.9	171	261	96	2.1
Corn Bread	2" x 4" piece	180	4.7	27.6	5.5	0.9	1.6	154	97	121	1.2
Cranberry Bread	½" slice	136	2.4	25.1	3.2	0.4	1.5	40	67	14	0.5
Fruit and Nut Muffins	1 muffin	82	1.4	14.9	2.2	0.3	1.1	37	66	12	0.3
Grandma Kirschner's Date Nut Bread	½" slice	209	3.3	42.6	3.8	0.4	2.5	83	222	29	1.0
Hearty Corn Bread	2" x 4" piece	197	5.9	37.2	2.8	0.7	2.8	168	185	100	1.8
Honey Wheat Bread	½" slice	121	3.9	22.7	2.2	0.4	2.9	17	122	19	1.0
Lemon Nut Bread	½" slice	153	3.3	24.2	5.0	0.8	1.0	113	77	54	0.6
Natural Bran Muffins	1 muffin	97	3.1	17.0	3.0	0.5	3.3	87	129	30	1.3
Old-Style Wheat Biscuits	1 biscuit	86	2.3	11.5	3.6	0.6	1.1	81	76	51	0.5
Pita Bread	1 pita	158	5.6	33.3	0.7	0.1	3.4	30	157	22	1.4
Pizza Crusts, Thin	3½" x 3½" piece	64	2.1	13.0	0.7	0.1	1.8	<1	45	5	0.4
Pizza Crusts, Thick	3" x 3" piece	107	3.4	22.6	0.4	0.1	1.7	90	68	62	0.9
Pumpkin Harvest Loaf	½" slice	163	3.1	29.8	3.6	0.5	1.1	119	98	45	1.0
Quick Wheat Bread	1/16 recipe	107	4.1	20.5	1.3	0.4	1.9	118	159	71	0.9
Soft Pretzels	1 pretzel	193	5.2	35.3	3.1	0.5	1.0	80	158	46	1.2
Whole Wheat French Bread	1/5 loaf	125	4.5	26.3	0.5	0.1	2.7	52	157	10	1.1
Whole Wheat Muffins	1 muffin	135	3.5	19.5	5.0	0.8	1.5	111	85	67	0.6
Whole Wheat Refrigerator Roll Dough	1 roll	106	3.5	20.9	1.2	0.2	2.2	26	123	9	0.9
Whole Wheat Tortillas	1 tortilla	101	3.5	21.3	0.4	0.1	2.2	1	69	83	0.9

Breakfasts and Brunches

Recipes	Amount	Calories	Protein (gm)	Carbohydrate (gm)	Total Fat (gm)	CSI* (units)	Dietary Fiber (gm)	Sodium (mg)	Potassium (mg)	Calcium (mg)	Iron (mg)
Apple Dumplings	1 dumpling	428	8.5	82.6	9.6	1.7	9.1	626	447	217	3.1

* Cholesterol-Saturated Fat Index.
† Calculation includes rice or other grain, potatoes, pasta or bread.

Recipes	Amount	Calories	Protein (gm)	Carbohydrate (gm)	Total Fat (gm)	CSI* (units)	Dietary Fiber (gm)	Sodium (mg)	Potassium (mg)	Calcium (mg)	Iron (mg)
Breakfast Volcanos	1 volcano	238	17.6	17.8	10.8	3.7	1.3	840	275	114	1.9
Crepe Blintzes	1 blintz	239	11.6	32.9	7.1	3.6	1.5	281	341	93	0.6
German Oven Pancake	½ pancake	373	16.8	55.2	10.2	1.8	3.2	355	585	152	2.7
Homemade Egg Substitute	¼ cup	70	6.5	2.8	3.5	0.6	0.0	99	140	58	0.0
Morning Rice	1 cup	173	5.1	36.1	1.5	0.9	2.7	42	223	87	0.8
Muesli	1 cup	292	8.5	53.7	6.4	1.2	6.1	46	437	115	2.1
Mushroom Strata	1/9 recipe	176	10.2	24.0	5.2	1.5	2.7	442	434	138	1.9
Oatmeal Buttermilk Pancakes	4″ pancake	76	3.7	13.6	1.0	0.3	1.8	145	115	45	0.7
Orange Pancakes with Orange Sauce	⅙ recipe	393	12.7	69.9	9.8	4.8	5.0	236	430	289	1.5
Our Granola	1 cup	409	9.4	70.2	12.4	1.8	6.8	97	445	74	5.4
Spanish Omelet	⅙ recipe	93	11.7	9.3	1.0	0.2	2.1	170	278	39	1.5
Sunrise Cake	1/16 recipe	161	3.3	28.8	4.1	0.9	1.5	132	148	38	1.0
Vegetable Frittata	½ recipe	232	20.6	24.8	6.5	1.9	5.8	410	464	189	4.4
Waffles	7″ waffle	192	6.7	24.6	7.7	1.6	2.2	274	179	136	0.9
Chicken, Turkey and Rabbit											
Acapulco Enchiladas†	1 enchilada	193	17.0	21.6	4.7	3.1	2.0	573	380	148	1.8
Basic Stir-Fried Chicken	¼ recipe	142	15.4	9.3	5.1	2.4	3.4	300	367	55	1.4
Cashew Chicken	¼ recipe	242	21.0	20.5	9.7	3.5	3.5	391	868	60	2.8
Chicken and Mushroom Crepes—Filling	1/12 recipe	78	8.8	3.8	2.8	1.8	0.1	71	181	67	0.6
Chicken and Tomatoes in Black Bean Sauce	⅓ recipe	165	18.5	11.6	4.9	2.9	1.3	176	499	20	1.6
Chicken and Vegetables Provençale	¼ recipe	198	29.8	14.6	3.0	3.7	5.3	279	990	97	3.3
Chicken Braised in Wine	⅙ recipe	226	28.4	10.6	7.3	5.7	2.1	216	498	48	2.3
Chicken Cacciatore	¼ recipe	222	27.8	13.4	6.3	4.2	1.8	212	749	37	3.3

* Cholesterol-Saturated Fat Index.
† Calculation includes rice or other grain, potatoes, pasta or bread.

Recipes	Amount	Calories	Protein (gm)	Carbohydrate (gm)	Total Fat (gm)	CSI* (units)	Dietary Fiber (gm)	Sodium (mg)	Potassium (mg)	Calcium (mg)	Iron (mg)
Chicken Italian	⅙ recipe	214	28.2	6.7	7.8	5.7	2.1	151	430	48	2.1
Chicken Madeira	¼ recipe	214	27.3	19.4	2.6	3.7	1.0	97	543	30	1.6
Chicken Nepal	⅙ recipe	274	32.0	16.8	8.7	6.2	3.1	180	850	92	3.2
Chicken Salad with Yogurt-Chive Dressing	⅙ recipe	252	29.6	21.4	5.1	4.9	1.2	136	564	129	1.9
Cornish Game Hens à La Crock†	¼ recipe	410	33.4	54.2	6.3	5.4	4.5	485	443	53	3.7
Country Captain	¼ recipe	279	28.0	29.5	6.5	4.2	4.2	65	980	44	3.3
Couscous†	⅕ recipe	396	31.4	48.1	9.2	4.5	8.1	413	1009	131	9.5
Cracked Chicken	⅙ recipe	213	29.5	10.0	5.6	5.4	0.7	286	612	39	2.1
Curried Chicken Quickie†	⅙ recipe	415	24.8	68.8	4.1	3.3	0.7	149	479	142	4.7
Easy Oven Lasagna†	⅛ recipe	277	18.2	33.4	8.4	4.1	2.8	258	578	169	2.5
Far East Chicken	⅙ recipe	234	21.9	27.5	4.5	3.4	1.4	110	528	41	1.9
Homemade Raviolis†	12	366	17.2	55.1	9.8	1.9	5.0	119	1101	73	4.7
Lemony Chicken Kabobs	¼ recipe	203	27.0	10.2	6.1	4.2	2.7	158	745	43	2.0
Orange Baked Chicken	⅙ recipe	224	28.3	14.5	5.3	5.3	0.6	283	524	37	2.0
Parmesan Yogurt Chicken	⅙ recipe	235	30.1	5.8	9.5	6.8	0.2	212	325	97	2.0
Pollo Tepehuano†	⅙ recipe	404	33.8	55.5	4.9	4.2	5.0	528	890	87	3.4
Portland Fried Chicken	⅙ recipe	187	27.5	5.8	5.3	5.3	0.2	154	274	30	2.7
Rabbit Fricassee	⅙ recipe	247	37.5	4.0	9.2	6.6	0.2	127	487	42	8.7
Simply Wonderful Turkey Salad†	⅙ recipe	233	11.2	34.0	6.0	1.9	2.6	460	414	56	2.8
South Seas Chicken	⅙ recipe	174	28.2	2.3	5.2	5.3	0.0	637	315	22	2.0
Spicy Chicken with Spinach	¼ recipe	221	29.6	11.5	6.7	4.3	5.1	440	725	167	4.3
Tangerine Chicken	⅙ recipe	146	24.9	1.5	3.9	3.9	0.5	169	279	20	1.3
Texas Hash†	¼ recipe	424	24.1	66.4	7.3	3.1	5.2	149	1064	75	4.4
Turkey Lettuce Stir-Fry	¼ recipe	147	12.5	14.8	4.8	2.1	5.4	191	554	74	1.9

* Cholesterol-Saturated Fat Index.
† Calculation includes rice or other grain, potatoes, pasta or bread.

Recipes	Amount	Calories	Protein (gm)	Carbohydrate (gm)	Total Fat (gm)	CSI* (units)	Dietary Fiber (gm)	Sodium (mg)	Potassium (mg)	Calcium (mg)	Iron (mg)
Turkey-Mushroom Spaghetti Sauce	1 cup	148	15.5	16.6	2.9	2.4	3.0	55	886	43	3.4
Turkey-Vegetable Chowder	2 cups	280	21.4	37.9	6.6	3.2	8.2	433	1145	128	5.0

Desserts

Recipes	Amount	Calories	Protein (gm)	Carbohydrate (gm)	Total Fat (gm)	CSI* (units)	Dietary Fiber (gm)	Sodium (mg)	Potassium (mg)	Calcium (mg)	Iron (mg)
All Season Shortcake	3" x 3" piece	292	6.9	60.9	2.8	1.0	2.4	141	390	178	1.5
Angel Quickie	1/2 cake	155	4.5	33.4	0.8	0.5	1.3	171	124	10	0.4
Apple Crisp	1/6 recipe	153	1.2	29.0	4.4	0.8	2.4	54	146	22	0.8
Apple Loaf Cake	1/24 recipe	179	2.3	30.4	5.7	0.8	1.3	53	62	8	0.6
Apricot Bavarian	1/10 recipe	186	6.5	38.8	1.2	0.9	2.5	65	324	114	0.5
Apricot Meringue Bars	2" x 2" bar	91	1.3	14.6	3.2	0.5	0.3	42	25	5	0.4
Baba au Rhum	1/24 recipe	190	3.4	32.0	2.6	0.5	0.6	67	81	18	0.7
Baked Apples	1 apple	125	0.4	31.8	0.8	0.1	3.5	5	211	22	0.9
Baked Doughnut Holes	1 doughnut hole	59	1.0	10.8	1.3	0.2	0.1	39	17	26	0.2
Bananas en Papillote	1 banana	127	1.2	32.1	0.5	0.2	2.3	1	438	7	0.3
Blueberry Ice	1 cup	250	1.5	62.1	0.4	0.0	2.6	24	108	9	0.2
Carob Cookies	1 cookie	83	1.4	10.7	3.9	0.6	0.6	23	39	13	0.3
Chewy Wheat Germ Brownies	2" x 2" piece	97	3.4	13.6	3.5	0.5	0.4	41	116	47	0.6
Chocolate Pudding	1/2 cup	115	3.1	25.1	0.6	0.4	0.6	43	162	103	0.3
Chocolate Zucchini Cake	2" x 2" piece	142	2.5	22.6	5.0	0.9	1.5	54	87	15	0.6
Cocoa Cake	3" x 3" piece	205	2.4	37.7	5.3	1.1	1.2	92	56	6	0.8
Crème de Menthe Cheesecake	1/12 of 10" cake	210	8.0	25.4	7.5	4.6	0.0	156	105	160	0.4
Crepes	1 crepe	62	2.6	9.2	1.5	0.3	0.3	41	71	18	0.3
Crispy Spice Cookies	1 cookie	62	0.7	9.1	2.6	0.4	0.2	36	9	4	0.3
Depression Cake	3" x 3" piece	263	3.6	57.2	3.6	0.6	3.2	135	298	37	2.0
Forgotten Kisses	1 cookie	23	0.3	4.4	0.6	0.1	0.1	12	17	1	0.0
Fresh Fruit Crepes Filling	3 Tbsp.	22	0.9	4.1	0.3	0.2	0.4	10	51	21	0.2
Frozen Fruit Yogurts	1 cup	184	6.9	35.3	1.9	1.5	1.2	96	209	139	0.2

* Cholesterol-Saturated Fat Index.

383

Recipes	Amount	Calories	Protein (gm)	Carbohydrate (gm)	Total Fat (gm)	CSI* (units)	Dietary Fiber (gm)	Sodium (mg)	Potassium (mg)	Calcium (mg)	Iron (mg)
Fruit Salad Alaska	¼ recipe	164	3.6	36.5	0.6	0.0	4.0	41	304	39	1.0
Gingies	1 cookie	110	1.9	22.6	1.6	0.3	1.2	59	169	41	1.3
Graham Cracker Crust	9" crust	854	12.7	149.7	28.8	7.3	3.9	1054	624	66	5.7
Hot Fudge Pudding Cake	2¼" x 3" piece	194	2.3	40.0	3.8	0.9	1.5	70	155	74	1.3
Lebkuchen	1 cookie	58	0.8	12.7	0.5	0.1	0.2	11	52	13	0.4
Molasses Orange Bars	2" x 2" bar	123	1.7	21.7	3.5	0.6	0.9	90	179	25	0.9
Northwest Harvest Bars	2¼" x 2¼" bar	102	1.7	18.0	3.0	0.5	0.8	109	150	23	0.7
Oatmeal Cookies	1 cookie	93	1.1	13.9	3.8	0.9	0.7	18	54	7	0.4
Party Carrot Cake	2" x 2" piece	224	3.1	40.5	5.9	1.6	1.4	130	104	15	0.7
Peach Cardinal	1 peach	160	1.2	39.9	0.4	0.0	4.3	1	267	18	0.5
Pears in Wine	1 pear	244	1.7	56.0	3.3	0.3	5.7	8	338	42	1.3
Pinto Fiesta Cake	1/16 recipe	182	3.5	33.5	4.7	0.7	3.5	101	220	22	1.2
Poppy Seed Cake	½" slice	180	4.4	27.3	6.5	1.0	1.9	88	135	131	1.0
Pumpkin Bread Pudding	½ cup	184	6.3	40.5	0.8	0.3	2.8	164	390	119	2.4
Pumpkin Pie	1/8 of 9" pie	245	6.9	48.2	3.9	1.0	2.3	206	419	165	2.0
Rhubarb Buckle	1/8 recipe	160	3.0	38.0	0.1	0.0	2.0	58	253	81	0.7
Ricotta Cheesecake	1/12 of 10" cake	211	8.5	30.2	7.1	4.2	0.2	179	146	169	0.6
Strawberry Ice	1 cup	240	0.8	59.3	0.5	0.0	2.1	4	185	22	1.1
Strawberry Yogurt Pie	1/10 of 9" pie	182	8.7	29.4	4.3	1.7	1.3	268	222	80	1.2
Vanilla Pudding	½ cup	111	4.2	23.3	0.2	0.3	0.0	68	252	162	0.5
Walnut Squares	1½" square	40	0.9	6.5	1.4	0.2	0.2	21	41	9	0.3

Fish and Shellfish

Recipes	Amount	Calories	Protein (gm)	Carbohydrate (gm)	Total Fat (gm)	CSI* (units)	Dietary Fiber (gm)	Sodium (mg)	Potassium (mg)	Calcium (mg)	Iron (mg)
Alphabet Seafood Salad†	1 cup	242	15.3	36.3	3.4	1.8	1.1	243	231	52	2.0
Baked Herbed Fish	¼ recipe	189	28.8	2.7	4.9	5.4	0.3	253	736	31	1.0
Baked Snapper with Spicy Tomato Sauce	¼ recipe	214	33.5	9.2	5.4	5.9	1.9	229	971	48	1.7
Baked Snapper with Wine and Veggies	¼ recipe	196	32.9	5.0	5.2	5.9	0.9	185	805	39	1.5
Bean Sprout Tuna Chow Mein	1 cup	91	10.3	7.4	2.7	1.2	1.7	285	370	33	1.0

* Cholesterol-Saturated Fat Index.
† Calculation includes rice or other grain, potatoes, pasta or bread.

Recipes	Amount	Calories	Protein (gm)	Carbohydrate (gm)	Total Fat (gm)	CSI* (units)	Dietary Fiber (gm)	Sodium (mg)	Potassium (mg)	Calcium (mg)	Iron (mg)
Bouillabaisse	1 cup	82	11.6	4.6	2.1	1.9	0.9	281	424	23	0.9
Cioppino	1 cup	133	16.1	9.0	3.2	3.5	1.6	100	566	92	2.6
Clam Pilaff	¼ recipe	357	26.8	44.9	7.3	5.6	2.5	468	416	108	8.3
Clam Sauce for Pasta	1 cup	222	24.7	6.4	10.2	8.0	0.2	274	246	143	6.0
Cod Curry	¼ recipe	189	32.8	3.2	5.2	5.9	0.9	303	865	65	1.1
Creole Salmon	⅙ recipe	169	16.1	5.0	10.0	5.4	0.9	91	435	32	1.1
Creole Shrimp	⅙ recipe	107	12.6	7.3	3.7	4.1	1.4	84	500	165	2.0
Fillet of Fish Florentine	⅙ recipe	171	24.5	7.6	5.1	4.4	1.9	294	721	121	1.7
Fillet of Sole Oregon	⅙ recipe	184	23.9	6.6	7.1	5.5	1.2	175	495	52	1.5
Fish Almondine with Dilly Sauce	¼ recipe	248	36.2	8.5	8.3	6.8	1.1	255	790	123	1.5
Fish à la Mistral	¼ recipe	203	32.9	7.0	5.3	5.9	1.2	274	1006	42	1.6
Fish à L'Orange	¼ recipe	171	31.8	1.1	4.4	5.8	0.1	209	638	29	0.9
Fish Fillets with Walnuts	¼ recipe	246	34.6	3.3	10.9	6.6	0.5	460	712	43	1.4
Fish Hampton	¼ recipe	138	28.9	2.5	1.6	4.9	0.3	159	605	36	1.1
Hearty Fish Soup	1 cup	106	10.7	7.9	2.7	1.8	1.6	117	593	26	1.1
Lively Lemon Roll-Ups†	⅙ recipe	281	38.8	20.2	5.9	7.3	5.0	351	910	166	1.9
Medallion of Cod	¼ recipe	196	39.7	2.6	2.7	6.4	0.0	408	686	77	1.1
Pacific Stew Pot	1 cup	68	10.2	5.5	0.8	1.8	1.0	151	438	65	1.3
Portuguese Casserole†	⅙ recipe	268	14.9	41.9	5.7	1.3	7.1	508	1044	82	4.3
Salmon and Red Pepper Pasta†	¼ recipe	444	19.9	66.7	10.8	4.5	3.5	85	546	93	3.5
Salmon Loaf	⅙ recipe	174	16.9	10.9	7.3	2.8	1.2	498	348	128	2.1
Salmon Mousse	⅛ recipe	175	18.2	4.9	9.2	3.5	0.1	582	223	84	1.5
Savory Fish Fillets	¼ recipe	228	32.9	5.7	8.4	6.4	0.8	389	683	60	1.6
Scallops in Creamy Sauce	¼ recipe	218	22.5	9.1	6.4	3.9	0.8	318	691	127	3.2
Sesame Halibut	¼ recipe	176	29.7	7.6	3.3	5.1	0.4	382	646	33	1.3
Shrimp and Asparagus Crepe—Filling	2 Tbsp.	52	6.0	4.0	1.6	1.5	0.5	92	206	102	0.7

* Cholesterol-Saturated Fat Index.
† Calculation includes rice or other grain, potatoes, pasta or bread.

Recipes	Amount	Calories	Protein (gm)	Carbohy-drate (gm)	Total Fat (gm)	CSI* (units)	Dietary Fiber (gm)	Sodium (mg)	Potassium (mg)	Calcium (mg)	Iron (mg)
Skinny Sole	¼ recipe	227	25.1	13.5	8.1	5.1	1.3	128	480	20	1.4
Stuffed Sole	⅙ recipe	221	34.3	12.8	4.2	5.9	2.2	349	797	59	1.9
Sweet 'n' Sour Supper	1 cup	155	14.6	15.6	4.2	2.1	1.8	345	408	25	1.8
Tandoori Fish	¼ recipe	139	24.6	6.1	2.0	4.4	0.2	257	666	89	0.8
Tangy Snapper	¼ recipe	142	19.6	8.9	3.4	3.6	1.4	174	501	108	1.4
Tuna Noodle Casserole†	1 cup	146	10.4	21.2	2.1	1.3	2.4	164	281	43	1.7
Vegetable-Topped Fish Fillets	¼ recipe	242	36.0	9.0	7.2	7.4	0.9	471	896	129	1.6
Main Dishes Featuring Vegetables, Grains and Beans											
Acapulco Bean Casserole†	1 cup	236	13.9	28.3	8.6	4.5	8.8	626	486	144	2.8
Bean Lasagna†	1/12 recipe	220	17.0	28.6	4.6	2.6	3.0	420	517	151	2.4
Bean Stroganoff	⅙ recipe	196	12.6	32.0	3.2	1.2	9.7	175	700	129	3.3
Brazilian Black Beans and Rice†	1 cup	175	6.2	32.9	2.7	0.4	6.0	44	423	42	2.4
Broccoli Lasagna Rolls†	1 roll	200	12.3	30.1	4.9	2.2	3.7	198	453	270	8.9
Broccoli with Rice†	1 cup	157	4.3	25.6	4.5	1.6	2.8	495	204	72	1.0
Bryani†	1/12 recipe	197	6.4	33.9	4.8	1.2	4.0	87	366	76	1.4
Cabbage Rolls†	1 roll	80	3.1	16.6	0.9	0.1	2.2	70	334	44	1.3
Calzones†	1 calzone	362	22.5	50.3	9.0	5.9	6.3	332	450	375	3.6
Cauliflower Curry	1 cup	129	8.9	10.1	6.4	3.5	1.9	195	357	200	0.9
Cheese-Stuffed Manicotti†	1 manicotti	135	9.7	17.2	3.5	1.9	1.4	216	304	95	1.2
Chile Relleno Casserole†	¼ recipe	310	16.8	46.3	8.1	4.3	10.4	217	931	252	3.6
Creamy Enchiladas†	1 enchilada	179	12.9	24.2	4.1	2.5	2.2	687	362	190	1.4
Curried Lentils	1 cup	99	6.2	18.9	1.0	0.1	4.8	79	377	23	1.5
Garbanzo Goulash†	1 cup	208	8.9	37.5	2.8	0.4	3.5	135	367	46	2.9
Herbed Lentil Casserole†	1 cup	145	7.4	27.1	1.7	0.7	4.2	98	384	54	1.6
Kidney Bean Gumbo	1 cup	94	5.0	15.4	2.3	0.4	3.9	103	378	50	1.9

* Cholesterol-Saturated Fat Index.
† Calculation includes rice or other grain, potatoes, pasta or bread.

Recipes	Amount	Calories	Protein (gm)	Carbohydrate (gm)	Total Fat (gm)	CSI* (units)	Dietary Fiber (gm)	Sodium (mg)	Potassium (mg)	Calcium (mg)	Iron (mg)
Lentils over Rice†	1 cup	149	8.7	24.3	3.4	0.5	5.6	259	543	40	2.5
Macaroni Bake†	1 cup	246	14.9	35.2	4.7	1.7	1.0	381	321	139	1.6
Mexican Bean Pot	1 cup	147	8.5	25.1	3.0	0.5	5.5	236	578	63	3.2
Moroccan Vegetable Stew†	1 cup	81	2.4	14.6	2.0	0.3	3.6	14	464	31	1.2
Moussaka	1/12 recipe	108	9.2	11.4	3.3	1.6	3.1	233	367	96	1.3
No-Meat Enchiladas†	1 enchilada	202	14.1	21.3	7.3	3.5	2.8	371	286	204	1.4
Pasta Primavera†	1 cup	128	5.4	21.1	2.6	1.0	2.0	87	223	79	1.2
Pinto Bean Chow Mein	1 cup	96	5.3	16.2	2.0	0.3	4.1	416	372	42	1.7
Plymouth-Style Baked Beans	1 cup	180	9.9	32.1	3.1	0.6	12.6	48	657	76	3.7
Rick's Chili	1 cup	126	7.1	21.2	2.9	0.5	4.5	189	659	51	2.8
Romano Rice and Beans†	1 cup	158	6.4	27.9	3.1	1.1	5.5	109	435	98	2.0
Spanish Beans	1 cup	177	11.6	23.6	5.4	2.5	5.0	324	529	153	2.9
Spicy Cheese Pizza—Topping	1/8 recipe	101	7.5	11.0	3.7	2.8	2.1	128	420	158	1.6
Spinach Lasagna†	1/12 recipe	223	13.1	30.3	5.8	3.3	3.0	172	493	212	2.6
Summer Squash Delight†	1 cup	162	7.2	24.5	4.3	1.1	2.8	95	256	114	0.9
Sweet and Sour Vegetables with Tofu	1 cup	157	5.1	30.1	3.1	0.5	1.9	142	330	91	1.8
Tostadas†	1 tostada	119	6.2	17.3	3.5	1.5	4.0	281	284	107	1.5
Vegetable Creole	1 cup	136	6.9	19.4	4.4	0.7	6.6	53	497	53	2.9
Vegetable Crepes—Filling	5 Tbsp.	27	1.0	3.6	1.3	0.2	1.0	25	180	12	0.5
Zucchini Pie	1/8 recipe	188	13.1	18.0	7.4	4.9	2.8	317	342	255	1.2
Zucchini Spaghetti Dinner†	1 cup	176	5.3	30.5	4.6	0.6	4.8	177	793	62	1.8
Salads											
Carrot-Raisin Salad	1 cup	166	3.6	36.9	1.7	0.7	4.7	80	621	83	1.5
Chili Bean Salad	1 cup	255	13.1	43.7	5.3	0.8	9.3	353	752	86	4.7

* Cholesterol-Saturated Fat Index.
† Calculation includes rice or other grain, potatoes, pasta or bread.

Recipes	Amount	Calories	Protein (gm)	Carbohydrate (gm)	Total Fat (gm)	CSI* (units)	Dietary Fiber (gm)	Sodium (mg)	Potassium (mg)	Calcium (mg)	Iron (mg)
Chinese Cucumber Salad	½ cup	38	0.8	6.5	1.3	0.2	1.1	166	151	17	0.5
Chinese Salad Rich Style	1 cup	77	5.0	6.7	3.8	0.8	1.8	255	264	32	0.9
Confetti Appleslaw	1 cup	55	1.8	11.2	1.0	0.3	2.2	25	216	42	0.5
Crunchy Rice Salad†	1 cup	167	4.2	24.3	6.3	1.4	2.5	139	307	66	0.8
Cucumber Cumin Salad	½ cup	32	3.1	3.7	0.6	0.4	0.8	95	161	36	0.3
Five Veggie Salad	1 cup	102	2.6	10.6	6.1	0.9	2.8	10	506	31	1.4
Four Star Pasta Salad with Green Sauce†	1 cup	154	5.4	25.7	3.4	0.6	1.8	53	249	50	1.6
Greek Salad	1 cup	55	3.2	6.0	2.6	0.6	2.2	86	269	48	1.0
Layered Vegetable Platter	1 cup	87	2.6	9.9	5.2	0.9	3.0	53	318	52	1.3
Lentil Salad	½ cup	127	5.3	15.6	5.9	0.9	3.8	62	356	25	1.4
Montana Pasta Salad†	1 cup	169	5.4	30.0	3.9	0.5	3.4	121	374	60	2.1
Party Pasta Salad†	1 cup	196	9.1	34.5	2.3	1.2	1.7	58	203	70	1.8
Pasta Salad Italiano†	1 cup	187	6.5	33.1	3.0	0.6	1.4	76	176	51	1.5
Picnic Salad†	1 cup	204	10.5	34.6	2.3	1.0	0.9	88	174	45	1.7
Potato Salad†	1 cup	206	7.1	36.7	3.9	1.1	3.6	306	602	66	1.2
Salata	1 cup	48	1.7	8.0	1.6	0.2	2.1	20	295	25	1.0
South of the Border Salad†	1 cup	193	6.8	36.9	2.2	0.5	2.3	27	198	43	1.6
Spicy Soybean Salad	½ cup	104	6.5	7.9	5.8	0.9	1.3	47	405	49	1.7
Sunshine Spinach Salad	1 cup	51	1.4	7.6	2.1	0.3	2.0	175	234	44	1.1
Tabouli†	1 cup	178	3.9	25.3	7.5	1.0	3.9	12	306	42	2.4
Waldorf Salad	½ cup	98	2.5	13.1	4.9	0.8	1.8	41	222	41	0.6
Wild Broccoli Salad†	1 cup	180	7.5	30.2	3.8	1.1	3.3	331	346	84	1.8
Sandwiches											
Baked Bean Special Sandwich†	½ sandwich	374	16.1	77.5	2.5	0.5	11.0	698	846	141	6.2
"Egg" Salad Sandwich Spread	½ cup	110	9.0	7.6	5.0	0.9	0.2	274	132	48	1.2

* Cholesterol-Saturated Fat Index.
† Calculation includes rice or other grain, potatoes, pasta or bread.

Recipes	Amount	Calories	Protein (gm)	Carbohydrate (gm)	Total Fat (gm)	CSI* (units)	Dietary Fiber (gm)	Sodium (mg)	Potassium (mg)	Calcium (mg)	Iron (mg)
Falafel	¼ recipe	124	6.6	21.8	1.6	0.1	3.2	39	231	43	2.3
Tahini Dressing	¼ cup	67	2.9	2.7	5.8	0.8	1.6	77	156	15	0.9
Yogurt Dressing	¼ cup	37	3.1	4.3	0.9	0.7	0.1	90	157	71	0.1
Fruit-Nut Sandwich Spread	½ cup	162	10.4	14.8	7.1	1.6	1.4	279	224	57	0.6
Pita Pizza†	1 pizza	255	12.1	40.2	5.1	2.7	1.3	458	327	185	2.0
Tofu "Egg" Salad Sandwich Spread	½ cup	66	5.1	2.4	4.6	0.7	0.5	168	70	79	1.6
Tuna Salad Sandwich Spread	½ cup	111	18.5	3.8	2.0	2.5	0.4	285	255	41	1.1
Vegetable-Cottage Cheese Sandwich Spread	½ cup	68	9.5	4.0	1.3	1.1	0.3	287	114	52	0.2
Your Basic Bean Burrito†	1 burrito	269	12.3	45.2	5.4	2.2	9.1	221	518	153	4.1

Sauces, Gravies and Salad Dressings

Recipes	Amount	Calories	Protein (gm)	Carbohydrate (gm)	Total Fat (gm)	CSI* (units)	Dietary Fiber (gm)	Sodium (mg)	Potassium (mg)	Calcium (mg)	Iron (mg)
Basic White Sauce	1 cup	189	8.2	15.8	10.5	2.2	0.1	334	493	274	0.5
Dilly Sauce	1 Tbsp.	15	0.8	1.4	0.7	0.3	0.0	20	25	19	0.1
Glorious Blueberries	¼ cup	49	1.2	10.6	0.4	0.2	0.8	15	49	24	0.1
Light Mushroom Sauce for Pasta	1 cup	140	10.0	14.9	5.0	2.0	1.3	312	859	238	1.5
Marinara Sauce	1 cup	117	4.4	19.0	4.4	0.5	3.9	41	799	35	2.3
Mock Hollandaise Sauce	¼ cup	90	3.4	2.6	7.4	2.2	0.1	310	67	61	0.2
Oriental Sauce for Fish	¼ cup	32	1.1	7.6	0.2	0.0	0.5	234	180	28	0.9
Red French Salad Dressing	1 Tbsp.	34	0.1	4.3	2.0	0.3	0.0	56	23	1	0.1
Russian Salad Dressing	1 Tbsp.	21	0.1	0.8	2.0	0.3	0.2	1	13	2	0.0
Strawberry or Raspberry Sauce	¼ cup	31	0.3	7.4	0.2	0.0	0.8	1	64	8	0.4
Tangy Salad Dressing	1 Tbsp.	14	0.6	1.2	0.7	0.3	0.0	22	17	14	0.0
Tartar Sauce	1 Tbsp.	10	1.2	0.9	0.2	0.2	0.0	41	16	8	0.0

* Cholesterol-Saturated Fat Index.
† Calculation includes rice or other grain, potatoes, pasta or bread.

Recipes	Amount	Calories	Protein (gm)	Carbohydrate (gm)	Total Fat (gm)	CSI* (units)	Dietary Fiber (gm)	Sodium (mg)	Potassium (mg)	Calcium (mg)	Iron (mg)
Thousand Island Salad Dressing	1 Tbsp.	15	1.2	1.2	0.6	0.2	0.0	65	19	9	0.0
Tomato-Mushroom Spaghetti Sauce	1 cup	97	5.7	16.3	2.1	1.2	2.9	118	769	113	2.9
Turkey Gravy	1 Tbsp.	8	0.2	0.8	0.5	0.1	0.9	34	25	2	0.1
Vinaigrette Salad Dressing with Greens	1/3 recipe	42	0.1	0.7	4.4	0.6	0.0	21	12	2	0.1
Western Salad Dressing	1 Tbsp.	12	0.6	1.1	0.6	0.2	0.0	28	28	15	0.0
Yogurt Dessert Sauce	1/4 cup	61	3.0	10.4	0.9	0.7	0.0	40	82	68	0.1
Side Dishes											
Basic Stir-Fried Vegetables	1 cup	76	3.5	7.7	4.0	0.6	3.0	281	364	37	1.0
Bulgur Pilaf†	1/4 recipe	156	5.6	29.7	1.9	0.4	3.6	208	175	14	2.3
Classic Baked Beans	1/2 cup	115	5.5	23.0	1.0	0.2	6.8	122	460	59	2.4
Corn Bake	1/4 recipe	118	4.4	26.8	0.9	0.1	7.0	139	391	15	1.3
Cottage Spinach	1/6 recipe	101	14.4	5.6	2.7	2.0	3.1	390	366	197	1.9
"Creamed" Vegetables	1/4 recipe	110	5.3	12.8	4.7	0.9	3.5	178	446	160	0.9
Curried Rice†	1/6 recipe	111	1.6	21.6	2.7	0.4	1.9	6	170	13	0.7
Eggplant Parmesan	1/6 recipe	124	6.1	14.2	6.0	2.0	4.1	146	571	122	1.9
Eggplant Szechuan Style	1/4 recipe	72	2.5	6.5	4.4	0.7	1.8	426	205	14	0.9
Garden Peas	1/4 recipe	122	7.7	19.1	2.3	0.5	6.6	96	271	38	3.0
Gourmet Pasta Pilaf†	1/4 recipe	82	2.1	11.6	3.0	0.5	0.6	40	93	10	0.6
Homemade Tatertots†	1/4 recipe	120	4.0	16.8	4.4	1.5	1.6	244	266	76	0.6
Mashed Potatoes†	1 cup	111	3.7	24.1	0.2	0.1	3.2	79	574	35	0.8
Mexican Corn Medley	1/6 recipe	71	3.4	16.3	0.5	0.0	6.6	6	377	48	1.2
Millet Vegetable Casserole†	1/9 recipe	122	4.5	19.5	2.7	0.7	1.1	196	245	47	0.9
Mushroom Barley Pilaf†	1/8 recipe	196	6.5	37.7	2.4	0.4	4.3	223	381	18	1.5

* Cholesterol-Saturated Fat Index.
† Calculation includes rice or other grain, potatoes, pasta or bread.

Recipes	Amount	Calories	Protein (gm)	Carbohydrate (gm)	Total Fat (gm)	CSI* (units)	Dietary Fiber (gm)	Sodium (mg)	Potassium (mg)	Calcium (mg)	Iron (mg)
Onion Squares†	3" x 3" piece	140	4.3	19.6	5.4	1.2	2.7	121	161	88	0.8
Potato Puff†	1/6 recipe	142	7.2	25.5	1.5	1.1	3.3	223	711	101	0.9
Ratatouille Provençale	1/8 recipe	72	3.6	10.5	2.4	0.6	2.7	30	374	63	1.1
Refried Beans	1 cup	225	12.7	35.0	5.8	1.0	15.8	12	684	83	4.4
Scalloped Potatoes†	1/6 recipe	219	8.2	42.4	2.3	0.6	5.2	150	1083	143	1.5
Skinny "French Fries"†	1/4 recipe	134	3.0	23.1	3.7	0.5	3.2	101	583	10	0.8
Spanish Rice†	1 cup	149	3.2	28.2	2.8	0.4	1.6	75	351	22	1.5
Spinach and Rice Casserole†	1/8 recipe	174	13.3	21.6	4.1	1.5	3.3	343	367	118	1.9
Stir-Fried Mushrooms and Broccoli	1/8 recipe	69	2.5	8.3	3.4	0.5	2.1	120	262	32	0.7
Stuffed Acorn Squash†	1/2 squash	200	5.8	36.9	4.3	1.2	5.7	99	579	65	1.5
Stuffed Zucchini Boats	1 boat	66	3.3	6.4	3.6	1.2	2.9	74	285	89	0.9
Super Stuffed Potatoes†	1/2 potato	113	4.9	18.4	2.5	1.3	3.1	94	501	79	0.7
Tomatoes "Provençale"	1 tomato	73	2.4	10.7	2.9	0.4	1.7	31	412	17	1.1
Twice-Baked Potatoes, Cottage Style†	1/2 potato	107	6.5	19.0	0.7	0.5	2.5	175	527	46	0.7
Zucchini Mexicali	1/6 recipe	81	3.9	9.2	3.9	1.4	3.3	216	347	92	1.0

Soups

Recipes	Amount	Calories	Protein (gm)	Carbohydrate (gm)	Total Fat (gm)	CSI* (units)	Dietary Fiber (gm)	Sodium (mg)	Potassium (mg)	Calcium (mg)	Iron (mg)
Bean and Basil Soup	1 cup	165	7.5	27.9	3.5	1.3	4.7	184	518	96	2.7
French Onion Soup	1 cup	109	4.8	14.7	3.7	1.6	1.8	203	175	78	0.7
Gazpacho (cold)	1 cup	99	3.3	8.9	6.2	1.0	4.0	264	542	25	1.3
Greek Lentil Soup	1 cup	149	9.8	27.7	1.4	0.2	6.8	67	491	22	2.1
Greek-Style Garbanzo Soup	1 cup	156	7.2	25.3	3.6	0.4	4.2	240	424	52	2.9
Homemade "Cream" Soup Mix	1/9 recipe	131	9.5	19.4	1.4	0.6	0.3	728	456	201	0.7
Hot and Sour Soup	1 cup	68	6.7	4.8	2.5	0.5	0.6	468	178	59	1.3
Icy Olive Soup (cold)	1 cup	83	5.4	6.5	4.0	1.3	0.6	467	223	97	0.7

* Cholesterol-Saturated Fat Index.
† Calculation includes rice or other grain, potatoes, pasta or bread.

Recipes	Amount	Calories	Protein (gm)	Carbohydrate (gm)	Total Fat (gm)	CSI* (units)	Dietary Fiber (gm)	Sodium (mg)	Potassium (mg)	Calcium (mg)	Iron (mg)
Minestrone Soup	1 cup	81	3.5	13.4	2.0	0.3	3.8	102	326	38	1.1
Navy Bean Soup	1 cup	79	5.0	14.8	0.9	0.2	6.4	49	373	41	1.8
Potato Leek Soup	1 cup	61	2.1	10.6	1.2	0.2	1.4	68	280	36	0.4
Red Root Soup	1 cup	81	5.5	12.7	1.0	0.3	2.8	434	456	99	1.2
Simple Vegetable Soup	1 cup	74	2.5	12.1	2.3	0.3	2.8	93	294	19	1.1
Split Pea Soup	1 cup	106	7.0	19.6	1.0	0.1	5.1	91	408	23	1.7
Tomato Soup	1 cup	55	4.2	9.5	0.3	0.1	1.2	299	388	118	0.6
Zucchini and Basil Soup	1 cup	63	4.7	7.6	1.6	0.4	1.4	384	280	91	0.6

* Cholesterol-Saturated Fat Index.

INDEX